CELL BIOLOGY RESEARCH PROGRESS SERIES

CELL DIVISION: THEORY, VARIANTS AND DEGRADATION

CELL BIOLOGY RESEARCH PROGRESS SERIES

Tumor Necrosis Factor
Toma P. Rossard (Editor)
2009. ISBN: 978-1-60741-708-8

Tumor Necrosis Factor
Toma P. Rossard (Editor)
2009. ISBN: 978-1-61668-276-7 (Online book)

Cell Determination During Hematopoiesis
Geoffrey Brown and Rhodri Ceredig (Editors)
2009. ISBN: 978-1-60741-733-0

Handbook of Cell Proliferation
Andre P. Briggs and Jacob A. Coburn (Editors)
2009. ISBN: 978-1-60741-105-5

Handbook of Cell Proliferation
Andre P. Briggs and Jacob A. Coburn (Editors)
2009. ISBN: 978-1-60876-854-7 (Online book)

Daughter Cells of Microalgae
Dilwyn J. Griffiths
2010. ISBN: 978-1-60876-787-8

Handbook of Free Radicals: Formation, Types and Effects
Dimitri Kozyrev and Vasily Slutsky (Editors)
2010. ISBN: 978-1-60876-101-2

Endocytosis: Structural Components, Functions and Pathways
Brynn C. Dowler (Editor)
2010. ISBN: 978-1-61668-189-0

Endocytosis: Structural Components, Functions and Pathways
Brynn C. Dowler (Editor)
2010. ISBN: 978-1-61668-717-5 (Online book)

Cell Respiration and Cell Survival: Processes, Types and Effects
Gijsbert Osterhoudt and Jos Barhydt (Editors)
2010. ISBN: 978-1-60876-462-4

Handbook of Molecular Chaperones: Roles, Structures and Mechanisms
Piero Durante and Leandro Colucci (Editors)
2010. ISBN: 978-1-60876-366-5

Cell Division: Theory, Variants and Degradation
Yuri N. Golitsin and Mikhail C. Krylov (Editors)
2010. ISBN: 978-1-60876-986-5

Basophil Granulocytes
Paul K. Vellis (Editor)
2010. ISBN: 978-1-60741-797-2

Daughter Cells: Properties, Characteristics and Stem Cells
Ayane Hitomi and Masuyo Katoaka (Editors)
2010. ISBN: 978-1-60876-790-8

Cytoskeleton: Cell Movement, Cytokinesis and Organelles Organization
Sébastien Lansing and Tristan Rousseau (Editors)
2010. ISBN: 978-1-60876-559-1

Prostaglandins: Biochemistry, Functions, Types and Roles
Gillian M. Goodwin (Editor)
2010. ISBN: 978-1-61668-272-9

Prostaglandins: Biochemistry, Functions, Types and Roles
Gillian M. Goodwin (Editor)
2010. ISBN: 978-1-61668-645-1 (Online book)

Lipids: Categories, Biological Functions and Metabolism, Nutrition and Health
Paige L. Gilmore (Editor)
2010. ISBN: 978-1-61668-464-8

Lipids: Categories, Biological Functions and Metabolism, Nutrition and Health
Paige L. Gilmore (Editor)
2010. ISBN: 978-1-61668-522-5 (Online book)

CELL BIOLOGY RESEARCH PROGRESS SERIES

CELL DIVISION: THEORY, VARIANTS AND DEGRADATION

YURI N. GOLITSIN
AND
MIKHAIL C. KRYLOV
EDITORS

Nova Science Publishers, Inc.

New York

For permission to use material from this book please contact us:
Telephone 631-231-7269; Fax 631-231-8175
Web Site: http://www.novapublishers.com

LIBRARY OF CONGRESS CATALOGING-IN-PUBLICATION DATA

Available upon request.

ISBN: 978-1-60876-986-5

Published by Nova Science Publishers, Inc. ✝ New York

CONTENTS

PREFACE

Cell division is a highly coordinated process by which the living organisms grow, develop and reproduce. This book presents original research results on the leading edge of cell division research. Each article has been carefully selected in an attempt to present substantial research results across a broad spectrum.

Chapter 1 - Which genes are important, or even essential, for cyanobacterial cell division? One tool that should be able to provide an answer to this question is forward genetics, which aims to identify and clone mutant genes responsible for a phenotype of an interest. By using forward genetics approaches first we conduct mutant screens of a new quality and quantity and then proceed to new gene identification. Reverse genetic analysis for cyanobacterial genes encoding cell division proteins could be also applied after comparative genomic and proteomic analysis. Identification and functional studies of cyanobacterial mutants and genes that are involved in cell division and cell differentiation can enhance understanding of the regulation of morphogenesis of bacteria and plant chloroplasts.

Chapter 2 - Laboratory populations of microalgae are widely used as sensitive test objects for the phytotoxicity of chemicals and wastewater streams evaluation. The laboratory cultures of freshwater green alga *Scenedesmus quadricauda* (Turp.) Breb. and marine diatom alga *Thalassiosira weissflogii* (Grunow) Fryxell et Hastle were studied under pollution impact. As toxicants we used heavy metals (chromium and silver as a part of water-dissolved salt, experiments both with freshwater and marine algae) and pesticide (imazalil sulfate, experiments only with freshwater algae).

The simultaneous presence of two groups of *S. quadricauda* cells ("large", 4.0-4.5 μm in width, mainly in the composition of two-cellular coenobia, and "small", 3.0 μm in width in the composition of four-cellular coenobia) proved to be a specific feature of the dimensional-age structure of the control population at different stages of its growth. This structure allows analyzing any possible changes in cell population both in normal and toxicant pressure conditions and to predict which cell cycle stage is disturbed. The dimensional-age structure analysis for diatom alga culture is complicated significantly because of their propagation features.

At low metal concentrations (0.0001, 0.001 and 0.01 mg/L) and low pesticide concentration (0.001 mg/L) the total cell number decreased as compare to the control one. The reason of possible population growth delay under low-level toxic exposure was the arrest of proliferation of some cells (probably, the most sensitive cells within heterogeneous population) rather than cell cycle slowdown in all cells. Notice, that the differences between control and sample cultures at low concentrations were reversible during the period of experiment. At medium toxicant concentrations (0.05 mg/L silver, 0.1 mg/L chromium and 0.1 mg/L imazalil) the effect varied from indifferent to toxic according to algal species and season. At concentration of 0.1 mg/L chromium and imazalil the division of cells resumed within 1-2 days of intoxication. At concentrations of the toxicants over 0.05 mg/L for silver and over 1.0 mg/L for chromium and imazalil a total cell number and proportion of living cells decreased. Imazalil sulfate at concentration 1.0 mg/L was found to inhibit the division of cells and imparted to them anomalous increase in size and the formation of gigantic cells. Such state of algae was reversible: giant cells rapidly resumed their division after being transferred to a toxicant-free medium. At the concentration 3.0 mg/L chromium we observed both undividing and proliferating cells. At high toxicant concentrations (0.1 and 0.5 mg/L silver; 10.0 mg/L chromium; 5.0, 10.0 and 20.0 mg/L imazalil) cell division stimulation preceded the fast death of algal population and the small immature cells predominated in the beginning of the treatment. Only the high-level toxicant treatment caused photosynthetic efficiency reducing twice as compared to the control level.

On the whole, the freshwater algae were found to be more sensitive to heavy metal action than marine algae. It was shown the existence of algostatic effect of silver after the growth of algal cultures in the presence of high toxicant concentrations. In this case the cell number stayed particularly unchangeable during the period of the experiment.

S. quadricauda adaptation to extreme environmental pressure was analyzed by using an experimental model of the multiple intoxication (triple 10.0 mg/L chromium intoxication and double 1.0 mg/L silver intoxication). The selection of the resistant algal cells in the presence of high toxicant concentrations was demonstrated. These cells could restore the algal population. It is concluded that there are initial resistant cell number within the heterogenous algal population is 3-7 % (depending on toxicant) of initial cell number.

A modified fluctuation analysis was performed to distinguish resistant cells within *S. quadricauda* and *T. weissflogii* laboratory cultures that had originated as a result of random spontaneous pre-selective mutations (prior to chromium exposure) from those arising through acquired post-selective adaptation (during the exposure to chromium).

The changes of population structure of freshwater green alga *S. quadricauda* and marine diatom alga *T. weissflogii* were studied under different regimens of chromium exposure.

Data on the cell number, their photosynthetic characteristics, population structure and share of alive and dead cells will be appropriate for use to predict the most sensitive ecosystem responses and indicate the permissible amount of toxicants in the environment. These data may have important implications for design and interpretations of the bioassay, especially within the context of the hazard/risk assessment.

Chapter 3 - Homologues to actin are ubiquitous in nature, and actin-based cellular skeletons are crucial for the maintenance of prokaryotic and eukaryotic cellular morphology. Regarding the prokaryotes, MreB actin-homologues sustain the peptidoglycan (PG) synthesis along the lateral cell wall of most rod-shaped bacteria; FtsA actin-homologues are essential for cell division in *Escherichia coli* or *Bacillus subtilis*. However, the rod-shaped actinomycete *Corynebacterium glutamicum* has lost during evolution any homologues to actin found in most of other bacteria. Instead, this bacterium elongates in a mycelium fashion, synthesizing PG at the cell poles sustained by internal structures made of a coiled-coil rich protein called DivIVA. This protein interacts with the molecular machinery involved in polar PG synthesis, mainly comprised by RodA, a transporter of PG-precursors, and the class A penicillin-binding proteins. The cell division of *C. glutamicum* is also accomplished by the absence of any actin-homologue. In fact, the cell division machinery of this bacterium is a minimalist version of other septum molecular structures described in most bacteria. Despite of the minimalism exhibited in such crucial processes, the coordination of cell growth, cell division and DNA partition of *C. glutamicum* have been elusive to researchers for a long period of time. This coordination must be tightly controlled since *C. glutamicum* is able to change its cellular morphology to a coco-bacillus shape depending on the environmental conditions. Nevertheless, recent reports have characterized some of the molecular factors involved in the spatio-temporal regulation of cell division and cell growth in this bacterium. This regulation implicates protein phosphorylation, which is also exceptional in bacterial cell-shape acquisition. In summary, *Corynebacterium glutamicum* is able to generate a rod-shaped cell by using in a different way the molecular mechanisms that are generally accepted as involved in bacterial morphogenesis.

Chapter 4 - Cell division is a highly coordinated process by which living organisms grow, develop and reproduce. It starts in the zygote, is essential during embryogenesis and lasts for the entire life as a source of new cells for repairing purposes. The molecular mechanisms underlying mitotic cell division is under intense investigation due to their key role in the discovery of potential molecular targets for cell therapy. For cell cycle entry and commitment to completion, the exposure to growth factors is required. After receptor activation, signals transmit by phosphorylating substrates leading to the trigger of a number of early signaling cascades, including activation of tyrosine kinases (Tyr K), Ras, and phospholipase C, among others. These proteins subsequently activate secondary effectors that regulate transcription factors such as c-Myc. Cell cycle orchestration is guided by molecular mechanisms that govern crucial irreversible transitions assuring that steps take place in the right order. Progress has been made toward the understanding of cell cycle regulation through better characterization of the cyclin role, the promoting anaphase complex (APC), and the functions of cyclin kinases. Disruptions in such mechanisms can trigger cell transformations and contribute to tumorigenesis. Cell cycle checkpoint deficiencies have also been proposed as events whereby cells lose their ability to avoid division until the optimal conditions are reached. Humans are exposed to a large range of disruptors, from their own physiology to environmental substances which are constantly challenging their cells and potentially inciting disturbances in the cell cycle and division mainly by virtue of a series of DNA injuries.

Chapter 5 - In animal cells and fungi, cytokinesis is achieved by constriction of an actomyosin-based ring assembled during mitosis. The fission yeast *Schizosaccharomyces pombe* is an excellent model organism for unraveling cell division controls by combining molecular genetics with cell biology approaches. Once spatially defined, the ring assembly site is the place of sequential incorporation of a set of proteins during mitotic progression, most of which are evolutionarily conserved. Then, fission yeast divides medially to produce equally sized daughter cells. In the past years, several studies have explored mechanisms of division site determination. It has been demonstrated that positive signals for division plane positioning originate from the central region. Position of the predivided nucleus and the anilin-related protein Mid1 give spatial cues to establish the place of ring formation. In addition, negative signals controlled by the DYRK Pom1 kinase and emanating from the cell ends restrict ring formation in the central region. This dual system prevents illegitimate cell division outside the centre of the cell and subsequent polyploid cell formation. Recently, it has been shown that the mitotic regulator Cdr2 kinase is intrinsically involved in division plane specification by binding to Mid1 at the cell equator during interphase. Moreover, nuclear-to-cytoplasm shuttling of Mid1 is another independent crucial mechanism that couples nuclear position with the actomyosin ring assembly site late in the G2 phase. Kin1, another kinase that regulates morphogenesis and intracellular organization, shares an essential function with Pom1 in cytokinesis. Recent advances have also identified distinct pathways involved in completion of CAR formation. Therefore, multiple regulatory mechanisms act in parallel to accurately specify and build up the actomyosin ring at the centre of the cell. Concomitant inhibition of these pathways dramatically affects cytokinesis and cell viability. Here we present these redundant pathways that contribute to faithful distribution of the genetic material into daughter cells.

Chapter 6 - Regulation of eukaryotic cell division is under tight control and includes several checkpoints. The controlling elements consist of cyclin-dependent kinases (CDKs) and their activators (cyclins) and inhibitors (INK4 and CIP/KIP). As the cell progresses through the cell cycle, various cyclins appear and bind to specific CDKs. These heterodimeric protein kinases are responsible for shuttling the cell through different regulatory checkpoints along the cell cycle. The major checkpoints include the G1/S checkpoint, which regulates entrance into the S-phase and the duplication of DNA; the G2/M checkpoint, which regulates entrance into mitosis and the alignment of the chromosomes; and the metaphase checkpoint, which regulates entrance into anaphase resulting in chromosome splitting and eventually in cell division. The connection between the cell cycle checkpoints and carcinogenesis involves checkpoint misregulation. This misregulation can lead to unscheduled cell division and cell proliferation and to genomic and chromosome instability associated with tumorigenesis. It is often the product of CDK mutation, overexpression of cyclins, or inactivation of CDK inhibitors. Finally, the mechanism of checkpoint (mis)regulation provides ample targets for developing drugs to treat cancer and represents a fecund area for future therapeutic developments.

Chapter 7 - About a decade ago, a four-protein complex denominated the cohesin complex emerged as a key player on the control of sister chromatid cohesion during cell division. In addition, during the last 2-3 years, new findings have implicated the cohesin complex in the control of gene expression, development and other essential cell functions in mammals.

The function of cohesin complex in chromosome segregation is mediated by the formation of a ring-like structure, which entrapped replicated DNA. The dynamic of the cohesin ring is regulated by a more and more large number of cohesin-interacting proteins. Cohesin-regulators were essentially identified and studied in relation with the cohesion function of cohesin complexes. However, recent results on the phenotype of mouse KO models and the discovery that mutations in some cohesin-regulator genes are the molecular causes of Cornelia de Lange and Roberts syndrome/Phocomelia human disorders suggested that these proteins are also involved in other important biological tasks of cohesins.

Chapter 8 - The known function of the evolutionary conservative NXF1 (Nuclear eXport Factor) is the nuclear-cytoplasmic transport of the most mRNAs. On our data Dm NXF1 is involved in control of cell division. By immunostaining of early embryos with antibodies to C-terminal part of Dm NXF1 we have shown that the intensity of the staining depends on the cell cycle stage. The cytoplasmic Dm NXF1 is abundant on prometaphase and it almost disappears on anaphase. It is possible that Dm NXF1 can be involved in RNP-complexes including mRNAs which translation is regulated during cell cycle. Such complexes dissociate to resolve the translation of according mRNAs.

Chapter 9 - Division in cyanobacteria, ancient phototrophic relatives of chloroplasts, may serve as a model for study of plant chloroplast division. Cyanobacterial mutants impaired in cell division were identified after chemical mutagenesis, by random cassette mutagenesis and by transposon mutagenesis. Analysis of such mutants appears to be an effective strategy for investigating cyanobacterial cell division. In addition, the availability of the complete genomic sequences of many cyanobacteria, bacteria, some plants and algae facilitates comparative genomic analysis. Some of the cyanobacterial cell division genes have homologues among cyanobacteria, green algae and higher plants, some genes are specific only for cyanobacteria. Finding of cyanobacterial *ftn2* gene, for example, helped to study the function of its plant homologoes that encoding Arc6 protein, a nuclear-encoded protein of chloroplast inner envelope membranes that is required for organelle division. Cell division is a highly co-ordinated and fine-tuned process, and the precise regulation and positioning of the cell division apparatus requires a number of both structural and regulatory components, of which many are still unidentified. Mutagenic disruption of proper regulation in the cell division machinery often leads to the formation of elongated and/or mini cells and may impose a strong internal stress, altering cell physiology. Metabolic pathways that are regulated by the cell cycle may also be affected. The first proteomic comparative study of two cyanobacterial cell division mutants has been initiated. Quantitative differences in the protein maps were detected and proteins with significant quantitative changes were identified. The upregulated proteins include proteins involved in cell division/cell morphogenesis, protein synthesis and processing, oxidative stress response, amino acid metabolism, nucleotide biosynthesis, and glycolysis, as well as unknown proteins. Among the downregulated proteins are those involved in chromosome segregation, protein processing, photosynthesis, redox regulation, carbon dioxide fixation, nucleotide biosynthesis, the biosynthetic pathway to fatty acids, and energy production. Identification of such differentially expressed proteins provides new targets for future studies that will allow assessment of their physiological roles and significance in cyanobacterial cell division.

In: Cell Division: Theory, Variants and Degradation
Editors: Y. N. Golitsin, M. C. Krylov, pp. 1-28
ISBN: 978-1-60876-986-5

Chapter 1

DIRECT AND REVERSE GENETICS FOR CYANOBACTERIAL CELL DIVISION STUDIES IN GENOMIC AND PROTEOMIC ERA

Olga A. Koksharova
A.N. Belozersky Institute of Physico-Chemical Biology, M.V. Lomonosov Moscow State University, Moscow 119992, Russian Federation.

ABSTRACT

Which genes are important, or even essential, for cyanobacterial cell division? One tool that should be able to provide an answer to this question is forward genetics, which aims to identify and clone mutant genes responsible for a phenotype of an interest. By using forward genetics approaches first we conduct mutant screens of a new quality and quantity and then proceed to new gene identification. Reverse genetic analysis for cyanobacterial genes encoding cell division proteins could be also applied after comparative genomic and proteomic analysis. Identification and functional studies of cyanobacterial mutants and genes that are involved in cell division and cell differentiation can enhance understanding of the regulation of morphogenesis of bacteria and plant chloroplasts.

INTRODUCTION

Most known bacteria divide symmetrically during normal growth. Although superficially simple, bacterial cell division is a complex regulatory process about which much is being learned. Discovery of bacterial *fts* and other genes [Bouche & Pichoff, 1998; Bramhill, 1997; Levin & Losick, 2000; Margolin, 2000; Shapiro & Losick, 2000; Howard & Kruse, 2005; Dajkovic & Lutkenhaus, 2006] has helped enhance understanding of cell division: how the bacterial cell forms the membrane-associated FtsZ ring that mediates septation, how a cell determines the site of division, how division is coordinated with chromosome replication, and how regulation of proteolysis assists cell division.

Despite their small size (typically 1-3 μm) and normal lack of the specialized organelles and cytoskeletal elements that are found in eukaryotic cells, bacterial cells are highly organized. It has become clear that many proteins and specific parts of the chromosome are localized to specific subcellular regions [Shapiro & Losick, 2000; Dajkovic & Lutkenhaus, 2006.]. Hirota *et al.* [Hirota *et al.*, 1968] identified conditionally lethal mutants of *E. coli* affected in cell division by screening for the formation of long, non-septate filaments at a restrictive temperature. This approach relied on the ability of the bacteria to continue elongation of the cylindrical portion of the cell in the absence of division. Later, additional such mutations and genes were described [Bramhill, 1997; Margolin, 2000]. Bacteria possess a number of cytoskeletal elements [Mayer, 2003], including FtsZ, a bacterial tubulin homologue [Carballido-López & Errington, 2003; Michie & Löwe, 2006; Klint *et al.*, 2007], MreB coiled structures similar to F-actin, the physiological polymer of eukaryotic actin [van den Ent *et al.*, 2001], MinCDE coiled arrays [Shih *et al.*, 2003] and intracellular protofilaments containing bacterial elongation factor Tu (EF-Tu) [Löwe *et al.*, 2004]. All of them may form cytoskeletal webs, which are important for the organization of intracellular structures and cell function [Mayer, 2003]. Dividing bacteria use a cytoskeletal structure at the division site for the mechanical constriction of the cell. The major component of this structure in most species is FtsZ [Bi & Lutkenhaus, 1991], a tubulin-like GTPase [Löwe & Amos, 1998] that shares many properties with eukaryotic cytoskeletal molecules. FtsZ assembles at the site of division and orchestrates cell division [Lutkenhaus & Addinall, 1997]. In the presence of GTP, purified FtsZ molecules self-assemble into long filamentous structures that are depolymerized rapidly when all of the GTP has been hydrolysed [Mukherjee & Lutkenhaus, 1998]. After a ring of molecules of FtsZ is formed, a dozen other cell-division proteins are recruited sequentially to the site of future division, forming additional ring structures [Rothfield, *et al.*, 1999; Dajkovic & Lutkenhaus, 2006]. In most bacterial species, the septum is formed at the midpoint of the cell. The mechanism of midsite selection is still not completely investigated, but in *E. coli*, the minicell genes *minC, minD* and *minE* are implicated in this process [de Boer, *et al.*, 1989; Jacobs & Shapiro, 1999; Raskin & de Boer. 1999a,b; Sullivan & Maddock, 2000; Jensen & Shapiro, 2000; Kruse *et al.*, 2007; Loose *et al.*, 2008]. Donachie and Begg [Donachie & Begg, 1996] confirmed that the number of septa formed per generation per *E. coli* cell length is fixed and that "division potential" is directly proportional to cell length. In a *minC* mutant, septa form with equal probability at the poles, centers, and 1/4- and 3/4-cell positions. These same authors showed that the time to next division is inversely related to cell length and that division is asynchronous in long cells, suggesting that a single cell can form only one septum at a time.

Since the discovery of the Z ring, immunofluorescence microscopy and fusion to green fluorescent protein (GFP) have been used for visualization of FtsZ and other cell division proteins. Most associate with the Z ring to form a complete septal apparatus (divisome or septal ring) capable of carrying out cell division [Lutkenhaus & Addinall, 1997; Errington *et al.*, 2003; Dajkovic & Lutkenhaus, 2006].

Cell-cycle processes, such as DNA replication, chromosome segregation and cell division must be strictly coordinated to ensure efficient proliferation. To understand how all of these processes are coordinately regulated in the bacterial cell, the complete set of related regulatory genes must be identified and their roles understood.

Cyanobacterial cell division mutants can aid in the search for such genes. Cyanobacteria, ancient relatives of chloroplasts and structurally similar to Gram-negative prokaryotes, perform plant-type photosynthesis; some of them are able to fix nitrogen and to cell differentiation. All methods of molecular biology are available for study of cyanobacteria [Koksharova & Wolk, 2002a]. Genomic DNA sequences are available for more than 40 different strains and species of cyanobacteria (http://www.ncbi.nlm.nih.gov/sutils/genom_table.cgi). However, the genetical control of cell division has been studied much less in cyanobacteria than it has in *Escherichia coli*, *Bacillus subtilis* or *Caulobacter crescentus*. Morphologically aberrant mutants of cyanobacteria presumably impaired in cell division, recovered with high frequency after chemical mutagenesis [Ingram & Thurston, 1970; Ingram & Van Baalen. 1970; Ingram, *et al.*, 1972; Ingram & Fisher, 1973a,b; Zhevner *et al.*, 1973; Ingram *et al.*,1975], were described several decades ago. During that time, only limited information has been obtained about cyanobacterial genes that are involved in the regulation of cell division. Study of cyanobacterial cell division can help to investigate molecular mechanisms of plastid division and plastid evolution. Genetic approach in a combination with genomics and proteomics could be applied for that study.

Genetical Approaches to Study Cyanobacterial Cell Division

Many genetic tools have been developed for unicellular and filamentous strains of cyanobacteria. These tools provide abundant opportunity for identifying novel genes; for investigating the structure, regulation and evolution of genes. Many vectors and other genetic tools have been applied for study of cyanobacteria. Transformation, electroporation, and conjugation are used for gene transfer. Diverse methods of mutagenesis allow the isolation of many sought-for kinds of mutants, including site-directed mutants of specific genes. Reporter genes permit measurement of the level of transcription of particular genes, and assays of transcription within individual colonies or within individual cells in a filament [for review Koksharova and Wolk, 2002a]. Complete genomic sequences have been obtained for today for the 43 strains and species of cyanobacteria. Genomic sequence data provide the opportunity for global monitoring of changes in genetic expression at transcriptional and translational levels in response to variations in environmental conditions. The availability of genomic sequences accelerates the identification, study, modification and comparison of cyanobacterial genes, and facilitates analysis of evolutionary relationships, including the relationship of chloroplasts to ancient cyanobacteria.

Which genes are important, or even essential, for cyanobacterial cell division? To answer this question forward and reverse genetics approaches could be applied (Table 1). Forward genetics permits to identify and clone mutant genes responsible for a phenotype of an interest. By using forward genetics approaches first we conduct mutant screens of a new quality and quantity and then proceed to new gene identification. Reverse genetic analysis for cyanobacterial genes encoding cell division proteins could be also applied after comparative genomic and proteomic analysis. Identification of cyanobacterial mutants and genes that are involved in cell division and cell differentiation can enhance understanding of the regulation of morphogenesis of bacteria and plant chloroplasts.

The first cyanobacterial mutants impaired in cell division were described many years ago [Ingram & Thurston, 1970; Ingram & Van Baalen. 1970; Ingram, *et al.*, 1972; Ingram & Fisher, 1973a,b; Zhevner *et al.*, 1973; Ingram *et al.*,1975]. Filamentous mutants showed two distinct phenotypes [Ingram & Fisher, 1973a]: septate filaments containing cross-walls apparently impaired in the terminal stages of cell separation; and serpentine forms that divide sporadically to produce multinucleoidal long cells. The gene mutated in a septate mutant of *Synechococcus* sp. strain PCC 7942 as a consequence of insertional inactivation [Dolganov & Grossman, 1993] was identified and characterized. Dolganov and Grossman by using "random cassette mutagenesis", i.e. the random insertion of an antibiotic resistance gene into the genome upon homologous recombination of genomic restriction fragments fused to that gene [Broedel & Wolf, 1990; Labarre, *et al.*, 1989], identified seven filamentous mutants of *Synechococcus* PCC 7942 as a result of insertional inactivation [Dolganov & Grossman, 1993]. In one of the mutants, the lesion may have been in an *flm3* region in *orf3* (Synpcc7942_*2006*), which encoded hypothetical protein. We applied transposon mutagenesis to the study of cell division. By use of transposon Tn*5*-692, which provides large numbers of transposon mutants in *Synechococcus* sp. PCC 7942, could have identified the mutants of the second, serpentine type [Koksharova & Wolk, 2002b; Miyagishima *et al.*, 2005].

Transposon mutagenesis and analysis of ftn genes, of Synechococcus sp. strain PCC 7942. Mutagenesis by transposition was first reported in *Synechococcus* sp. PCC 7942 (PCC 7942) when Tandeau de Marsac *et al.* [Tandeau de Marsac *et al.*, 1982] used transposition of Tn*901* from a plasmid to the chromosome to mutagenize a chromosomal locus. Transposon mutagenesis with Tn*901* from plasmid pUH24 of PCC 7942 [van den Hondel *et al.*, 1980] has been used to identify a cluster of genes involved in nitrate assimilation [Madueño, *et al.*, 1988; Luque, *et al.*, 1992]. Limiting the utility of Tn*901* is its low frequency of transposition [Golden, 1988]. Tn*5* was later used in *Anabaena* sp. strain PCC 7120 [Borthakur & Haselkorn, 1989], but became much more effective with the introduction of variants, e.g., Tn*5*-1058 and its progeny, that had (i) a much stronger promoter driving the antibiotic-resistance operon, (ii) enhanced transposition, and (iii) an *Escherichia coli* origin of replication within the transposon that facilitates recovery of the mutated gene. This vector allows the cloning of sequences contiguous with the transposon, by cutting genomic DNA with a restriction endonuclease that does not cut within the transposon, recircularizing *in vitro* and transforming *E. coli* with the resulting ligation mixture [e.g., Wolk *et al.*, 1991; Cohen *et al.*, 1998]. We introduce the use of transposon Tn*5*-692, whose ca. 100-fold increase in the rate of transposition provides large numbers of transposon mutants of *Anabaena variabilis* strain ATCC 29413 (PCC 7937) (C.P. Wolk & O.A. Koksharova, unpublished data) and of *Synechococcus* sp. PCC 7942. Two new transposition-derived cell division mutants of PCC 7942 have been characterized and two new cell division genes have been sequenced (GenBank accession AF421196 and AF421197) [Koksharova & Wolk, 2002b].

When *Synechococcus* sp. strain PCC 7942 was mutagenized with transposon Tn*5*-692, ca. 3000 Em^rSp^r, dense, round mutant colonies with regular margins were accompanied by 39 spreading colonies with irregular borders (Figure 1) that were comprised of very elongated cells. In classical studies of *f*ilamentous *t*emperature-*s*ensitive mutants of *E. coli* affected in cell division [Bramhill, 1997], the corresponding genes were designated *fts*; by analogy, we designated the mutants that we isolated, FTN-mutants (Filamentous, TransposoN-derived) and the corresponding genes, *ftn*. Two such mutants, FTN2 and FTN6, whose irregular colonies are composed of cells that are longer than wild-type cells have been selected for further inquiry. Cells of mutants FTN2 and FTN6 of *Synechococcus* sp. strain PCC 7942 have the appearance of long filaments that divide occasionally, at variable positions along the cell (Figure 2). The cells of both mutants usually divided asymmetrically. It appears that inactivation of *ftn2* or *ftn6* blocks cell division at an early stage or, alternatively, that the coordination of cell elongation and cell division is disrupted. Mutants FTN2 and FTN6 of *Synechococcus* sp. PCC 7942 are completely segregated. In FTN2 and FTN6, the transposon was inserted in single-copy open reading frames that we denote *ftn2* and *ftn6*. *ftn2* predicts a 631-amino acid protein that shows greatest similarity to the predicted products of other cyanobacterial and plants (Table 2).

The InterProScan program (http://www.ebi.ac.uk/interpro/scan.html) shows the presence in Ftn2 of a DnaJ N-terminal domain (aa 6-70) and a single TPR repeat (aa 136-169) in *Synechococcus* sp. PCC 7942. The Prosite-Protein against PROSITE program (http://ca.expasy.org/tools/scnpsite.html/) shows the presence in Ftn2 of a leucine zipper pattern (aa 234-255; Table 2). Ftn2 and its cyanobacterial and plant orthologs show the presence of a DnaJ N-terminal domain, but are otherwise, as are Ftn6 and its orthogs, dissimilar from the products of known division-related genes [Bramhill, 1997]. *ftn6* predicts a 152-amino acid protein and specific to cyanobacteria (Table3).

Table 1. Comparison of the "forward" and "reverse" genetics approaches.

"Forward»" genetics	"Reverse" genetics
1. P redicted function/phenotype 2. Mutant selection after chemical or transposon mutagenesis 3. New gene identification	1. The gene is known (after genomic or proteomic studies) 2. Mutant obtaining as result of gene inactivation by insertion of antibiotic resistance cassette in the gene 3. Gene function study

Table 2. Ftn2-like proteins and their accession numbers.

Organism	Accession Number/Open Reading Frame Name
Synechococcus sp PCC 7942	AF421196/Synpcc7942_*1943*
Thermosynechococcus elongatus BP-1	NP_681547/ *tlr0758*
Synechococcus sp. WH 7803	YP_001225456/SynWH7803_*1733*
Synechocystis sp PCC 6803	NP_441990/*Sll0169*
Anabaena/Nostoc sp PCC 7120	NP_486747/*all2707*
Nostoc punctiforme PCC 73102	YP_001868827/Npun_*R5579*
Anabaena variabilis ATCC 29413	YP_324769/Ava_*4275*
Trichodesmium erythraeum IMS101	YP_724444/Tery_*5067*
Protochlorococcus marinus MIT 9211	YP_001551219/P9211_*13341*
Protochlorococcus marinus MT9313	NP_894181/PMT*0348*
Chlamydomonas reinhardtii	XP_001690917/CHLREDRAFT_*169875*
Paulinella chromatophora	YP_002048788/PCC_*0126*
Arabidopsis thaliana	AAQ18646/*ARC6*
Oryza sativa	DAA01472/*Arc6*
Zea mays	ACF86369.1/BT041364.1:53…2338

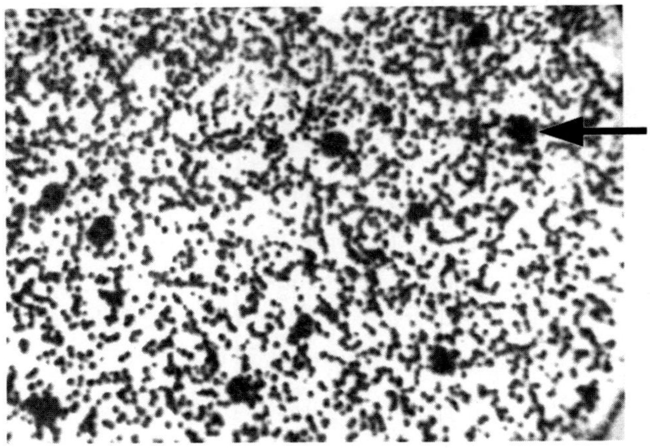

Figure 1. When the unicellular cyanobacterium, *Synechococcus* sp. strain PCC 7942, was mutagenized with transposon Tn5-692, dense, round mutant colonies with regular margins were accompanied by spreading colonies with irregular borders (one of them is indicated by an arrow).

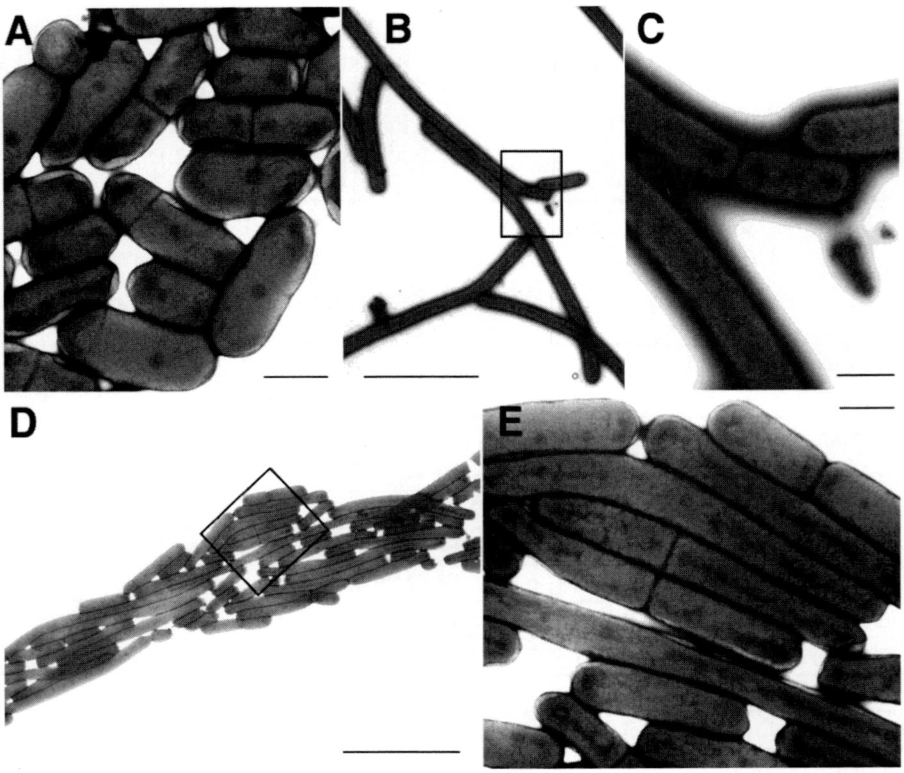

Figure 2. Structure of wild-type PCC 7942 (A), and of mutants FTN2 (C, see box in panel B) and FTN6 (E, see box in panel D), negatively stained with uranyl acetate, and examined by electron microscopy. The cells of both mutants usually divided asymmetrically. Scale bars represent 1 μm (A,C,E) or 10 μm (B,D) [Koksharova & Wolk, 2002b].

The presence of a DnaJ domain, a (single) tetratricopeptide repeat (TPR) and a leucine zipper motif suggest that Ftn2 may function as part of a complex with one or more other proteins and may be regulatory. DnaJ domains are characteristic of a family of chaperonins.

Proteins in this family, from bacterial to human, have three distinct domains: (i) a highly conserved J domain of approximately 70 amino acids, often found near the N-terminus, which mediates interaction of DnaJ (a.k.a., Hsp40) with Hsp70 (DnaK) and regulates the ATPase activity of the latter; (ii) a glycine and phenylalanine (G/F)-rich region of unknown function that may act as a flexible linker; and (iii) a cysteine-rich region (C domain) that contains four CXXCXGXG motifs, and resembles a zinc-finger domain [Ohtsuka & Hata, 2000]. Although not originally identified as an *fts* gene, *dnaJ* shares with *fts* genes the property that its inactivation leads to a filamentous phenotype [Paciorek *et al.*, 1997]. Cheetham and Caplan [Cheetham & Caplan, 1998] classified DnaJ/Hsp40 homologs into three groups: type I have all three of these domains; type II have only the J and G/F domains; and type III, like Ftn2, have only a J domain. DnaK proteins are highly versatile chaperones that assist a large variety of processes [Bukau, 1999; Bukau & Horwich, 1998; Bukau & Walker, 1989; Fink, 1999; Gething, 1997; Hartl, 1996], from folding of newly synthesized proteins to facilitation of proteolytic degradation of unstable proteins [Laufen *et al.*, 1999]. This functional diversity requires that DnaK proteins associate promiscuously with misfolded proteins or selectively with folded substrates, including with regulatory proteins of low abundance.

The tetratricopeptide repeat (TPR) of, typically, 34 amino acids was first described in the yeast cell division cycle regulator Cdc23p [Sikorski *et al.*, 1990] and was later found in many other proteins [Das *et al.*, 1998, Goebl & Yanagida, 1991; Lamb *et al.*, 1995]. TPRs are frequently present in tandem arrays of 3-16 copies, although single (as in Ftn2) or paired TPRs are also common [Lamb *et al.*, 1995]. Processes involving TPR proteins include cell-cycle control, repression of transcription, response to stress, protein kinase inhibition, mitochondrial and peroxisomal protein transport, and neurogenesis [Goebl & Yanagida, 1991]. There appears to be no common biochemical function connecting TRP-containing proteins, although the TRP forms scaffolds that mediate protein-protein interactions and, often, the assembly of multiprotein complexes.

A web-based program (http://HypothesisCreator.net/iPSORT/) predicts that an *Arabidopsis* ortholog of *ftn2* has a chloroplast transit peptide (MEALS HVGIG LSPFQ LCRLP PATTK LRRSH); according to ProfileScan (http://www.isrec.isb-sib.ch/software/PFSCAN_form.html), this protein possesses a DnaJ domain profile; and according to InterProScan (http://www.ebi.ac.uk/interpro/scan.html), the protein possesses a Myb DNA-binding domain. A role of this ortholog in chloroplast cell division has been shown [Vitha *et al.*, 2003].

Reverse genetic analysis for homologous cyanobacterial genes encoding cell division proteins Ftn2 [Koksharova & Wolk, 2002b; Mazouni *et al.*, 2004] and Ftn6 [Koksharova & Wolk, 2002b] in *Anabaena* sp. PCC 7120 and in *Synechocystis* sp. PCC 6803 has been applied. Mutants show significant cell division defects. However, in contrast to *Synechococcus* sp. PCC 7942 FTN2 mutant, corresponding mutants of *Anabaena* and *Synechocystis* failed to segregate completely [Koksharova & Wolk, 2002b; Mazouni *et al.*, 2004]. The presence of the greatly enlarged cells, which by their shape and frequent contiguity to heterocysts somewhat resemble akinetes, suggests that *Anabaena* sp. PCC 7120 Ftn2 and Ftn6 homologues may be involved not only in the regulation of cell growth, but also in cellular differentiation [Koksharova & Wolk, 2002b].

In order to identify other genes involved in cyanobacterial cell division, *Synechococcus* sp. PCC 7942 has been mutagenized [Miyagishima *et al.*, 2005] by the introduction of pRL692, which carries a derivative of transposon Tn5 (Tn5-692; [Koksharova & Wolk, 2002b]). Seven loci have been selected for study. These included *ftn2* (Synpcc7942_*1943*) and *minE* (Synpcc7942_*0897*), whose roles in cyanobacterial cell division have been lately investigated [Koksharova & Wolk, 2002b; Mazouni *et al.*, 2004]; *flm3* region *orf3* (Synpcc7942_*2006*) and *ftn6* (Synpcc7942_*1707*), previously identified as possible cell division loci [Dolganov & Grossman, 1993; Koksharova & Wolk, 2002b]; and three genes, Synpcc7942_*0653*, Synpcc7942_*0644* and Synpcc7942_*2059*, not previously associated with cell division in cyanobacteria [Miyagishima *et al.*, 2005]. Synpcc7942_*0644* encodes CikA, a regulator of the *Synechococcus elongatus* PCC 7942 circadian clock [Schmitz *et al.*, 2000; Mutsuda *et al.*, 2003]. Synpcc7942_*0653* (named as *cdv1*, [Miyagishima *et al.*, 2005]) encodes *p*eptidyl-prolyl cis-trans isomerase and Synpcc7942_*2059* (named as *cdv2*, [Miyagishima *et al.*, 2005] encodes cell division protein SepF.

Now all these genes and several new ones are placed on the list of the known genes that control of cyanobacteria cell proliferation (Table3). By using Tn mutagenesis as a molecular genetical experimental tool we can add more new cell division genes to this list in the nearest future.

Table 3. Genes involved in cell division by the example of *Synechococcus* sp. PCC 7942.

Gene	Protein	Function	Reference	Bacterial homolog	Plant homolog (in *Arabidopsis* genome)
Synpcc7942_*2378*	FtsZ	GTP-binding cell division protein; septum ring formation	Bi & Lutkenhaus. 1991	FtsZ	FtsZ1-1 AT5G55280 FtsZ2-1 AT2G36250
Synpcc7942_*2377*	FtsQ	cell division protein that is part of the divisome complex	van den Ent *et al.*, 2008	FtsQ	absent
Synpcc7942_*0580* Synpcc7942_*0482*	FtsI	peptidoglycan glycosyltransferase	Pogliano *et al.*, 1997	FtsI	absent
Synpcc7942_*0564* Synpcc7942_*1414*	FtsE	cell division protein	Corbin etal., 2007	FtsE	absent
Synpcc7942_*2580* Synpcc7942_*2468* Synpcc7942_*2073*	dnaK molecular chaperone	Heat shock protein 70; assists in folding of nascent polypeptide chains; refolding of misfolded proteins.	Bukau & Walker, 1989; Nimura *et al.*,2001	dnaK	CPHSC70-1 (chloroplast heat shock protein 70-1 NP_194159.1
Synpcc7942_*1943*	Ftn2	may function in a chaperone system	Koksharova & Wolk, 2002b; Vitha *et al.*, 2003	absent	Arc6 AAQ18646/ARC6
Synpcc7942_*1707*	Ftn6	hypothetical protein	Koksharova & Wolk, 2002b	absent	absent
Synpcc7942_*1633*	hypothetical protein	hypothetical protein	Koksharova, this work	absent	absent
Synpcc7942_0706	precorrin-6B methylase	catalyzes the formation of precorrin-8x from precorrin-6y	Koksharova, this work	absent	absent
Synpcc7942_*0897*	MinE	cell division topological specificity factor	Lutkenhaus, 2007; Loose *et al.*, 2008	MinE	AtMinE1 AT1G69390 BAB79236
Synpcc7942_*0896*	MinD	septum site-determining protein	Lutkenhaus, 2007; Kerr *et al.*, 2006; Loose *et al.*, 2008	MinD	MIND AT5G24020

Table 3. (Continued)

Gene	Protein	Function	Reference	Bacterial homolog	Plant homolog (in *Arabidopsis* genome)
Synpcc7942_*1104* Synpcc7942_*0324*	FtsW	cell division protein	Mercer & Weiss, 2001	FtsW	absent
Synpcc7942_*2001*	MinC	septum formation inhibitor	Lutkenhaus, 2007; Zhou & Lutkenhaus, 2005; Loose *et al.*, 2008	MinC	absent
Synpcc7942_*0653* *cdv1*	Peptidyl-prolyl cis-trans isomerase (rotamase) - cyclophilin family-like	unknown	Miyagishima *et al.*, 2005	*Bacillus* sp. B14905 ZP_01724138.1	CYP38 (Cyclophilin 38); peptidyl-prolyl cis-trans isomerase AT3G01480
Synpcc7942_*0644*	CikA GAF sensor hybrid histidine kinase	a regulator of the *Synechococcus elongatus* PCC 7942 circadian clock	Schmitz *et al.*, 2000 Miyagishima *et al.*, 2005	Several histidine kinases (Score 98-160 bits)	AHK3 NP_564276
Synpcc7942_*2059* *cdv2*	hypothetical protein; cell division protein SepF	Cell division protein that is part of the divisome complex and is recruited early to the Z-ring. Probably stimulates Z-ring formation, perhaps through the cross-linking of FtsZ protofilaments. Its function overlaps with FtsA.	Miyagishima *et al.*, 2005	BSU15390 *B subtilis*	absent
Synpcc7942_*2006* *cdv3*	hypothetical protein	unknown	Dolganov & Grossman, 1993; Miyagishima *et al.*, 2005	absent	absent
S 6803 slr1471 Synpcc7942_1617	Putative inner membrane protein translocase component YidC NP441564.1	member of the Alb3/Oxa1/YidC protein family	Fulgosi et al., PNAS, 2002,99:11501-11506	absent	ARTEMIS locus of Arabidopsis (NP_173858) envelope membrane integrase
Slr1223 S6803 Synpcc7942_2477	SulA cell division inhibitor	Predicted nucleoside-diphosphate sugar epimerase	Raynaud et al, 2004	SulA	(GC1) (Giant chloroplast1); NP_565505

Table 3. (*Continued*)

Gene	Protein	Function	Reference	Bacterial homolog	Plant homolog (in *Arabidopsis* genome)
murC Synpcc7942_1741	UDP-N-acetylmuramate--L-alanine ligase	involved in cell wall formation; peptidoglycan synthesis;	Smith, 2006; Deva et al., 2006; El Zoeiby et al., 2003; Meroueh et al., 2006	E. coli ZP_03071496	absent
murE Synpcc7942_1484	UDP-N-acetylmuramoylalanyl-D-glutamate-2,6-diaminopimelate ligase	involved in cell wall formation; peptidoglycan synthesis; catalyzes the addition of meso-diaminopimelic acid to the nucleotide precursor UDP-N-aceylmuramoyl-l-alanyl-d-glutamate		NP_414627.1	absent
murD Synpcc7942_1667	UDP-N-acetylmuramoyl-L-alanyl-D-glutamate synthetase			NP_414630	absent
murI Synpcc7942_2361	glutamate racemase	involved in peptidoglycan biosynthesis; catalyzes the addition of glutamate to the nucleotide precursor UDP-N-acetylmuramoyl-L-alanine during cell wall formation converts L-glutamate to D-glutamate, a component of peptidoglycan		NP_418402	absent
Synpcc7942_2360	N-acetylmuramoyl-L-alanine amidase	is an autolysin that hydrolyzes the amide bond between N-acetylmuramoyl and L-amino	Koksharova, this work	Escherichia coli HS YP_001459220.1	absent

GENOMIC AND PROTEOMIC STUDIES OF CYANOBACTERIAL CELL DIVISION GENES

By mutational and comparative analysis, the list of genes known or predicted to influence cell division in *Synechococcus* sp. PCC 7942 has been extended. The availability of whole bacterial genome sequences has revealed that cyanobacteria encode homologues of cell division genes originally identified in *E. coli*: *ftsE, ftsI, ftsK, ftsQ, ftsW, ftsZ, minC, minD* and *minE* [Doherty & Adams, 1995; Mazouni *et al.*, 2004; Miyagishima *et al.*, 2005]. Studies in *Synechococcus* and in *Synechocystis* have confirmed a role for six further cell division genes, *ftn2, ftn6, cdv1, cdv2* and *cdv3, sulA*, [Koksharova *et al.*, 2002; Raynaud *et al.*, 2004; Miyagishima *et al.*, 2005] (Table 3). A cyanobacterial gene that encodes an ortholog of cell division protein FtsZ has been cloned and sequenced so far from *Anabaena* PCC 7120 [Doherty & Adams, 1995; Zhang, *et al.*, 1995]. This protein, present in vegetative cells [Kuhn, *et al.*, 2000], forming a ring structure [Sakr *et al.*, 2006; Klint *et al.*, 2007], as well as some amount of FtsZ present in non-dividing, differentiated cells called heterocysts. This protein may have a cytoskeletal function [Klint *et al.*, 2007]. FtsZ gene was insertion-inactivated in *Synechococcus* sp. PCC 7942 and in *Synechocystis* sp. PCC 6803 [Sarcina & Mullineaux, 2000]. Mutation was lethal, only heteroplasmic (that is, they retained both wild-type and transformed chromosomes) cells can survive. One more example of the successful application of reverse genetics in the characterization of chloroplast functions is the targeted mutagenesis of plant homologues of the bacterial cell division protein FtsZ [Osteryoung *et al.*, 1998; Strepp *et al.*, 1998; Stokes *et al.*, 2000]. This protein was shown to have a functional chloroplast targeting transit peptide, and subsequent studies demonstrated that, by contrast with most bacteria encoding a single FtsZ protein, *Arabidopsis* and other plant species harbour two families of plastid-targeted FtsZs. FtsZ proteins from both of these families were found to co-localize into a Z ring at the division site in *Arabidopsis*, pea, and tobacco [Fujiwara & Yoshida, 2001; McAndrew *et al.*, 2001; Vitha *et al.*, 2001].

Comparative genomic approach permitted to discover some new common cyanobacterial and plastid division genes. Cell division in cyanobacteria serves as a model for the study of chloroplast division. The morphological similarities between dividing cyanobacteria and dividing chloroplasts are striking and knowledge of cyanobacterial division will undoubtedly benefit plastid division research. Plastids are descended from a cyanobacterial symbiosis which occurred over 1.2 billion years ago. However only 100 years ago the first clear exposition of the hypothesis that plastids are derived from endosymbiotic cyanobacteria had been made by Mereschkowsky C. [Mereschkowsky, 1905; Martin & Kowallik, 1999]. During the course of endosymbiosis, most genes were lost from the cyanobacterium's genome and many were relocated to the host nucleus through endosymbiotic gene transfer (EGT) [Raven & Allen, 2003]. According recent estimations, 16-18% of plant nucleus genes are transferred from cyanobacteria [Martin *et al.*, 2002; Deusch *et al.*, 2008]. Among them some chloroplast division genes/proteins have been found: Arc6; ARTEMIS and GC1 (also called AtSulA) (Table 3) [Koksharova & Wolk, 2002b; Vitha *et al.*, 2003; Fulgosi *et al.*, 2002; Raynaud *et al.*, 2004; Maple *et al.*, 2004], ptCpn60α and ptCpn60β [Suzuki *et al.*, 2009].

Plant nuclear gene *arc6* is a descendant of the cyanobacterial cell division gene *ftn2* [Koksharova & Wolk, 2002; Vitha *et al.*, 2003], and ARC6 and its orthologs are only found in cyanobacteria, eukaryotic algae and higher plants. ARC6 was originally identified through cloning of the arc6 mutant [Pyke *et al.*, 1994; Vitha *et al.*, 2003]. ARC6 is an inner envelope membrane protein that acts as a positive regulator of Z-ring formation [Vitha *et al.*, 2003]. ARC6-GFP localizes to a ring-like structure at the mid-plastid [Vitha *et al.*, 2003]. ARC6 and Ftn2 proteins possess a conserved region at their N-termini with sequence similarity to J-domains, implicating them as possible Hsp70-associated co-chaperones. arc6 mutants have short FtsZ filaments within a single large chloroplast. In plants overexpressing ARC6, FtsZ filaments are more numerous and form spiral patterns around the enlarged chloroplast. These phenotypes suggest that ARC6 could play a role in bundling of short FtsZ filaments into a ring at the chloroplast division site. The N-terminus of ARC6 resides in the stroma [Vitha *et al.*, 2003] and a conserved N-terminal segment of ARC6 interacts with FtsZ2-1 but not FtsZ1-1 [Maple *et al.*, 2005]. ARC6 has been shown to interact with the CORE domain of AtFtsZ2-1 [Maple *et al.*, 2005]. In *E. coli*, the CORE domain of FtsZ mediates the interaction with both FtsA and ZipA proteins. FtsA and ZipA could be involved in controlling the FtsZ polymerization. No homologues of these bacterial proteins have been identified in the genomes of cyanobacteria or higher plants and ARC6 may play a role analogous to that of FtsA and ZipA, stabilizing or anchoring the Z-ring [Maple & Møller, 2007.]. Actually Z-ring formation by either FtsZ protein is dependent on functional ARC6 since in the *arc6* background both AtFtsZ1-1 and AtFtsZ2-1 form short filaments [Vitha *et al.*, 2003]. This is especially interesting in connection with the discovery that ARC6 interacts specifically with AtFtsZ2-1, and it is possible that inner membrane-bound AtFtsZ2-1 is stabilized though its interactions with ARC6 and that, subsequently, AtFtsZ1-1 polymerizes and interacts with AtFtsZ2-1, allowing further protein recruitment to the site of division. Quantitative yeast two-hybrid assays using truncated forms of the ARC6 stromal domain revealed that the conserved domain was sufficient for the interaction between ARC6 and AtFtsZ2-1 and that this interaction was not dependent on the presence of the J-domain [Maple *et al.*, 2005]. In contrast, Ftn2 is reported to require the J-domain for interaction with cyanobacterial FtsZ [Mazouni *et al.*, 2004] but the significance of this difference is not yet understood.

Protein ARTEMIS (*Arabidopsis thaliana* envelope membrane integrase) was identified in a search for proteins involved in chloroplast biogenesis [Fulgosi *et al.*, 2002]. The role of ARTEMIS in chloroplast division was discovered from studies using transposon insertion *Arabidopsis* plants with greatly reduced levels of the ARTEMIS protein [Fulgosi *et al.*, 2002]. These plants have similar growth characteristics to wild-type plants, but ultrastructural analysis revealed extended, duplicated, or triplicated, undividing chloroplasts. Whereas the envelope membranes fail to complete constriction, the thylakoid membranes are visibly constricted at the centre of the chloroplasts and are apparently portioned between the two halves of the organelle. ARTEMIS protein has a unique molecular structure combining a C-terminal domain similar to the Alb3 and Oxa1 proteins with conserved YidC translocase elements and an N-terminal region similar to receptor protein kinases. Using the YidC/Alb3-like translocase domain, a homologue of ARTEMIS has been identified in *Synechocystis* PCC6803 (*slr147*). Deletion mutant for this gene has altered cell morphology, with the formation of tetrameric or hexameric clusters of cells indicative of late cell division arrest [Fulgosi *et al.*, 2002]. Cells also seem to initiate their fission events unevenly, leading to cells of irregular shape. The evolutionary conservation of ARTEMIS has been demonstrated by the rescue of wild-type division characteristics in the *slr1471* cyanobacterial mutant with the YidC/Alb3-like domain of ARTEMIS [Fulgosi *et al.*, 2002].

Protein GC1 (Giant Chloroplast 1, also called AtSulA) was originally identified based on its similarity to putative cell division inhibitor SulA proteins in *Anabaena* sp. PCC 7120 (*all2390*) and *Synechocystis* sp. PCC 6803 (*slr1223*), although no function had been reported for the cyanobacterial proteins [Maple *et al.*, 2004; Raynaud *et al.*, 2004]. Gene encoding GC1 is located on chromosome II and encodes a protein of 347 amino acids which has an N-terminal plastid-targeting transit peptide absent in the cyanobacterial protein. Phylogenetic analysis of GC1 homologues indicates a clear cyanobacterial origin of GC1. The analysis of a *Synechocystis slr1223* deletion mutant, showing that *slr1223* is essential for cell survival as complete segregaton of this mutant could not be achieved [Raynaud *et al*, 2004]. Microscopic analysis of heteroploid clones revealed that up to 40% initiated but failed to complete cell division, resulting in cloverleaf-like structures, demonstrating that *slr1223* is required for correct cell division in *Synechocystis.* GC1 was shown to be associated with the inner envelope and is likely to be a key regulator of the division process, although its exact function is still unknown. In a subset of bacterial systems, induction of SulA is one of many responses to DNA damage; SulA inhibits cell division by binding directly to FtsZ and occluding the protofilament interface, preventing FtsZ polymerization [Mizusawa & Gottesman, 1983; Cordell *et al.*, 2003]. However, unlike SulA, GC1 does not appear to possess an FtsZ-binding domain identical to that in *Pseudomonas aeruginosa* SulA [Cordell *et al.*, 2003] nor does it bind FtsZ1 or FtsZ2 directly [Maple *et al.*, 2004]. Although SulA inhibits cell division in bacteria, the published effects of GC1 on chloroplast division are contradictory: work from one group suggests that GC1 acts as a positive regulator of chloroplast division [Maple *et al.*, 2004]; while work from another indicates that it acts as a negative regulator [Raynaud *et al.*, 2004]. Further work on GC1 is needed to clarify its role in the division process.

Chaperonin proteins ptCpn60α and ptCpn60β are required for proper plastid division in *A. thaliana.* These new plastid division proteins have been identified recently by characterizing plastid division mutants obtained by using forward genetics approach [Suzuki *et al.*, 2009]. Phylogenetic analysis showed that both ptCpn60 proteins are derived from ancestral cyanobacterial proteins and have a similarity with chaperonin GroEL. Early it has been shown that the filamentous phenotypes were observed in GroEL-depleted *Escherichia coli* [Fujiwara & Taguchi, 2007], *Caulobacter crescentus* and *Streptococcus* mutans, suggesting [Susin *et al.*, 2006; Lemos *et al.*, 2007] that GroEL plays a universal role in cell division in bacteria. Notably, a level of Gro EL protein has been upshifted in the proteomes of the FTN2 and FTH6 cell division mutants of *Synechococcus* sp. PCC 7942 [Koksharova *et al.*, 2007] (see also below). No more cell division function had been reported for the cyanobacterial GroEL proteins so far.

Despite its significance to our understanding of plastid division, till now only a few studies have identified components of the cyanobacterial cell division apparatus [Koksharova& Wolk, 2002; Fulgosi *et al.*, 2002; Raynaud *et al.*, 2004; Miyagishima at al., 2005]. It is important that the identification and analysis of division components may be more efficient in cyanobacteria rather than *Arabidopsis* or other model systems because of the easy cultivation, the short cyanobacterial generation time, the ability to obtain a near-synchronous culture, availability of many genetic tools [Koksharova & Wolk, 2002a]. One more of the experimental tools for functional study cyanobacterial cell division could be comparative proteomic analysis.

Cell division is a highly co-ordinated and fine-tuned process, and the precise regulation and positioning of the cell division apparatus require a number of both structural and regulatory components, of which many are still unidentified. Mutagenic disruption of proper regulation in the cell division machinery often leads to the formation of elongated and/or mini cells and may impose a strong internal stress altering the cellular physiology. In addition, metabolic pathways, which are regulated by the cell cycle, will be affected. Also, compensatory mechanisms to overcome the impaired cell division are expected. Although the cell division is impaired, for example, in the FTN2 and FTN6 cell division mutants, they have comparable growth rates [Koksharova & Wolk, 2002; Miyagishima *et al.,* 2005].

Fueled by ever-growing DNA sequence information, proteomics – the large scale analysis of proteins – has become one of the most important disciplines for characterizing gene function, for building functional linkages between protein molecules, and for providing insight into the mechanisms of biological processes in a high-throughput mode. In particular, proteomic analysis is vital, as the observed phenotype is a direct result of the action of the proteins rather than the genome sequence. Two-dimensional polyacrylamide gel electrophoresis (2-D gels) is the pre-eminent tool for monitoring proteomic changes for example during bacterial stress responses [for review Neidhardt & VanBogelen, 2000]. However, proteomic studies of stress responses in cyanobacteria, including the potentially stressful condition that a blocked cell division may impose, are so far limited. Proteome analysis has been successfully used for identifying periplasmic proteins of salt-stressed *Synechocystis* sp. strain PCC 6803 cells, and resulted in the identification of proteins responding strongly to salt stress [Fulda *et al.*, 2000; Fulda *et al*, 2006; Huang *et al.*, 2006]. Proteomic analysis of the heat shock response of wild-type and a mutant of the histidine kinase 34 gene has been performed in the cyanobacterium *Synechocystis* sp. strain PCC 6803 [Slabas *et al.*, 2006]. Moreover, 2-D gel electrophoresis with *in vivo* [^{35}S] methionine labelling has been applied for investigating long-term chlorotic cells of *Synechococcus* [Sauer *et al.*, 2001].

The unicellular *Synechococcus* sp. strain PCC 7942 belongs to the ancient cyanobacterial group of photoautotrophic prokaryotes [Rippka *et al.,* 1979], and has been used as a model organism for studying the genetic control of cyanobacterial cell division [Dolganov & Grossman, 1993; Koksharova & Wolk, 2002; Miyagishima *et al.,* 2005] as well as plastid division in higher plants [Vitha *et al.*, 2003]. In *Synechococcus* sp. strain PCC 7942, the first proteomic overview has been initiated recently [Koksharova *et al.*, 2006]. The proteome was analyzed by two-dimensional gel electrophoresis with subsequent MALDI-TOF mass spectroscopy and database analysis. Of the 140 analyzed protein spots, 110 were successfully identified as 62 different proteins, many of which occurred as multiple spots on the gel. The identified proteins participate in the major metabolic and cellular processes in cyanobacterial cells during the exponential growth phase. In addition, 14 proteins which were previously either unknown or considered to be hypothetical were shown to be true gene products in *Synechococcus* sp. strain PCC 7942 [Koksharova *et al.*, 2006]. These results may be helpful for the annotation of the sequenced genome of this cyanobacterium, as well as for biochemical and physiological studies of *Synechococcus.*

In the next proteomic study of this cyanobacteria [Koksharova *et al.*, 2007] proteomes of the two cell division mutants FTN2 and FTN6 mutants were compared to the wild-type in order to widen our knowledge about the cell division machinery using a new approach. Quantitative differences in the protein maps were detected and proteins with significant quantitative changes were identified.

Two new cell division genes, *ftn2* and *ftn6*, were discovered in *Synechococcus* sp. strain PCC 7942 by transposon Tn5-692 mutagenesis, followed by mutant DNA cloning and sequencing [Koksharova & Wolk, 2002]. The Ftn2 protein contains a DnaJ domain, a single tetratricopeptide repeat (TPR) and a leucine zipper pattern suggesting that Ftn2 may associate as a component in a protein complex and have a regulatory function. The Ftn6 protein was found to be specific for cyanobacteria and, as no detectable conserved domains have been found within the protein, knowledge about its precise function is still lacking [Koksharova & Wolk, 2002; Miyagishima *et al.,* 2005]. Occasionally FTN2 and FTN6 mutant cells divide and septum formation takes place irregularly [Koksharova & Wolk, 2002] but only a slight and diffuses localization of the key cell division protein FtsZ, homologous of tubulin [Bi & Lutkenhaus, 1991], has been detected at these rare cell division constriction sites. However, only a small difference in FtsZ protein levels could be detected between the mutants and the wild-type strain using immunoblot analysis of total soluble protein extracts [Koksharova, Klint, Rasmussen, 2003, unpublished results; Miyagishima *et al.,* 2005]. Therefore it has been suggested that these mutants are defective in recruitment of FtsZ to the division site or in subsequent assembly of the Z ring. Investigations of the Ftn2 protein orthologs in *Arabidopsis thaliana* (ARC6) and in the cyanobacterium *Synechocystis* sp. strain PCC 6803 (ZipN) have shown that a direct interaction between Ftn2 and FtsZ is most likely [Vitha *et al.*, 2003; Mazouni *et al.*, 2004]. Ftn2 may function in a chaperone system, probably to stabilize FtsZ filaments. Whether the Ftn6 protein in cyanobacteria interacts directly or indirectly with FtsZ is not known, but a loss of the *ftn6* gene results in aberrant cell division, similar to the FTN2 mutant [Koksharova & Wolk, 2002; Mazouni *et al.*, 2004; Miyagishima *et al.,* 2005].

For the first proteomic study of cyanobacterial cell division total soluble proteins extracted from the wild-type *Synechococcus* sp. strain PCC 7942 and the two cell division mutants FTN2 and FTN6 were analyzed by separation on 2-D gels in the pH range 3-10 and 4-7, followed by staining with SYPRO Ruby. Fluorescent chromophore-staining (SYPRO Ruby) dye is very sensitive [Berggren *et al.*, 2000] and permits to obtain digital image of the gel that can be analyzed by using PDQuest software. More than 800 protein spots on each gel were visualized, among which 76 protein spots in total were changed in quantity between the wild-type and the mutants as resolved by using the PDQuest software. These protein spots were subjected to MALDI-TOF mass spectroscopy resulting in the identification of 53 protein spots representing 44 unique proteins, which were grouped into seven main functional categories. Fifteen proteins were up-shifted or induced in both cell division mutants, and 13 proteins were down-shifted or repressed. The changed proteins included a general increased level of proteins involved in cell cycle and regeneration as well as protein synthesis, posttranslational processing and modification. Besides of eliciting common responses, the inactivation of *ftn2* and *ftn6* in the mutants may result in different responses in protein levels between the mutants [Koksharova *et al.*, 2007]. Among identified differentially affected proteins, 80% (8/10) of the spots affected in the FTN2 mutant were up-shifted, whereas in the FTN6 mutant 70% (7/10) of the affected protein spots were down-shifted. These results indicate that the Ftn2 protein may have a negative effect and the Ftn6 protein may have a positive effect on the level of some proteins in *Synechococcu*s sp. PCC 7942, either directly or indirectly. Mutations in genes *ftn2* and *ftn6* influence on level of 44 idetified proteins that are represent different physiological processes, among them are cell cycle and morphogenesis, synthesis and modification of proteins, photosynthesis, oxidative stress defense, CO2 fixation and carbon concentrating mechanism, energy production and different biosynthetic processes, as well as processes that involve unknown and hypothetical proteins. Possible functions of some of these proteins are discussed below to assess the impact of impaired cell division at the protein level.

Several proteins involved in cell cycle control were affected in the cell division mutants FTN2 and FTN6. The beta subunit (DnaN) of the multi-chain enzyme, DNA polymerase III, a key enzyme in the replicative synthesis of bacteria, was two fold up-shifted in the FTN2 mutant (Table 4) DnaN is required for the initiation of DNA replication and regulates the chromosomal replication cycle [Katayama *et al.*, 1998]. The rhythmical expression of *dnaN* gene in *Synechococcus* sp. strain PCC 7942 suggests that DNA replication could be under circadian control in this organism [Liu & Tsinoremas, 1996]. Chromosome replication and cell division are highly co-coordinated processes, and the early stages of DNA replication play a key role in the precise positioning of the Z ring at mid-cell and between replicating daughter chromosomes [Harry *et al.*, 1999]. In *Escherichia coli*, the function of DnaA is negatively regulated by DnaN [Katayama *et al.*, 1998], and an interaction between the replication initiator DnaA and DnaN is required to regulate the chromosomal replication cycle [Katayama *et al.*, 1998; Kawakami *et al.*, 2001]. It is likely that the increased amount of DnaN in cells of the FTN2 mutants may affect DNA replication and consequently disturbs cell division.

A protein identified as chromosome segregation ATPases was two fold down-shifted in the FTN6 mutant (Table 4). However, how the chromosome segregation ATPase contributes to the process of cyanobacterial chromosome segregation and how it can be connected functionally with Ftn6 protein are presently unknown. Since MreB was also affected in the mutants (see below), the processes of chromosome segregation and cell septation may be co-regulated at some level in cyanobacteria *Synechococcus* sp. PCC 7942.

Chromosome segregation has been well studied in the heterotrophic bacteria *E. coli, Bacillus subtilis,* and *Caulobacter crescentus* [Kruse *et al.*, 2003; Sherratt, 2003] where proteins such as the Min system [Åkerlund *et al.*, 2002], Par A and Par B [Easter & Gober, 2002], DivIVA [Thomaides *et al.*, 2001], SMC proteins [Graumann, 2001], and SpoIIIE [Bath *et al.*, 2000] have been proposed to be involved. Cell division normally follows the completion of each round of chromosome replication in *Escherichia coli*. Transcription of the essential cell division genes clustered at the *mra* region (*ftsL, ftsI, ftsW, ftsQ, ftsA*) is shown to depend on continuing chromosomal DNA replication [Liu *et al.*, 2001]. W.D.Donachie and his colleagues suggested the existence of SOS-independent co-ordination of cell division and chromosome replication. In *Caurobacter crescentus* response regulator of the cell cycle, CtrA, coordinates the cell cycle-dependent expression of genes including *ftsZ* [Wortinger *et al.*, 2000]. Little is known about cyanobacterial cell cycle and about a coordination of DNA replication and cell division. In some cyanobacteria these processes are reported to be under the control of a circadian clock [Sweeney & Borgese.1989; Mori *et al.*, 1996; Kondo *et al.*, 1997]. Study of expression of cell cycle-related genes (*ftsZ* and *dnaA*) in synchronized cultures of *Prochlorococcus* sp. strain PCC 9511 has shown that both genes exhibited clear expression patterns with mRNA maxim a during the replication (S) phase. Western blot experiments indicated that the peak of FtsZ concentration occurred at night, i.e., at the time of cell division. Thus, the transcript accumulation of genes involved in replication and division is coordinated in *Prochlorococcus* sp. strain PCC 9511 [Holtzendorff *et al.*, 2001]. Other study was performed for the bloom forming cyanobacteria *Microcystis aeruginosa* [Yoshida T. *et al.*, 2005]. In this research authors have shown that when either nalidixic acid (an inhibitor of DNA gyrase) or hydroxyurea (an inhibitor of ribonucleotide reductase) was added to a synchronized culture of *Microcystis aeruginosa* to block DNA replication, cell division did not occur and FtsZ transcription was repressed. However, the increased amount of DNA, in DAPI-DNA-stained tubulin inhibitor, such as thiabendazole (TBZ), treated *Synechococcus* 7942 cells, indicates that DNA replication still occurs in the presence of TBZ, which block cell division [Sarcina & Mullineaux, 2000].

MreB, an actin homologue, is involved in shape determination in rod-shaped prokaryotic cells [Wachi *et al.*, 1987; Jones *et al.*, 2001; Figge *et al.*, 2004; Gitai *et al.*, 2004] and may or may not be involved in DNA replication in some bacterial species [Kruse *et al.*, 2003, 2006; Gitai *et al.*, 2005; Hu *et al.*, 2007]. Very little is known about MreB function in cyanobacterial cells. Recently it has been suggested [Hu *et al.*, 2007] that in *Anabaena* sp. PCC 7120 this protein involved in shape determination, but not in DNA segregation. A previous study revealed that cell division in *E. coli* is under negative control of the *mreB* gene [Wachi & Matsuhashi, 1989]. While overexpression of wild-type MreB has been shown to inhibit cell division but not perturb chromosome segregation, overexpression of mutant forms of MreB causes, in addition to the inhibition of cell division, abnormal MreB filament morphology and induces severe localization defects of the nucleoid in *E. coli* [Kruse *et al.*, 2003]. This fact, together with enhanced expression of the cell division gene *ftsI* in *mreB* mutant *E. coli* cells [Wachi & Matsuhashi, 1989], may indicate a function of the *mreB* gene as a regulator for determining progression to cell division or elongation in *E. coli*. At the same time, in *Synechococcus* sp. strain PCC 7942, the upshift of the MreB protein in the two cell division mutants could reflect a direct or indirect negative regulation of MreB by the *ftn2* and *ftn6* genes and explain the filamentous phenotype of the mutant cells [Koksharova *et al.*, 2007].

Bacteria possess a number of cytoskeletal elements [Mayer, 2003], including FtsZ, a bacterial tubulin homologue [Carballido-López & Errington, 2003; Michie & Löwe, 2006; Klint *et al.*, 2007], MreB coiled structures similar to F-actin, the physiological polymer of eukaryotic actin [van den Ent *et al.*, 2001], MinCDE coiled arrays [Shih *et al.*, 2003] and intracellular protofilaments containing bacterial elongation factor Tu (EF-Tu) [Löwe *et al.*, 2004]. All of them may form cytoskeletal webs, which are important for the organization of intracellular structures and cell function [Mayer, 2003]. Two of these proteins, MreB and EF-Tu were notably upshifted in the cell division mutants FTN2 and FTN6 (Table 4). It is likely that filamentous cells of the mutants may require an extended cytoskeletal web.

A molecular chaperone, heat shock protein Hsp70 was up-regulated in the FTN2 mutant (Table 4). This 634 amino acid protein has an N-terminal MreB (amino acid 1-371) region, and the protein show 94% sequence identity with the chaperone protein K2 (heat shock protein 70-2) of *Synechococcus* sp. strain PCC 7942 (gi|1706478|sp|P50021|DNK2_SYNP7). Overproduction of DnaK2 has resulted in defects in cell septation and formation of cell filaments [Nimura *et al.*, 2001], suggesting an interaction with key cell septation protein(s).

An outer membrane protein containing one transmembrane helix in the N-terminus was up-regulated in both cell division mutants (Table 4). This protein show homology with the chloroplast import-associated channel IAP75 protein of *Synechocystis* sp. PCC 6803 (Gene ID: 954135 IAP75) and with *Arabidopsis thaliana* outer envelope protein of 80 kDa (Gene ID: 832082 OEP80), wich involved in protein import as one of the translocation channel protein at the chloroplast outer envelope membrane [Baldwin *et al.*, 2005]. The location of this protein in the outer membrane may suggest its involvement in cyanobacteria cell envelope biogenesis and/or secretion. Presumably, elongated mutant cells require an increased synthesis of cell membrane as well as an intensive intracellular traffic.

In the cell division mutants, three proteins involved in posttranslational protein processing and modifications (chaperonin GroEL, molecular chaperone GrpE, and periplasmic protease) were up-shifted (Table 4). GroEL and GrpE are chaperones, which may additionally reflect that the mutants are under a stressed condition; notably chaperonin GroEL was exclusively found in the mutant cells (Table 4). The GroEL/GroES system is a major chaperone system in all bacteria and its involvement in cyanobacterial stress responses have been extensively studied [Hihara *et al.*, 2001; Kovacs *et al.*, 2001; Mary *et al.*, 2004]. Some new data appeared suggesting involvement of GroEL in bacterial cell division [Kerner *et al.*, 2005; Susin *et al.*, 2006; Fujiwara & Taguchi, 2007; Lemos *et al.*, 2007]. In addition, new plastid division proteins, ptCpn60α and ptCpn60β, have been identified recently [Suzuki *et al.*, 2009]. These two proteins have a similarity with cyanobacterial chaperonin GroEL. It is possible that cyanobacterial chaperonin GroEL also may be involved in cell division and therefore in the mutants FTN2 and FTN6 its level noticeably increased due to impaired cell division.

The two fold up-shift of periplasmic protease was only obvious for the FTN2 mutant (Table 4).

One protein, identified as TPR repeat-containing protein was distinctly up-shifted in the FTN6 (Table 4). The tetratricopeptide repeat (TPR) is a degenerate 34-amino-acid sequence, present in tandem arrays of 1–16 motifs mediating protein–protein interactions, was found for the first time by Sikorski and co-authors in the cell division control protein Cdc23 [Sikorski *et al.*, 1990]. TPR motifs are important for the function of chaperones, cell-cycle, transcription, and protein-transport complexes [Blatch & Lässle, 1999]. Interestingly, the TPR repeat is present also in the cell division protein Ftn2 in *Synechococcus* sp. strain PCC 7942 [Koksharova & Wolk, 2002b].

Two proteins, possibly involved in protein-protein interactions and protein processing/degradation, were, in contrast to the other proteins in this group, down-shifted in both mutants. One, the leucyl aminopeptidase (Table 4), was only detected in the wild-type. A second protein, containing the FHA domain, was absent in FTN6 mutant and down-shifted in cells of FTN2 mutant (Table 4). FHA domains are implicated in many bacterial processes, including the regulation of cell shape, type III secretion, sporulation, pathogenic and symbiotic host-bacterium interactions, carbohydrate storage and transport, signal transduction [Pallen *et al.*, 2002].

Reverse genetic analysis for some of the identified proteins/genes may permit to study their specific functions in cyanobacterial cell division.

Table 4. Some of the identified proteins that are differently expressed in the wild-type and cell division mutants of *Synechococcus* sp. strain PCC 7942.

NCBI Acces. no.	Gene no.	Encoded protein	Protein level (arbitrary units)*		
			WT	FTN2	FTN6
Group 1. Cell cycle/cell morphogenesis					
974615	0001	DNA polymerase III β subunit	1474	3005	1911
46129703	1139	Chromosome segregation ATPase	557	621	274
81299111	0300	Actin-like ATPase involved in cell morphogenesis (MreB)	1857	3094	3291
46130530	2468	Molecular chaperone (Hsp70)	4781	6240	5158
46129574	0928	Outer-membrane protein	138	482	281
Group 2. Protein synthesis and processing					
46129550	0884	GTPase translation elongation factor	3687	7040	6077
46130513	2440	Polyribonucleotide nucleotidyltransferase	0	1123	541
22002498	1591	Ribosomal protein S1	1313	1974	2121
45512376	0790	RNA-binding protein (RRM domain)	1673	5300	293
53762838	0685	Chaperonin GroEL	0	372	127
45513516	2072	Molecular chaperone GrpE	2726	5463	3667
53762820	0712	Periplasmic protease	1257	2627	1328
53762940	0531	TPR domain	1133	1352	2154
46129730	1190	Leucyl aminopeptidase	1201	0	0
53762913	0565	FHA domain	715	444	0

* These values were calculated by PDQuest software as an average from three independent experiments [Koksharova *et al.*, 2007]

Conclusion

Cyanobacteria, structurally Gram-negative prokaryotes and ancient relatives of chloroplasts, can assist analysis of cell division and its regulation more easily than can studies with higher plants. Gene transfer systems are available, as are many cloning vectors, transposons, methods of mutagenesis, reporter genes, and genomic sequences. These tools provide abundant opportunity for identifying novel genes; for investigating the structure, regulation and evolution of genes. Identification and study of cyanobacterial genes could help to discover their plant homologues and to study functions of these genes. A fruitful genetical approach to understanding of the division process in both cyanobacteria and chloroplasts is created. High efficient transposon mutagenesis helps to identified new cell division genes. The availability of the complete genomic sequences of many cyanobacteria, bacteria, some plants and algae facilitates comparative genomic and proteomic analysis. The results show that mutations only in two cell division genes *ftn2* and *ftn6* affect the cellular quantity of many different proteins. Identification of these proteins provides the new targets for coming studies that will allow assessments of their functions and importance in cell division of cyanobacteria. Many questions remain to be answered. This work just has started. For a deeper understanding of molecular biology of cyanobacterial cell division, integration of genetical, genomic, proteomic and future transcriptomic data are required.

Acknowledgements

This work was supported in part by grant from the Russian Foundation for Basic Research 08-04-00878.

References

Åkerlund, T., Gullbrand, B. & Nordström, K. (2002). Effects of the Min system on nucleoid segregation in *Escherichia coli. Microbiology, 148*, 3213-3222.

Baldwin, A., Wardle, A., Patel, R., Dudley, P., S. Ki Park, Twell, D., Inoue, K. & Jarvis, P. (2005). A molecular-genetic study of the *Arabidopsis* Toc75 gene family. *Plant Physiology, 138*, 715-733.

Bath, J., Wu, L. J., Errington, J. & Wang, J. C. (2000). Role of *Bacillus subtilis* SpoIIIE in DNA transport across the mother cell-prespore division septum. *Science, 290*, 995-997.

Berggren, K., Chernokalskaya, E., Steinberg, T. H., Kemper, C., Lopez, M. F., Diwu, Z., Haugland, R. P. & Patton, W. F. (2000). Background-free, high sensitivity staining of proteins in one- and two-dimensional sodium dodecyl sulfate-polyacrylamide gels using a luminescent ruthenium complex. *Electrophoresis, 21*, 2509-2521.

Bi, E. & Lutkenhaus, J. (1991). FtsZ ring structure associated with division in *Escherichia coli. Nature*, *354*, 161-164.

Blatch, G. L. & Lässle, M. (1999). The tetratricopeptide repeat: a structural motif mediating protein-protein interactions. *Bioessays, 21*, 932-939.

Borthakur, D. & Haselkorn, R. (1989). Tn*5* mutagenesis of *Anabaena* sp. strain PCC 7120: isolation of a new mutant unable to grow without combined nitrogen. *J. Bacteriol, 171*, 5759- 5761.

Bouche, J. P. & Pichoff, S. (1998). On the birth and fate of bacterial division sites. *Mol. Microbiol. 29*, 19-26.

Bramhill, D. (1997). Bacterial cell division. *Annu. Rev. Cell. Dev. Biol, 13*, 395-424.

Broedel, S. E. & Wolf, R. E. (1990). Genetic tagging, cloning, and DNA sequence of the *Synechococcus* sp. strain PCC 7942 gene (*gnd*) encoding 6-phosphogluconate dehydrogenase. *J. Bacteriol., 172*, 4023-4031.

Bukau, B. (1999). Molecular Chaperones and Folding Catalysts-Regulation, Cellular Function and Mechanisms. Amsterdam. Hardwood.

Bukau, B. & Horwich, A. L. (1998). The Hsp70 and Hsp60 chaperone machines. *Cell, 92*, 351-366.

Bukau, B. & Walker, G. C. (1989). Cellular defects caused by deletion of the *Escherichia coli dnaK* gene indicate roles for heat shock protein in normal metabolism. *J. Bacteriol., 171*, 2337- 2346.

Carballido-López, R. & Errington, J. (2003). A dynamic bacterial cytoskeleton. *Trends Cell Biol, 13*, 577-583.

Cheetham, M. E. & Caplan, A. J. (1998). Structure, function and evolution of DnaJ: conservation and adaptation of chaperone function. *Cell Stress Chaperones*, *3*, 28-36.

Cohen, M. F., Meeks, J. C., Cai, Y. A. & Wolk, C. P. (1998). Transposon mutagenesis of heterocyst-forming filamentous cyanobacteria. *Methods Enzymol.*, *297*, 3-17.

Corbin, B. D., Wang, Y., Beuria, T. K. & Margolin, W. (2007). Interaction between cell division proteins FtsE and FtsZ. *J. Bacteriol.*, *189*, 3026-3035.

Cordell, S. C., Robinson, E. J., Lowe, J. (2003).Crystal structure of the SOS cell division inhibitor SulA and in complex with FtsZ. *Proc Natl Acad Sci U S A*; *100*, 7889-7894.

Dajkovic, A. & Lutkenhaus, J. (2006). Z ring as executor of bacterial cell division. *J. Mol. Microbiol. Biotechnol.*, *11*, 140-151.

Das, A. K., Cohen, P. W. & Barford, D. (1998). The structure of the tetratricopeptide repeats of protein phosphatase 5: implications for TPR-mediated protein-protein interactions. *EMBO J.*, *17*, 1192-1199.

de Boer, P. A., Crossley, R. E. & Rothfield, L. I. (1989). A division inhibitor and a topological specificity factor coded for by the minicell locus determine proper placement of the division septum in *E. coli*. *Cell*, *56*, 641-649.

Deusch, O., Landan, G., Roettger, M., Gruenheit, N., Kowallik, K. V., Allen, J. F., Martin, W. & Dagan, T. (2008). Genes of cyanobacterial origin in plant nuclear genomes point to a heterocyst-forming plastid ancestor. *Mol. Biol. Evol.*, *25*, 748-761.

Deva, T., Baker, E. N., Squire, C. J. & Smith, C. A. (2006). Structure of *Escherichia coli* UDP-N-acetylmuramoyl: L-alanine ligase (MurC). *Acta Crystallogr D Biol Crystallogr*, *62*, 1466-1474.

Doherty, H. M. & Adams, D. G. (1995). Cloning and sequence of *ftsZ* and flanking regions from the cyanobacterium *Anabaena* PCC 7120. *Gene*, *163*, 93-99.

Dolganov, N. & Grossman, A. R. (1993). Insertional inactivation of genes to isolate mutants of *Synechococcus* sp. strain PCC 7942: isolation of filamentous strains. *J. Bacteriol.*, *175*, 7644-7651.

Donachie, W. D. & Begg, K. J. (1996). "Division potential" in *Escherichia coli*. *J. Bacteriol.*, *178*, 5971-5976.

Easter, J. & Gober, J. W. (2002). ParB-stimulated nucleotideexchange regulates a switch in functionally distinct ParA activities. *Mol Cell*, *10*, 427-434.

El Zoeiby, A., Sanschagrin, F. & Levesque, R. C. (2003). Structure and function of the Mur enzymes: development of novel inhibitors. *Mol Microbiol*, *47*, 1-12.

Errington, J., Daniel, R. A. & Scheffers, D. J. (2003). Cytokinesis in bacteria. *Microbiol Mol Biol Rev*, *67*, 52-65.

Figge, R. M., Divakaruni, A. V. & Gober, J. W. (2004). MreB, the cell shape-determining bacterial actin homologue, co-ordinates cell wall morphogenesis in *Caulobacter crescentus*. *Mol Microbiol*, *51*, 1321-1332.

Fink, A. (1999). Chaperone-mediated protein folding. *Physiological Rev*. 79, 425-449.

Fujiwara, K. & Taguchi, H. 2007. Filamentous morphology in GroE-depleted *Escherichia coli* induced by impaired folding of FtsE. *J.Bacteriol.*, *189*, 5860-5866.

Fujiwara, M. & Yoshida, S. (2001). Chloroplast targeting of chloroplast division FtsZ2 proteins in *Arabidopsis*. *Biochemical and Biophysical Research Communications*, *287*, 462-467.

Fulda, S., Huang, F., Nilsson, F., Hagemann, M. & Norling, B. (2000). Proteomics of *Synechocystis* sp. strain PCC 6803. Identification of periplasmic proteins in cells grown at low and high salt concentrations. *Eur J Biochem*, *267*, 5900-5907.

Fulda, S., Mikkat, S., Huang, F., Huckauf, J., Marin, K., Norling, B. & Hagemann, M. (2006). Proteome analysis of salt stress response in the cyanobacterium *Synechocystis* sp. strain PCC 6803. *Proteomics*, *6*, 2733-2745.

Fulgosi, H., Gerdes, L., Westphal, S., Glockmann, C. & Soll, J. (2002). Cell and chloroplast division requires ARTEMIS. *Proceedings of the National Academy of Sciences USA*, *99*, 11501-11506.

Gething, M. J. (1997). Protein folding. The difference with prokaryotes. *Nature*, *388*, 329-331.

Gitai, Z., Dye, N. A. & Shapiro, L. (2004). An actin-like gene can determine cell polarity in bacteria. *Proc Natl Acad Sci U S A*, *101*, 8643-8648.

Gitai, Z., Dye, N. A., Reisenauer, A., Wachi, M. & Shapiro, L. (2005). MreB actin-mediated segregation of a specific region of a bacterial chromosome. *Cell*, *120*, 329-341.

Goebl, M. & Yanagida, M. (1991). The TPR snap helix: a novel protein repeat motif from mitosis to transcription. *Trends Biochem. Sci.*, *16*, 3-177.

Golden, S. S. (1988). Mutagenesis of cyanobacteria by classical and gene-transfer based methods. *Methods Enzymol.*, *167*, 714-727.

Graumann, P. L. (2001). SMC proteins in bacteria: condensation motors for chromosome segregation? *Biochimie*, *83*, 53-59.

Harry, E. J., Rodwell, J. & Wake, R. G. (1999). Co-ordinating DNA replication with cell division in bacteria: a link between the early stages of a round of replication and mid-cell Z ring assembly. *Mol Microbiol*, *33*, 33-40.

Hartl, F. U. (1996). Molecular chaperones in cellular protein folding. *Nature*, *381*, 571-579.

Hihara, Y., Kamei, A., Kanehisa, M., Kaplan, A. & Ikeuchi, M. (2001). DNA microarray analysis of cyanobacterial gene expression during acclimation to high light. *Plant Cell*, *13*, 793-806.

Hirota, Y., Ryter, A. & Jacob, F. (1968). Thermosensitive mutants of *E. coli* affected in the processes of DNA synthesis and cellular division. *Cold Spring Harb. Symp. Quant. Biol.*, 33, 677-693.

Holtzendorff, J., Partensky, F., Jacquet, S. J., Bruyant, F., Marie, D., Garczarek, L., Mary, I., Vaulot, D. & Hess, W. R. (2001). Diel expression of cell cycle-related genes in synchronized cultures of *Prochlorococcus* sp. strain PCC 9511. *J. Bacteriol. 183*, 915-920.

Howard, M. & Kruse, K. (2005). Cellular organization by self-organization: mechanisms and models for Min protein dynamics. *J Cell Biol*, *168*, 533-536.

Hu, B., Yang, G., Zhao, W., Zhang, Y. & Zhao, J. (2007). MreB is important for cell shape but not for chromosome segregation of the filamentous cyanobacterium *Anabaena* sp. PCC 7120. *Mol Microbiol*, *63*, 1640-1652.

Huang, F., Fulda, S., Hagemann, M. & Norling, B. (2006). Proteomic screening of salt-stress-induced changes in plasma membranes of *Synechocystis* sp. strain PCC 6803. *Proteomics*, *6*, 910-920.

Ingram, L. O. & Thurston, E. L. (1970). Cell division in morphological mutants of *Agmenellum quadruplicatum*, strain BG-1. *Protoplasma*, *71*, 55-75.

Ingram, L. O. & Van Baalen, C. (1970). Characteristics of a stable, filamentous mutant of a coccoid blue-green alga. *J. Bacteriol.*, *102*, 784-789.

Ingram, L. O., Van Baalen C. & Fisher, W. D. (1972). Cell division mutations in the blue-green bacterium *Agmenellum quadruplicatum* strain BG1: a comparison of the cell wall. *J. Bacteriol.*, *11*, 614-621.

Ingram, L. O. & Fisher, W. D. (1973a). Novel mutant impaired in cell division: evidence for a positive regulating factor. *J. Bacteriol.*, *113*, 999-1005.

Ingram, L. O. & Fisher, W. D. (1973b). Mechanism for the regulation of cell division in *Agmenellum. J. Bacteriol.*, *113*, 1006-1014.

Ingram, L. O., Olson, G. J. & Blackwell, M. M. (1975). Isolation of a small-cell mutant in the blue-green bacterium *Agmenellum quadruplicatum. J. Bacteriol.*, *123*, 743-746.

Jensen, R. B. & Shapiro, L. (2000). Proteins on the move: dynamic protein localization in prokaryotes. *Trends Cell. Biol.*, *10*, 483-488.

Jacobs, C. & Shapiro, L. (1999). Bacterial cell division: a moveable feast. *Proc. Natl. Acad. Sci. USA*, *96*, 5891-5893.

Jones, L. J., Carballido-Lopez, R. & Errington, J. (2001). Control of cell shape in bacteria: helical, actin-like filaments in *Bacillus subtilis. Cell, 104*, 913-922.

Katayama, T., Kubota, T., Kurokawa, K., Crooke, E. & Sekimizu, K. (1998). The initiator function of DnaA protein is negatively regulated by the sliding clamp of the *E. coli* chromosomal replicase. *Cell, 94*, 61-71.

Kawakami, H., Iwura, T., Takata, M., Sekimizu, K., Hiraga, S. & Katayama, T. (2001). Arrest of cell division and nucleoid partition by genetic alterations in the sliding clamp of the replicase and in DnaA. *Mol Genet Genomics*, *266*, 167-179.

Kerner, M. J., Naylor, D. J., Ishihama, Y., Maier, T., Chang, H. C., Stines, A. P, Georgopoulos, C., Frishman, D., Hayer-Hartl, M., Mann, M. & Hartl, F. U. (2005). Proteome-wide analysis of chaperonin-dependent protein folding in *Escherichia coli. Cell, 122*, 209-220.

Kerr, R. A., Levine, H., Sejnowski, T. J. & Rappel, W. J. (2006). Division accuracy in a stochastic model of Min oscillations in *Escherichia coli. Proc Natl Acad Sci USA*, *103*, 347-352.

Klint, J., Rasmussen, U. & Bergman, B. (2007). FtsZ may have dualroles in the filamentous cyanobacterium *Nostoc/Anabaena* sp. strain PCC 7120. *J Plant Physiol*, *164*, 11-18.

Koksharova O. A. & Wolk, C. P. (2002a). Genetic tools for cyanobacteria. *Appl Microbiol Biotechnol.*, 58, 123-137.

Koksharova, O. A. & Wolk, C. P. (2002b). A novel gene that bears a DnaJ motif influences cyanobacterial cell division. *J Bacteriol*, *184*, 5524-5528.

Koksharova, O. A., Klint, J. & Rasmussen, U. (2006). The first protein map of *Synechococcus* sp. strain PCC 7942. *Mikrobiologiia*, *75*, 765-774.

Koksharova, O. A., Klint, J. & Rasmussen, U. (2007). Comparative proteomics of cell division mutants and wild-type of *Synechococcus* sp. strain PCC 7942. *Microbiology*, *153*, 2505-2517.

Kondo,T., Mori, T., Lebedeva, N. V., Aoki, S., Ishiura, M. & Golden, S. S. (1997). Circadian rhythms in rapidly dividing cyanobacteria. *Science*, *275,* 224-227.

Kovacs, E., van der Vies, S. M., Glatz, A., Torok, Z., Varvasovszki, V., Horvath, I. & Vigh, L. (2001). The chaperonins of *Synechocystis* PCC 6803 differ in heat inducibility and chaperone activity. *Biochem. Biophys Res Commun*, *289*, 908-915.

Kruse, K., Howard, M. & Margolin, W. (2007). An experimentalist's guide to computational modelling of the Min system. *Molecular Microbiology, 63,* 1279-1284.

Kruse, T., Möller-Jensen, J., Löbner-Olesen, A. & Gerdes, K. (2003). Dysfunctional MreB inhibits chromosome segregation in *Escherichia coli. EMBO J, 22,* 5283-5292.

Kruse, T., Blagoev, B., Løbner-Olesen, A., Wachi, M., Sasaki, K., Iwai, N., Mann, M. & Gerdes, K. (2006). Actin homolog MreB and RNA polymerase interact and are both required for chromosome segregation in *Escherichia coli. Genes Dev., 20,* 113-124.

Kuhn, I., Peng, L., Bedu, S. & Zhang, C. C. (2000). Developmental regulation of the cell division protein FtsZ in *Anabaena* sp. strain PCC 7120, a cyanobacterium capable of terminal differentiation. *J. Bacteriol., 182,* 4640-4643.

Labarre, J., Chauvat, F. & Thuriaux, P. (1989). Insertional mutagenesis by random cloning of antibiotic resistance genes into the genome of the cyanobacterium *Synechocystis* strain PCC 6803. *J. Bacteriol., 171,* 3449-3457.

Lamb, J. R., Tugendreich, S. & Hieter, P. (1995). Tetratrico peptide repeat interactions: to TPR or not to TPR? *Trends Biochem. Sci., 20,* 257-259.

Laufen, T., Mayer, M. P., Beisel, C., Klostermeier, D., Mogk, A., Reinstein, J. & Bukau, B. (1999). Mechanism of regulation of Hsp70 chaperones by DnaJ cochaperones. *Proc. Natl. Acad. Sci. USA, 96,* 5452-5457.

Lemos, J. A., Luzardo, Y. & Burne, R. A. (2007). Physiologic effects of forced downregulation of dnaK and groEL expression in *Streptococcus* mutans. *J. Bacteriol., 189,* 1582-1588.

Levin, P. A. & Losick R. Asymmetric division and cell fate during sporulation in *Bacillus subtilis,* In Brun Y. V. & L. J. Shimkets, editors. (2000). Prokaryotic Development. Washington, DC: Am. Soc. Microbiol., 167-189.

Liu, G., Begg, K., Geddes, A. & Donachie, W. D. (2001). Transcription of essential cell division genes is linked to chromosome replication in *Escherichia coli. Mol. Microbiol. 40,* 909-916.

Liu, Y. & Tsinoremas, N. F. (1996). An unusual gene arrangement for the putative chromosome replication origin and circadian expression of *dnaN* in *Synechococcus* sp. strain PCC 7942. *Gene, 172,* 105-109.

Loose, M., Fischer-Friedrich, E., Ries, J., Kruse, K. & Schwille, P. (2008). Spatial regulators for bacterial cell division self-organize into surface waves in vitro. *Science, 320,* 789-792.

Löwe, J. & Amos, L. A. (1998). Crystal structure of the bacterial cell-division protein FtsZ. *Nature, 391,* 203-206.

Löwe, J., van den Ent, F. & Amos, L. A. (2004). Molecules of the bacterial cytoskeleton. *Annu Rev Biophys Biomol Struct, 33,* 177-198.

Luque, I., Herrero, A., Flores, E. & Madueño, F. (1992). Clustering of genes involved in nitrate assimilation in the cyanobacterium *Synechococcus. Mol. Gen. Genet., 232,* 7-11.

Lutkenhaus, J, & Addinall, S. G. (1997). Bacterial cell division and the Z ring. *Annu Rev Biochem, 66,* 93-116.

Lutkenhaus, J. (2007). Assembly dynamics of the bacterial MinCDE system and spatial regulation of the Z ring. *Annu Rev Biochem, 76,* 539-562.

Madueño, F., Borrias, W. E., van Arkel, G. A. & Guerrero, M. G. (1988). Isolation and characterization of *Anacystis nidulans* R2 mutants affected in nitrate assimilation: establishment of two new mutant types. *Mol. Gen. Genet., 213,* 223-228.

Maple, J, Aldridge, C, & Moller, S. G. (2005). Plastid division is mediated by combinatorial assembly of plastid division proteins. *Plant J*, *43*, 811-823.

Maple, J., Fujiwara, M. T., Kitahata, N., Lawson, T., Baker, N. R., Yoshida, S., Moller, S. G. (2004). GIANT CHLOROPLAST 1 is essential for correct plastid division in *Arabidopsis. Current Biology*, *14*, 776-781.

Maple, J. & Møller, S. G. (2007). Plastid division: evolution, mechanism and complexity. *Annals of Botany*, *99*, 565-579.

Margolin, W. (2000). Themes and variations in prokaryotic cell division. *FEMS Microbiol. Rev.*, *24*, 531-548.

Martin, W. & Kowallik, K. V. (1999). Annotated English translation of Mereschkowsky's 1905 paper Über Natur und Ursprung der Chromatophoren im Pflanzenreiche. *Eur J Phycol*, *34*, 287-295.

Martin, W., Rujan, T., Richly, E., Hansen, A., Cornelsen, S., Lins, T., Leister, D., Stoebe, B. , Hasegawa, M. , & Penny, D. (2002). Evolutionary analysis of *Arabidopsis*, cyanobacterial, and chloroplast genomes reveals plastid phylogeny and thousands of cyanobacterial genes in the nucleus. *Proc. Natl. Acad. Sci. USA*, *99*, 12246-12251.

Mary, I., Tu, C. J., Grossman, A. & Vaulot, D. (2004). Effects of highlight on transcripts of stress-associated genes for the cyanobacteria *Synechocystis* sp. PCC 6803 and *Prochlorococcus* MED4 and MIT9313. *Microbiology*, *150*, 1271-1281.

Mayer, F. (2003). Cytoskeletons in prokaryotes. *Cell Biol Int*, *27*, 429-438.

Mazouni, K., Domain, F., Cassier-Chauvat, C. & Chauvat, F. (2004). Molecular analysis of the key cytokinetic components of cyanobacteria: FtsZ, ZipN and MinCDE. *Mol Microbiol*, *52*, 1145-1158.

McAndrew, R. S, Froehlich, J. E, Vitha, S., Stokes, K. D, & Osteryoung, K. W. (2001). Colocalisation of plastid division proteins in the chloroplast stromal compartment establishes a new functional relationship between FtsZ1 and FtsZ2 in higher plants. *Plant Physiology, 127,* 1656-1666.

Mereschkowsky, C. (1905). Uber natur und ursprung der chromatophoren im pflanzenreiche. *Biol Centralbl*, *25*, 593-604.

Mercer, K. L. & Weiss, D. S. (2002). The *Escherichia coli* cell division protein FtsW is required to recruit its cognate transpeptidase, FtsI (PBP3), to the division site. *J Bacteriol.*, *184*, 904-912.

Meroueh, S. O., Bencze, K. Z., Hesek, D., Lee, M., Fisher, J. F., Stemmler, T. L. & Mobashery, S. (2006). Three-dimensional structure of the bacterial cell wall peptidoglycan. *Proc Natl Acad Sci USA*, *103*, 4404-4409.

Michie, K. A. & Löwe, J. (2006). Dynamic filaments of the bacterialcytoskeleton. *Annu Rev Biochem*, *75*, 467-492.

Miyagishima, S., Wolk, C. P. & Osteryoung, K. W. (2005). Identification of cyanobacterial cell division genes by comparative and mutational analyses. *Molecular Microbiology*, *56*, 126-143.

Mizusawa, S., Gottesman, S. (1983). Protein degradation in *Escherichia coli*: the *lon* gene controls the stability of sulA protein. *Proc Nat l Acad Sci U S A*, *80*, 358- 362.

Mori,T., Binder, B. & Johnson, C. H. (1996).Circadian gating of cell division in cyanobacteria growing with average doubling times of less than 24 hours. *Proc.Natl.Acad.Sci.USA*, *93*:10183-10188.

Mukherjee, A. & Lutkenhaus, J. (1998). Dynamic assembly of FtsZ regulated by GTP hydrolysis. *EMBO J.*, *17*, 462-469.

Mutsuda, M., Michel, K. P., Zhang, X., Montgomery, B. L. & Golden, S. S. (2003). Biochemical properties of CikA, an unusual phytochrome-like histidine protein kinase that resets the circadian clock in *Synechococcus elongatus* PCC 7942. *J Biol Chem*, *278*, 19102-19110.

Neidhardt, F. C. & VanBogelen, R. A. Proteomic analysis of bacterial stress responses. In: Storz, G. & Hengge-Aronis, R. editors. (2000). *Bacterial Stress Responses*, Washington, DC: ASM Press, 445-452.

Nimura, K., Takahashi, H. & Yoshikawa, H. (2001). Characterization of the *dnaK* multigene family in the cyanobacterium *Synechococcus* sp. strain PCC7942. *J Bacteriol*, *183*, 1320-1328.

Ohtsuka, K. & Hata, M. (2000). Molecular chaperone function of mammalian Hsp70 and Hsp40 - a review. *Int. J. Hyperthermia*, *16*, 231-245.

Osteryoung, K. W., Stokes, K. D., Rutherford, S. M., Percival, A. L. & Lee, W. Y. (1998). Chloroplast division in higher plants requires members of two functionally divergent gene families with homology to bacterial *ftsZ*. *The Plant Cell, 10,* 1991-2004.

Paciorek, J., Kardys, K., Lobacz, B. & Wolska, K. I. (1997). *Escherichia coli* defects caused by null mutations in *dnaK* and *dnaJ* genes. *Acta Microbiol. Pol.*, *46*, 7-17.

Pallen, M., Chaudhuri, R. & Khan, A. (2002). Bacterial FHA domains: neglected players in the phospho-threonine signalling game? *Trends Microbiol*, *10*, 556-563.

Pogliano, J., Pogliano, K., Weiss, D.S., Losick, R. & Beckwith, J. (1997). Inactivation of FtsI inhibits constriction of the FtsZ cytokinetic ring and delays the assembly of FtsZ rings at potential division sites.*Proc Natl Acad Sci USA*, *94*, 559-564.

Pyke, K. A., Rutherford, S. M, Robertson, E. J., Leech, R. M. (1994). *arc6*: a fertile *Arabidopsis* mutant with only two mesophyll cell chloroplasts. *Plant Physiology 106,* 1169-1177.

Raskin, D. M. & de Boer, P. A. (1999a). Rapid pole-to-pole oscillation of a protein required for directing division to the middle of *Escherichia coli. Proc. Natl. Acad. Sci. USA*, *96*, 4971-4976.

Raskin, D. M. & de Boer, P. A. (1999b). MinDE-dependent pole-to-pole oscillation of division inhibitor MinC in *Escherichia coli. J. Bacteriol.*, *181*, 6419-6424.

Raven, J. A. & Allen, J. F. (2003). Genomics and chloroplast evolution: what did cyanobacteria do for plants? *Genome Biology, 4, 209.1-209.5.*

Raynaud, C., Cassier-Chauvat, C., Perennes, C. & Bergounioux, C. (2004). An *Arabidopsis* homolog of the bacterial cell division inhibitor SulA is involved in plastid division. *The Plant Cell, 16*, 1801-1811.

Rippka, R., Deruelles, J., Waterbury, J. B., Herdman, M. & Stanier, R. Y. (1979). Generic assignments, strain histories and properties of pure cultures of cyanobacteria. *J. Gen. Microbiol.*, *111*, 1-61.

Rothfield, L., Justice, S. & Garcia-Lara, J. (1999). Bacterial cell division. *Annu Rev Genet*, *33*, 423-448.

Sauer, J., Schreiber, U., Schmid, R., Volker, U. & Forchhammer, K. (2001). Nitrogen starvation-induced chlorosis in *Synechococcus* PCC7942. Low-level photosynthesis as a mechanism of long-term survival. *Plant Physiol.*, *126*, 233-243.

Schmitz, O., Katayama, M., Williams, S. B., Kondo, T. & Golden, S. S. (2000). CikA, a bacteriophytochrome that resets the cyanobacterial circadian clock. *Science, 289,* 765-768.

Shapiro, L. & Losick, R. (2000). Dynamic spatial regulation in the bacterial cell. *Cell, 100,* 89-98.

Sherratt, D. J. (2003). Bacterial chromosome dynamics. *Science, 301,* 780-785.

Shih, Y. L., Le, T. & Rothfield, L. (2003). Division site selection in *Escherichia coli* involves dynamic redistribution of Min proteins within coiled structures that extend between the two cell poles. *Proc Natl Acad Sci U S A, 100,* 7865-7870.

Sikorski, R. S., Boguski, M. S., Goebl, M. & Hieter, P. (1990). A repeating amino acid motif in CDC23 defines a family of proteins and a new relationship among genes required for mitosis and RNA synthesis. *Cell, 60,* 307-317.

Slabas, A. R., Suzuki, I., Murata, M., Simon, W. J. & Hall, J. J. (2006). Proteomic analysis of the heat shock response in *Synechocystis* PCC6803 and a thermally tolerant knockout strain lacking the histidine kinase34 gene. *Proteomics, 6,* 845-864.

Smith, C. A. (2006). Structure, function and dynamics in the mur family of bacterial cell wall ligases. *J Mol Biol, 362,* 640-655.

Stokes, K. D., McAndrew, R. S., Figueroa, R., Vitha, S. & Osteryoung, K. W. (2000). Chloroplast division and morphology are differentially affected by overexpression of FtsZ1 and FtsZ2 genes in *Arabidopsis. Plant Physiology, 124,* 1668-1677.

Strepp, R., Scholz, S., Kruse, S., Speth, V. & Reski, R. (1998). Plant nuclear gene knockout reveals a role in plastid division for the homolog of the bacterial cell division protein FtsZ, an ancestral tubulin. *Proceedings of the National Academy of Sciences of the USA, 95,* 4368-4373.

Sullivan, S. M. & Maddock, J. R. (2000). Bacterial division: finding the dividing line. *Curr. Biol., 10,* 249-252.

Susin, M. F., Baldini, R. L., Gueiros-Filho, F. & Gomes, S. L. (2006). GroES/GroEL and DnaK/DnaJ have distinct roles in stress responses and during cell cycle progression in *Caulobacter crescentus. J. Bacteriol., 188,* 8044-8053.

Suzuki, K., Nakanishi, H., Bower, J., Yoder, D. W., Osteryoung, K. W. & Miyagishima, S. (2009). Plastid chaperonin proteins Cpn60alpha and Cpn60beta are required for plastid division in *Arabidopsis thaliana. BMC Plant Biology, 9,* 38 doi:10.1186/1471-2229-9-38

Sweeney, B. M. & Borgese, M. B. (1989). A circadian rhythm in cell division in a prokaryote, the cyanobacterium *Synechococcus* WH7803. *J.Phycol., 25,*183-186.

Tandeau de Marsac, N., Borrias, W. E., Kuhlemeier, C. J., Castets, A. M., van Arkel G. A. & van den Hondel, C. A. M. J. J. (1982). A new approach for molecular cloning in cyanobacteria: cloning of an *Anacystis nidulans met* gene using a Tn*901*-induced mutant. *Gene, 20,* 111-119.

Thomaides, H. B., Freeman, M., El Karoui, M. & Errington, J. (2001). Division site selection protein DivIVA of *Bacillus subtilis* has a second distinct function in chromosome segregation during sporulation. *Genes Dev, 15,* 1662-1673.

van den Ent, F., Amos, L. A. & Lowe, J. (2001). Prokaryotic origin ofthe actin cytoskeleton. *Nature, 413,* 39-44.

van den Ent, F., Vinkenvleugel, T. M., Ind, A., West, P., Veprintsev, D., Nanninga, N., den Blaauwen, T. & Löwe, J. (2008). Structural and mutational analysis of the cell division protein FtsQ. *Mol. Microbiol., 68,* 110-123.

van den Hondel, C. A. M. J. J., Verbeek, S., Van den Ende, A., Weisbeek, P. J., Borrias, W. E. & van Arkel, G. A. (1980). Introduction of transposon Tn*901* into a plasmid of *Anacystis nidulans*: preparation for cloning in cyanobacteria. *Proc. Natl. Acad. Sci. USA*, *77*, 1570-1574.

Vitha, S., McAndrew, R. S., Osteryoung, K. W. (2001). FtsZ ring formation at the chloroplast division site in plants. *Journal of Cell Biology, 153*, 111-119.

Vitha, S., Froehlich, J. E., Koksharova, O. A., Pyke, K. A., van Erp, H. & Osteryoug, K. W. (2003). ARC6 is a J-domain plastid division protein and an evolutionary descendant of the cyanobacterial cell division protein Ftn2. *Plant Cell*, *15*, 1918-1933.

Wachi, M., Doi, M., Tamaki, S., Park, W., Nakajima-Iijima, S. & Matsuhashi, M. (1987). Mutant isolation and molecular cloning of *mre* genes, which determine cell shape, sensitivity to mecillinam, and amount of penicillin-binding proteins in *Escherichia coli*. *J. Bacteriol.*, *169*, 4935-4940.

Wachi, M. & Matsuhashi, M. (1989). Negative control of cell division by *mreB*, a gene that functions in determining the rod shape of *Escherichia coli* cells. *J Bacteriol, 171*, 3123-3127.

Wolk, C. P., Cai, Y. & Panoff, J. M. (1991). Use of a transposon with luciferase as a reporter to identify environmentally responsive genes in a cyanobacterium. *Proc. Natl. Acad. Sci. USA*, *88*, 5355-5359.

Wortinger, M., Sackett, M. J. & Brun, Y. V. (2000). CtrA mediates a DNA replication checkpoint that prevents cell division in *Caulobacter crescentus*. *EMBO J.*, *19*, 4503-4512.

Yoshida, T, Maki, M., Okamoto, H. & Hiroishi, S. (2005). Coordination of DNA replication and cell division in cyanobacteria *Microcystis aeruginosa*. *FEMS Microbiology Letters*, *251*, 149-154.

Zhang, C. C., Huguenin, S. & Friry, A. (1995). Analysis of genes encoding the cell division protein FtsZ and a glutathione synthetase homologue in the cyanobacterium *Anabaena* sp. PCC 7120. *Res. Microbiol.*, *146*, 445-455.

Zhevner, V. D., Glazer, V. M. & Shestakov, S. V. (1973). Mutants of *Anacystis nidulans* with modified process of cell division. Mikrobiologiya, 42, 290-297 (in Russian).

Zhou H. & Lutkenhaus, J. (2005). MinC mutants deficient in MinD- and DicB-mediated cell division inhibition due to loss of interaction with MinD, DicB, or a septal component. *J. Bacteriol.*, *187*, 2846-2857.

In: Cell Division: Theory, Variants and Degradation
Editors: Y. N. Golitsin, M. C. Krylov, pp. 29-57
ISBN: 978-1-60876-986-5

Chapter 2

MICROALGAE CELL AND POPULATION PERFORMANCE UNDER POLLUTION IMPACT

Valeriya Yu. Prokhotskaya *
MV Lomonosov Moscow State University, Biology Institute,
Leninskie gory, 1-12, 199992, Moscow, Russia.

ABSTRACT

Laboratory populations of microalgae are widely used as sensitive test objects for the phytotoxicity of chemicals and wastewater streams evaluation. The laboratory cultures of freshwater green alga *Scenedesmus quadricauda* (Turp.) Breb. and marine diatom alga *Thalassiosira weissflogii* (Grunow) Fryxell et Hastle were studied under pollution impact. As toxicants we used heavy metals (chromium and silver as a part of water-dissolved salt, experiments both with freshwater and marine algae) and pesticide (imazalil sulfate, experiments only with freshwater algae).

The simultaneous presence of two groups of *S. quadricauda* cells ("large", 4.0-4.5 μm in width, mainly in the composition of two-cellular coenobia, and "small", 3.0 μm in width in the composition of four-cellular coenobia) proved to be a specific feature of the dimensional-age structure of the control population at different stages of its growth. This structure allows analyzing any possible changes in cell population both in normal and toxicant pressure conditions and to predict which cell cycle stage is disturbed. The dimensional-age structure analysis for diatom alga culture is complicated significantly because of their propagation features.

At low metal concentrations (0.0001, 0.001 and 0.01 mg/L) and low pesticide concentration (0.001 mg/L) the total cell number decreased as compare to the control one. The reason of possible population growth delay under low-level toxic exposure was the arrest of proliferation of some cells (probably, the most sensitive cells within heterogeneous population) rather than cell cycle slowdown in all cells. Notice, that the differences between control and sample cultures at low concentrations were reversible during the period of experiment. At medium toxicant concentrations (0.05 mg/L silver, 0.1 mg/L chromium and 0.1 mg/L imazalil) the effect varied from indifferent to toxic

* Corresponding author: E-mail: plera@mail.ru

according to algal species and season. At concentration of 0.1 mg/L chromium and imazalil the division of cells resumed within 1-2 days of intoxication. At concentrations of the toxicants over 0.05 mg/L for silver and over 1.0 mg/L for chromium and imazalil a total cell number and proportion of living cells decreased. Imazalil sulfate at concentration 1.0 mg/L was found to inhibit the division of cells and imparted to them anomalous increase in size and the formation of gigantic cells. Such state of algae was reversible: giant cells rapidly resumed their division after being transferred to a toxicant-free medium. At the concentration 3.0 mg/L chromium we observed both undividing and proliferating cells. At high toxicant concentrations (0.1 and 0.5 mg/L silver; 10.0 mg/L chromium; 5.0, 10.0 and 20.0 mg/L imazalil) cell division stimulation preceded the fast death of algal population and the small immature cells predominated in the beginning of the treatment. Only the high-level toxicant treatment caused photosynthetic efficiency reducing twice as compared to the control level.

On the whole, the freshwater algae were found to be more sensitive to heavy metal action than marine algae. It was shown the existence of algostatic effect of silver after the growth of algal cultures in the presence of high toxicant concentrations. In this case the cell number stayed particularly unchangeable during the period of the experiment.

S. quadricauda adaptation to extreme environmental pressure was analyzed by using an experimental model of the multiple intoxication (triple 10.0 mg/L chromium intoxication and double 1.0 mg/L silver intoxication). The selection of the resistant algal cells in the presence of high toxicant concentrations was demonstrated. These cells could restore the algal population. It is concluded that there are initial resistant cell number within the heterogenous algal population is 3-7 % (depending on toxicant) of initial cell number.

A modified fluctuation analysis was performed to distinguish resistant cells within *S. quadricauda* and *T. weissflogii* laboratory cultures that had originated as a result of random spontaneous pre-selective mutations (prior to chromium exposure) from those arising through acquired post-selective adaptation (during the exposure to chromium).

The changes of population structure of freshwater green alga *S. quadricauda* and marine diatom alga *T. weissflogii* were studied under different regimens of chromium exposure.

Data on the cell number, their photosynthetic characteristics, population structure and share of alive and dead cells will be appropriate for use to predict the most sensitive ecosystem responses and indicate the permissible amount of toxicants in the environment. These data may have important implications for design and interpretations of the bioassay, especially within the context of the hazard/risk assessment.

INTRODUCTION

Algae are a highly diverse group of photosynthetic organisms that play a vital role in aquatic ecosystems, e.g. unicellular algae floating in water make up the phytoplankton and macroscopic algae forming kelp beds on rocky shores. Algae are responsible for sustaining aquatic food webs and carry a large fraction of the aquatic biodiversity. Monitoring of the many species of algae is an essential part of water quality surveys. For the same reasons algae are used to evaluate the risk of new chemicals via laboratory research and these organisms are used for bio-assays to measure the toxicity of waste water streams.

Current procedures for dealing with water pollutants require that more trofic levels are represented that is a fish, a water flea and a microalga; occasionally supplementary bacterial or biochemical tests are added. Micro-algae hold great promise in this field because they can be identified in natural communities (serving as "indicator"), and can be used to measure toxicity (serving as "bioassay"). Algal bioassays can be simple and relatively inexpensive tests that are still very sensitive. The number of options for research and application of micro-algal tests are rapidly growing. The availability of advanced observation techniques is one aspect in addition to the use of the large biodiversity of algae, reflected in wide ranges of different sensitivities to toxicants. Only a few examples are given here. [Santos et al., 2002] applied microalgae encapsulated in gel beads to measure the toxicity of estuarine waters. [Ivorra et al., 2002] studied the selection of strains of diatoms that genetically adapt to large inputs of zinc and cadmium in a polluted river system. [Schäfer et al., 1994] combined algal tests and ciliate tests to derive long-term effects of pollution.

Laboratory populations of microalgae are widely used as sensitive test object for the evaluation of the phytotoxicity of chemicals and wastewater streams. Cell populations of microalgae are complex systems with resistant and sensitive cells. When pollutants are added to a dense microalgal culture, the cell density reduced after a few days due to the death of sensitive cells. However, after further incubations the culturesl sometimes increase its density again due to the growth of cell variant, which is resistant to the contaminants. Numerous studies have shown that heavy metals are extremely toxic to microalgae in both laboratory cultures and natural populations. It has also been reported that microalgae from contaminated sites appear to be adapted to high metal concentrations whereas algae from unpolluted sites remain sensitive [Knauer et al., 1999]. Rapid adaptation of microalgae to environmental changes resulting from water pollution has been demonstrated recently [Costas et al., 2001; López-Rodas et al., 2001]. Unfortunately, the evolution of microalgae subsequent to a catastrophic environmental change is insufficiently understood. Little is known about the mechanisms allowing algae to be adapted to such extreme conditions. Within limits, organisms survival in chemically-stressed environments is a result of two different processes: physiological adaptation (acclimation), usually resulting from modifications of gene expression; and, adaptation by natural selection if mutations provide the appropriate genetic variability [Belfiore & Anderson, 2001]. Because physiological adaptation is bounded by the types of conditions commonly encountered by organisms, it remains for genetic adaptation to overcome extreme environmental conditions [Hoffmann & Parsons, 1991].

Water pollutions are altering ecosystem, community, population, organism, cell, subcell and molecular level processes. It is causing structural-functional alteration in populations and communities and decreasing a biodiversity. Heavy metals, one of the most toxic pollutants, often occur in industrial effluents at very high concentrations. While many heavy metals are required micronutrients for biological systems, they become toxic to most aquatic life forms at only slightly higher concentrations than the minimum requirement. The presence of heavy metal ions in surface water continues to be the most pervasive environmental issues of present time. A wide range of pesticides are used to protect agricultural crops. Residuals of pesticides can be detected in aquatic environments. Herbicides are toxic to microalgae even in the micromolar concentration range [Nyström et al., 1999].

The cultures of freshwater green microalga *Scenedesmus quadricauda* (Turp.) Breb. and marine diatom *Thalassiosira weissflogii* (Grunow) Fryxell et Hastle were studied under the influence of different toxicants (heavy metals chromium and silver as a part of water-dissolved salt, pesticide imazalil sulfate). Population structure was used for quantifying signs on measurements of toxic action. The changes of population structure of freshwater green alga *Scenedesmus quadricauda* (Turp.) Breb. and marine diatom alga *Thalassiosira weissflogii* (Grunow) Fryxell et Hastle were studied under different regimens of heavy metal (chromium) exposure also. Adaptation of the algae to growth and survival in an extreme environment was analysed by using an experimental model.

The main contributions of this work are:

1. A new approach to the risk assessment and intensity/toxicity level evaluation on the base of *S. quadricauda* cell cycle (to be normal and under toxicity pressure) is proposed;
2. The technique of evaluation of the chromium contamination effect on microalgal populations under different regimens of chromium addition with respect to subsequent application as a model system in biotesting is implemented;
3. Determination of the chromium-resistant cells nature and origin is done;
4. The evaluation of the mutation rate from chromium sensitivity to chromium resistance on the base of fluctuation test is realized.

MATERIALS AND METHODS

1. Experimental Organisms

The culture of green chlorococcal alga *Scenedesmus qudricauda* (Turp.) Breb. (Moscow State University Biology Institute algal cultures collection, Microbiology Department, DMMSU, strain S-3) was grown non-axenically in Uspenskii medium N1 (composition, g/L: 0.025 KNO_3, 0.025 $MgSO_4$, 0.1 KH_2PO_4, 0.025 $Ca(NO_3)_2$, 0.0345 K_2CO_3, 0.002 $Fe_2(SO_4)_3$; pH 7.0-7.3) in conical flasks in luminostat under periodic illumination (12:12 h). Algal culture contained two- and four-cellular coenobia. The number of cells in the culture is doubled every 3-4 days.

The culture of diatom alga *Thalassiosira weissflogii* (Grunow) Fryxell et Hastle was grown non-axenically in Goldberg-Kabanova medium (composition, g/L: 0.2024 KNO_3, 0.007105 Na_2HPO_4; mg/l: 0.1979 $MnCl_2$, 0.2379 $CoCl_2$, 0.2703 $FeCl_3$).

2. Toxicity Tests

We investigated the toxic action of chromium (as $K_2Cr_2O_7$), well known as standart toxicant [Wang, 1997], silver (as Ag_2SO_4,) and pesticide imazalil sulfate ((1-[2-(2,4-dichlorophenyl)-2(2-propenyloxi)ethyl-1H-imidazole sulfate) in the long-term experiments (up to 36 days) in three replicates.

The laboratory algal cultures were exposed to increasing concentrations of the toxicants. The toxicant concentrations were varied by means of dilution of stock solutions (the toxicant concentration in stock solution was 1 mg/mL) by distilled water. The volume of the toxicants 1 mL was added in the algal cultures at a logarithmic phase of growth (initial cell number was about $2x10^5$ cells/mL) to a final concentrations of 0.001-10.0 mg/L.

Algal cells were counted with a Goryaev's hemocytometer under a light microscope. Cell linear sizes (width and length) were measured with a calibrated ocular micrometer (no less than 80 cells in each sample) with an accuracy of 0.1 μm. Cells were grouped according to their width into classes at 0.5 μm steps. And the cell size distribution was plotted as a percentage of the total cell number. Number of dead cells was counted with a luminescent microscope Axioskop 2FS (Carl Zeiss, Germany). Under illumination with UV and blue light, dead cells emit green light, whereas living cells emit red light.

3. Chromium Contamination Effect (Dose-Response Relationships)

We investigated the toxic effect of chromium on algae in view of maintenance of a constant dose of chromium per one cell during experiments in order to pass from concentration dependence to dose dependence. The experiments were performed both with single chromium addition at the start of experiment and with multiple additions during exposure time. The periods between toxicant additions approximately corresponded to doubling time for algae so that the dose of the toxicant per one cell was particularly the same as that at the initial day of experiment. The effect of chromium on *S. qudricauda* and *T. weissflogii* was estimated by calculating total cell number, a share of alive, dead and dying cells during exposure time (28 and 21 days, respectively). Cells were counted with a Goryaev's hemocytometer and Nazhotta cytometer under a light microscope. Number of alive, dead and dying dead cells was counted with luminescent microscope Axioskop 2FS (Carl Zeiss, Germany).

For experiment with *S. quadricauda* we used concentration of chromium: 0.001; 0.01; 0.1; 1.0; 5.0 and 10.0 mg/L. Concentration of toxicant in a stock solution was 1 mg/mL (counting per chromium). Initial number of cells after inoculation was 50 000 cells/mL. After that algal cultures grew during 5 days for reaching of logarithmic growth phase. Number of cells at this moment was $28\text{-}30 \cdot 10^4$ cells/mL. Experiment was performed in conical flasks in volume of 100 mL, volume of culture in which was 50 mL. We added toxicant to cultures at 0 day of experiment (single addition) and further at 3, 6, 10 and 17 day until necessary concentrations (multiple additions). Frequency of toxicant addition was defined by growth rate of cultures and rate of cell division. Average growth rate of culture (without chromium) was 0.33 division/day (cells were divided about one time for 3 days).

For experiment with *T. weissflogii* we used concentration of chromium: 0.001; 0.01; 0.1 and 1.0 mg/L. The initial number of cells taken for experimemt was 5 000 cells/mL. Experiment was performed in small phials with 10 mL of culture. Chromium was introduced into growth medium at 0 day of experiment until necessary concentrations (single addition). Further, in one series of culture we did not add the toxicant (conditionally named by us as "control") and in another series chromium was added at 3, 6, 10 and 13 day (multiple additions). Average growth rate of culture (without chromium) was 0.33 division/day.

Toxicant was introduced into the growth mediums proportionally to an increase of cell number of *S. quadricauda* and *T. weissflogii* so that the toxicant quantity per one cell (dose) was kept constant. Thus, the initial concentrations and the total final concentrations at the end of experiments were (the first value in every pair of values means initial concentration, the second one – the final concentration): 0.001 - 0.0033, 0.01 - 0.034, 0.1 - 0.34, 1 - 2.7, 5 - 7, 10 - 17.5 mg/L for *S. quadricauda* and 0.001 - 0.0055, 0.01 - 0.054, 0.1 - 0.55, 1 - 2.6 mg/L for *T. weissflogii*.

We determined total cell number, a share of alive, dead and dying cells of the cultures for an estimation of chromium toxic effect during exposure time (28 and 21 days, respectively). As the controls for these experiments, we used: (1) growth of the cultures in mediums without chromium (control); (2) growth of the cultures under single addition of chromium exposure (conditional "control").

4. The Photosynthetic Characteristics of Algal Cell

The functional state of the photosynthetic apparatus of the alga was characterized by *in vivo* measuring of delayed fluorescence (DF) of chlorophyll *a*. DF of 0.5 mL samples containing 1-3x10^5 cells was measured with a two-disk Becquerel phosphoroscope. Samples were illuminated with periodic 6-ms flashes of red light (wavelength range > 610 nm). DF imtensity was measured during a dark time between the flashes of excitation light for 3-18 ms. A flash light of 30 klx was attenuated when required with neutral optical filters. Irradiance necessary for light-saturated photosynthesis was determined from the dependency of DF intensity on excitation light. The thermal stability of thylakoid membranes was judged from the position of the maximum on temperature dependency plot of DF intensity. To accomplish this, DF was recorded while heating the cell suspension from 20 to 60 ^{0}C at a rate of 5 ^{0}C/min. The temperature of DF maximum was determined with an accuracy of 0.3 ^{0}C.

The amplitude of the DF decay phase during photosynthesis induction in dark preadapted samples was used to characterize the photosynthesis activity (η):

$$\eta = (I_{max} - I_s)/I_{max}.$$

Here, I_{max} is the DF intensity recorded immediately after the onset of illumination, when the photosynthetic rate is equal to zero (dark-adapted chloroplasts), and, I_s is the steady-state DF intensity, when photosynthetic rate is at its highest (light-adapted state).

The rate of non-cyclic electron transport was assessed from changes in the DF intensity, induced by the addition of an inhibitor of noncyclic electron transport diuron (DCMU):

$$ET = I_{+D}/I_{-D},$$

where I_{+D} and I_{-D} are DF intensities in the presence and in the absence of DCMU, respectively. DCMU herbicide blocks photosynthetic electron transport by binding the 32 kDa D1 popypeptide of photosystem II thylakoid membranes. The DF intensity measured in the presence of DCMU, when all the photosynthetic reaction centers are inactive, was used to assess the amount of photochemically active chlorophyll in algal cells.

5. Fluctuation Test: Analysis of Transformation from Chromium Sensitivity to Chromium Resistance

A modified Luria–Delbrück fluctuation analysis was performed in liquid medium as previously described [López-Rodas et al., 2001] to distinguish resistant cells that had originated as a result of random spontaneous pre-selective mutations (prior to chromium exposure) from those arising through acquired post-selective adaptation (during the exposure to chromium).

Two different sets of experimental cultures were prepared with both species of algae. The first set of experiments was performed in 52 (*S. quadricauda*) and 49 (*T. weissflogii*) parallel culture flasks with cell number $N_0 = 200$ cells and $N_t = 2.8{\cdot}10^4$ (*S. quadricauda*), $N_t = 10^5$ (*T. weissflogii*) cells; and treated with 2.5 (*S. quadricauda*), 1.5 (*T. weissflogii*) mg/L chromium after reaching N_t. For the second set of experiments, 30 aliquots of 10^4 (*S. quadricauda*) and 10^5 (*T. weissflogii*) cells from the same parental populations were separately transferred to flasks containing fresh liquid medium with 2.5 (*S. quadricauda*) and 1.5 (*T. weissflogii*) mg/L chromium. Cultures were observed for approximately 14 days, and the resistant cells in each culture (both in set 1 and set 2) were counted. The number of cells was counted by at least two independent observers.

If resistant cells arise by rare spontaneous mutations, each parallel culture in set 1 would have a given probability of generating resistant variants with each cell division. Then, inter-flask variation would not be consistent with the Poisson model. The number of cells from each flask in set 2 would show variation due only to random sampling; variation from flask to flask would be consistent with the Poisson model. If there is rare spontaneous mutation, the variance/mean $\text{ratio}_{\text{set1}}$ is usually many times higher than the variance/mean $\text{ratio}_{\text{set2}}$.

The method allows estimation of algal spontaneous mutation rate and the rate of appearance of resistant cells. The proportion of set 1 cultures showing no mutant cells after chromium exposure (P_0 estimator) was the parameter used to calculate the mutation rate (μ). The P_0 estimator [Luria & Delbrück, 1943] is defined as follows: $P_0 = e^{-\mu\,(Nt-No)}$, where P_0 is the proportion of cultures showing no resistant cells. Therefore, μ was calculated as:

$$\mu = -\ln P_0 / (N_t - N_0).$$

Results and Discussion

1. Intrapopulational Changes of Algae under Toxic Exposure

We investigated the culture growth in the presence of chromium and imazalil sulfate. The results of representative experiment with imazalil sulfate are demonstrated on the figure 1. Here the total cell number and a share of dead cells changes in the algal cultures are shown. The concentration-response curve for chromium has the similar view (figure is not shown).

As it can be seen from the figure, the algal population characteristics in the experimental cultures exposed to the toxicants for 4-7 days was changed in a complicated pattern. At low and high concentrations of imazalil and chromium the number of cells was less than in the control culture, whereas at moderate concentrations of the toxicants cell number had stimulation effect. Such concentration-response dependence we could observe during long-term experiment (up to 30 days). This type of the population number changes (so called "paradoxical reaction") is a usual behavior of biological systems in increasing of damaging factors intensity. The number of dead cells in the culture increased only at high toxicant concentration (Figure 1, curve 2). Therefore, the change in the relative cell number at low imazalil and chromium concentrations cannot be explained only by the summing of the process of cell division and death.

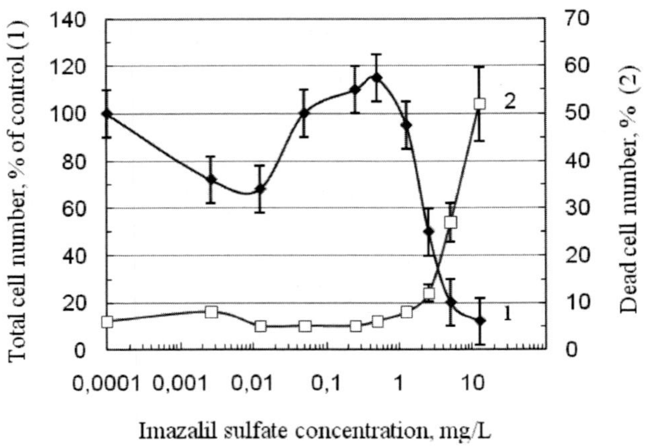

Figure. 1. Changes of the total cell number (1) and dead cell number (2) in the *S. quadricauda* culture as a function of imazalil sulfate concentrations on the 4th – 7th days of treatment.

It was supposed to be existence of certain principles of intrapopulational response to the toxic exposure, which does not depend on chemical nature of acting factor. These principles reflect the changes of structural and functional characteristics of algal population. We investigated the changes of population structure and average functional characteristics of *S. quadricauda* cells in the control cultures and in the presence of various concentrations of the toxicants.

1.1. Size-age distribution, coenobial composition and functional characteristics of S. quadricauda control culture.

The growth curve of the control culture had a stepwise shape apparently due to a partly synchronization of cell division under continuous light-dark periods. We can observe the simultaneous presence of two cell groups differing in size (large and small cells). That fact agrees completely with model previously described for population structure of chlorococcal alga *Chlorella* and *Scenedesmus* [Tamiya et al., 1953; Tamiya, 1966; Senger & Krupinska, 1986].

Figure 2 shows changes in the cell size distribution during growth of the control culture. Large cells (4.5 μm; length:width ratio is 1:0.5) composing two-cellular coenobia dominated before the cell number increasing. Small cells (3.0-3.5 μm; length:width ratio is 1:0.33) were rare and formed four-cellular coenobia. The increase of the cell number was accompanied by mirror changes in bimodal distribution: medium-sized (3.0 μm) cells formed a large maximum and large (4.5 μm) cells formed a lower maximum.

Notice, that the length of large and small cells remained rather constant (9.5-11.0 μm). So, in this particular case the cell volume was mainly determined by the cell width. The average width of small cells was 1.4-1.5 times less than the width of large cells; i. e. their volumes differed by a factor of two. Hence, it seems likely that large cells are ready for division and small cells are daughter young cells.

On the base of our data, the *S. quadricauda* cell cycle (in cultivation conditions described above) can be described in the following way: four-cellular coenobium with mature cells (4.0-4.5 μm, G_2 cell cycle phase) formes two two-cellular coenobia (without cell number changes); every mother cell (4.5 μm) produces two autospores (mitosis cell cycle phase). The young four-cellular coenobium (consisting from small cells, 3.0 μm in width) appeares. The total cell number is duplicated; small cells grow and turn into mature large cells (4.5 μm width, G_1 and S cell cycle phases). Then cell cycle is repeated.

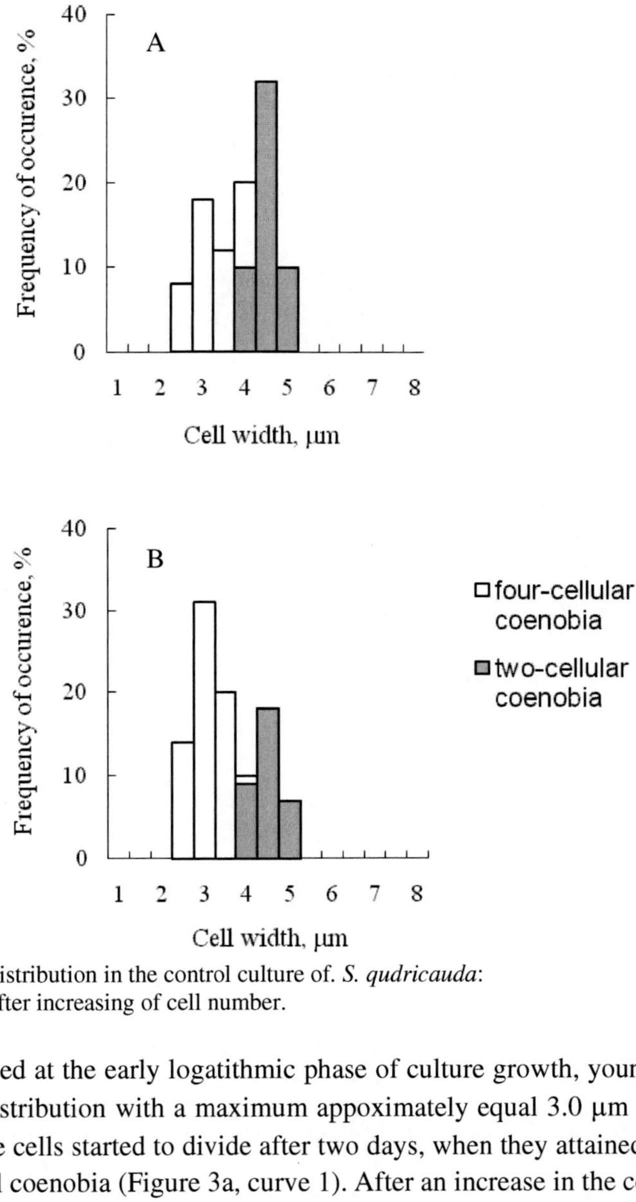

Figure. 2. Cell width distribution in the control culture of. *S. qudricauda*: (a) – before and (b) – after increasing of cell number.

When sedimented at the early logatithmic phase of culture growth, young cells displayed an unimodal size distribution with a maximum appoximately equal 3.0 μm and formed four-cell coenobia. These cells started to divide after two days, when they attained 4.5 μm in width and formed two-cell coenobia (Figure 3a, curve 1). After an increase in the cell number on the third day, a large maximum of small cells appeared in the cell size distribution.

The sedimented isolation of young cells from the mixed-aged (two-aged) culture revealed the functional differences between mature and young cells. In comprison to small cells, a higher DF level in large cells at a higher irradiance (higher amplitude of the millisecond component of DF) indicated an earlier light saturation of their photosynthesis. The efficiency of photosynthesis was slightly higher in small cells (η = 0.86±0.02) than in large cells (η =

0.80±0.02). The thermal stability of thylakoid membranes in small cells was higher than that of large cells (49.5 ^{0}C and 47.5 ^{0}C, respectively).

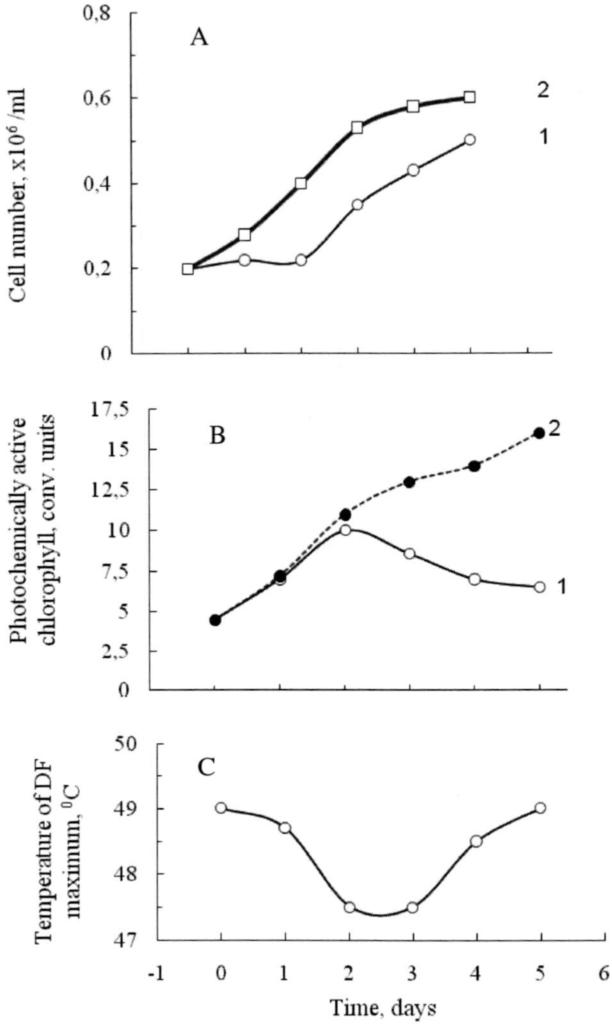

Figure 3. Characteristics of *S. quadricauda* culture growth:

(a) growth of the culture consisting primarily of (1) small or (2) large cells;

(b) Changes in the amount of photochemically active chlorophyll per cell during growth of algal culture consisting mostly of small cells (1) in the absence and (2) in the presence of imazalil at sublethal concentration 1.0 mg/L;

(c) changes in thermal stability of thylakoid membranes during growth of the culture which initially consisted of small cells.

By measuring DF intensity we followed cell cycle-dependent changes in the functional characteristics of the algae. Maturing of selected small cells was accompanied by a twofold increase in their DF per cell level (measured in the presence of DCMU), followed by DF decrease to the initial level after cell division (Figure 3b, curve 1). Hence, the amount of photochemically active chlorophyll also doubles upon doubling of cell volume. The initially high thermal stability of small cells decreased before cell division and then was restored (Figure 3c).

1.2. Effect of toxicants at low concentrations

The most evident effect of low toxicant concentrations (chromium at concentrations of 0.0001, 0.001, 0.01 mg/L and imazalil sulfate at concentration of 0.001 mg/L) was that the increase in cell number in the treated cultures lagged behind the control culture starting from the fourth day of experiments. Analysis of size-age distribution showed the appearance of large cells (4.5-5.5 μm) in two-cellular coenobia. Later, the cell size increased to 6.0-6.5 μm, and these cells became single and comprise about half of the total cell number. The size distribution of cells displayed two maxima, near 4.0 and 6.0-6.5 μm. The first (wide) maximum included proliferation cells both in four- and two-cell coenobia, and the second maximum comprised large single cells (Figure 4). By the 25th day of the experiment, large single cells transformed into single round "giant cells".

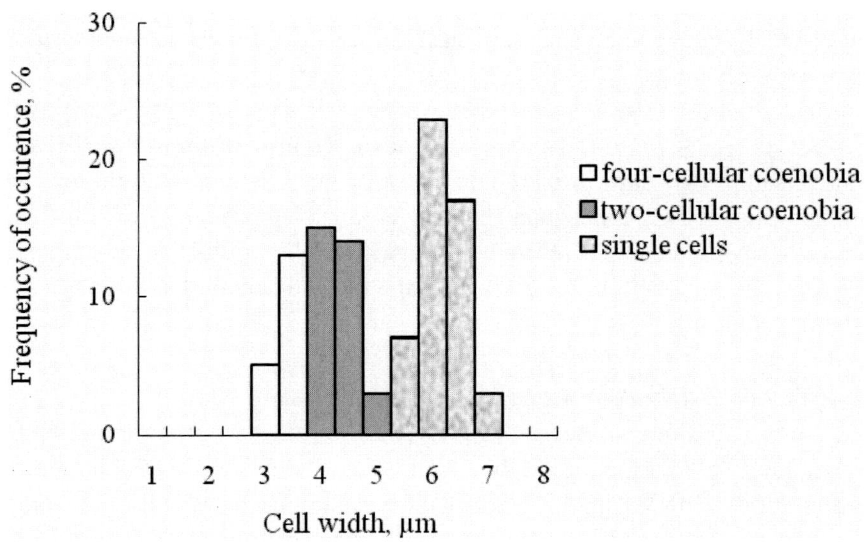

Figure 4. Size-age and coenobial structure of *S. quadricauda* population after imazalil 0.001 mg/L treatment.

Thus, the cause for the delay in culture growth at low concentrations of the toxicants was the arrest of proliferation of some cells rather than deceleration of cell cycle in all cells. The other part of the population did not respond to the presence of the toxicants and continue to proliferate. In other words, the response of the algae to low toxicant concentrations (or low intensity pollution impact) can be related with cell heterogeneity.

At low concentrations, the toxicant arrested cell division in a fraction of the population, but did not have a severe effect on the photosynthetic activity (η = 0.68±0.03 as compared to η = 0.82±0.02 in the control culture). It did not prevent biomass production, which is evident from the cell size increase. By the end of the third week, when large undividing cells comprised about half of the population, the thermal stability of photosynthetic membranes was 1.5 ^{0}C higher than that for the control culture.

Notice, that any differences between control and sample cultures at low concentrations disappeared after the toxic influence was ceased. It means that functional and morphological changes of algae due to weak toxic treatment were reversible.

1.3. Effect of toxicants at moderate concentrations

In the presence of moderate toxicant concentrations (0.1 mg/L of chromium and imazalil sulfate), the final effect (registered after the termination of the experiment) varied from indifferent to toxic according to algal species and season.

The response of algal cells to imazalil and chromium at concentrations of two orders of magnitude higher, than in the previous experiment was drastically different. Cell growth was blocked for two days, and the size of both large and small cells increased. The fraction of large (4.5-5.5 μm) cells in two-cellular coenobia increased. Then (on the third day), cell division resumed synchronously and on the fourth day the cell number in the culture grown in the presence of the fungicide only slightly differed from cell number in the control culture. The cell population mostly contained small cells organized in four-cellular coenobia. In the cell size distribution the maximum near 3.0-3.5 μm (which is characteristic of a control culture) was restored.

During the cell division arrest the efficiency of photosynthesis decreased only slightly to the level of $\eta = 0.70\pm0.02$ as compared to the control culture ($\eta = 0.82\pm0.02$), but it was restored within two days to the control level. The cells increased in size, and their thermal stability was 1.5 ^{0}C higher than that for the control culture. After cells are being resumed division, they retained the elevated thermal stability. Thus, an adaptive increase in cell resistance occurred within one cell cycle, and the cell acquired ability to grow in the presence of the fungicide.

1.4. Effect of toxicants at sublethal concentrations

At concentrations of the toxicants over 1.0 mg/L of chromium and imazalil, a total cell number and proportion of living cells decreased. At high chromium and imazalil concentrations (1.0-3.0 mg/L) we can observe long-term cell division inhibition and giant cells forming. Number of dead cells varied from 15 % in the presence of imazalil (1.0-3.0 mg/L) to 30 % in the presence of chromium (1.0-3.0 mg/L). At the concentration 3.0 mg/L of chromium the cell number was the same as initial one during the experiment. Analysis of size-age structure and functional characteristics of the cells showed that there were at least two reasons: delay of cell division of one cells and division and death of others. We observed both undividing and proliferating cells.

Sublethal concentrations of toxicants did not inhibit photosynthesis significantly (($\eta = 0.72\pm0.03$, as compared to $\eta = 0.80\pm0.02$ in the control culture). The increase of the cell volume was accompanied by an increase of the photochemically active chlorophyll amount (Figure 3b, curve 2). The thermal stability of thylakoid membranes in giant cells exceeded that of the control cells by 1.5 ^{0}C.

Division of single giant cells resumed after they had been washed of fungicide and transferred to a fresh nutrient medium. Two- and four-cellular coenobia with normal-sized cells reappeared in the culture.

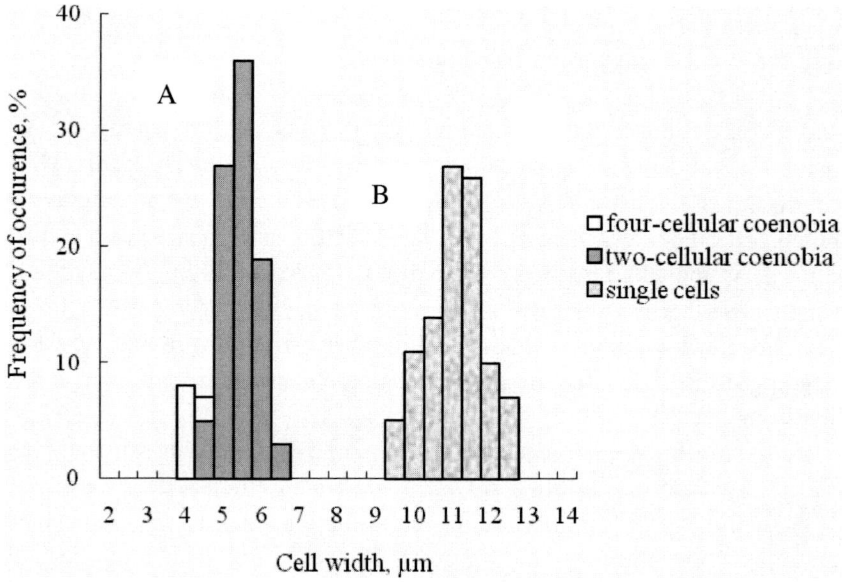

Figure 5. Size-age and coenobial structure of *S. quadricauda* population after imazalil 1.0 mg/L treatment: (a) – the 4th day of experiment; (b) – the 25-30th days of experiment.

1.5. Effect of toxicants at lethal concentrations

The lethal toxicant concentration induced cell death within 4-5 days, i. e. during the time period equal the cell cycle duration. However, in the mixed-aged (two-age) heterogenous algal culture the number of cells did not change during the first day.

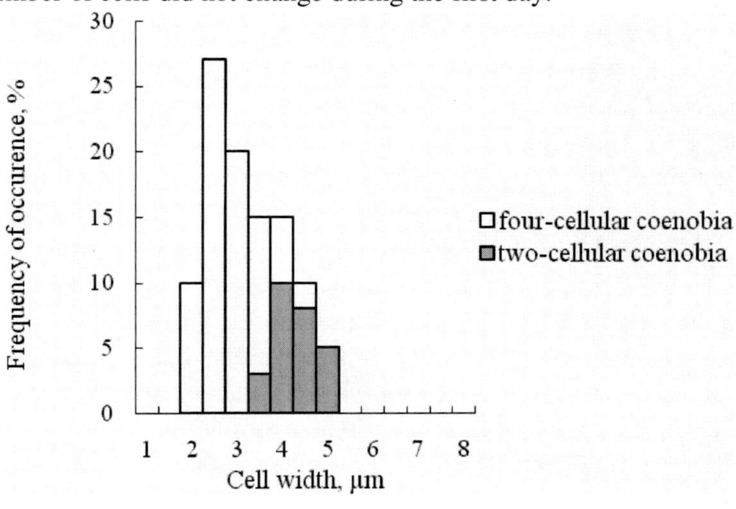

Figure 6. Size-age and coenobial structure of *S. quadricauda* population after imazalil 10.0 mg/L incubation, the 1st-2nd days of experiment.

Very small cells (width 2.0-2.5 µm) in four-cellular coenobia appeared in the cell size distribution with a simultaneous increase in the frequency of two-cellular coenobia. That implies that toxicants first initiated cell division in all cells, including those that had not attained the mature cell size (i. e., the size required for division). In the normal culture cells divided after attaining about 4.5 µm in diameter, whereas in the presence of toxicant they divided after attaining the size of 3.5 µm. Since the total cell number did not change, it is clear that a certain part of cells died. Therefore, the analysis of size-age population structure can find out the lethal effect earlier than counting of cell number.

Characteristics of DF monotonically changed under the action of lethal toxicant concentrations: the higher the concentrations, the faster they changed. After a 1-day incubation at a lethal concentration, the light curve of DF was changed (the DF level at high light intensity almost doubled, indicating the reduced efficiency of light energy used by cells). Photosynthetic efficiency was dropped to $\eta = 0.50 \pm 0.05$, as compared to $\eta = 0.80 \pm 0.02$ in the control culture. As indicated by the DF response to DCMU addition, noncyclic ET decreased almost to half. The thermal stability of thylacoid membranes decreased to 44-45 ^{0}C (against 48.5 ^{0}C in the control culture). These changes accelerated with an increase of toxicant concentrations within the lethal range (10-20 mg/L) and indicated that cell damage was irreversible.

Our data demonstrate the informational value of DF measuring for the analysis of algal response to the toxicants. It seems likely that integrated characteristic (a signal is obtained from 1-3x10^5 cells) is most appropriate for recording the responses of an asynchronous algal culture to lethal concentrations of pollutants. In this case, molecular mechanisms of the toxicants effect on energy metabilism can be assesed (more information can be obtained with a synchronous culture). At low toxicant concentrations DF characteristics are more due to the proportion of various cell types (resistant or sensitive) in the population.

1.6. S. quadricauda cell cycle changes after the toxic treatment

Available data on algal sige-age spectrum in the presence of toxicants sublethal and lethal concentrarions allow to suppose, which phase of cell cycle their action is realized on.

When sublethal amounts of chromium and imazalil were added to the culture with small cells (G_1 cell cycle phase) domination, population growth (cell number incresing) was ceased for a long period of time (Figure 7, curve 1). The cells increased in size (up to 4.5-5.0 μm within 3-4 days). However, they did not divide and had only one nucleus, clearly visible through the light microscope (objective x40). By the 7-8 day, the cell width was equal to 6.0-7.0 μm. By the end of experiment they became 11.0-12.0 μm. The coenobial envelope was disrupted, and only single spherical giant cells were present in the culture.

When large cells (G_2 cel cycle phase) dominated in the culture, they resumed their division in the presence of toxicants after a 1-day delay, and the cell number doubled within the next day (Figure 7, curve 2). So, the same amount of toxicants did not inhibit cell division process. But cell division took place only one time after the toxicant addition and then the cell number did not change. It seems likely that cessation of culture growth was due to the inability of young small cells to proliferate in the presence of toxicants. In other words, the sublethal toxicant concentrations cease the cell cycle in G_1 phase and inhibit DNA replication.

The lethal concentrations of toxicants caused the quick (during 4-5 days) cell death, i. e. during one cell cycle. As was mentioned above, at the first day of experiment the total cell number after the toxic treatment was close to the control one, but very small cells (2.0-2.5 μm) in four-cellular coenobia appeared in two-aged culture. It means that the toxicants induced immature cells (3.5 μm) division.

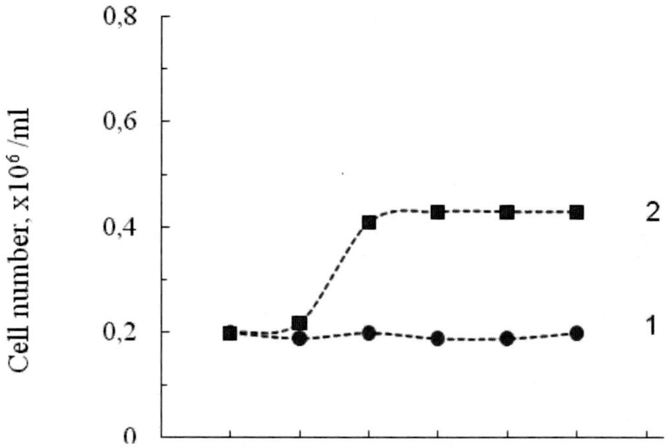

Figure 7. Growth of the *S. quadricauda* culture in the presence of imazalil at concentration 1.0 mg/L: (1) – growth of the culture consisting primarly of the small cells; (2) growth of the culture consisting primarly of the large cells.

In the one-age culture containing young cells which are not prepared for division (3.0 µm cells in four-cellular coenobia), the cell number also did not change for the 1st day in the presence of such amounts of toxicants. The toxicants did not prevent the increase in the cell size to 3.5 µm and more, which was accompanied by the appearance of two-cellular coenobia. However, on the next day, the cell number drastically decreased and the culture contained mainly four-cellular coenobia with very small cells (2.0-2.5 µm). The reduction in total cell number simultaneously with cell division signifies that cells died. It seems likely that immature cells died during the toxicant-induced division.

On the base of the cell death dynamics in one- and two-aged algal cultures in the presence of the lethal toxicant concentrations, it was supposed that small immature and large mature cells were dying within the different cell cycle phases. Small cells death occurred in the end of G_1 phase, large cells death occurred in the end of G_2 phase or during the mitosis.

Our data show that size-age population spectrum analysis allows determining the cell cycle target phase for toxicant action.

S. quadricauda cell cycle phases in the control culture and after toxic treatment are shown on the figure 8.

The paradoxical dependence of the relative cell number in a growing culture on the concentration of toxicants is an example of the fact that living systems do not obey a linear paradigm (the stronger the action, the greater the response). Causes for the nonlinear behavior of biological systems were investigated at various levels of biological organization in numerous works [Holzhutter & Quedenau, 1995; Calabrese & Balwin, 2001; Christofi et al., 2002; Calabrese & Balwin, 2003]. This is determined by the fact that pollution impact (such as radioactive elements, heavy metals, wastes of chemical industry, etc.) high concentration of which are harmful for the biota, may have a beneficial (therapeutic) effect in low doses. However, the causes and mechanisms of the nonlinear response of living system to changes in the factor strength are still unclear.

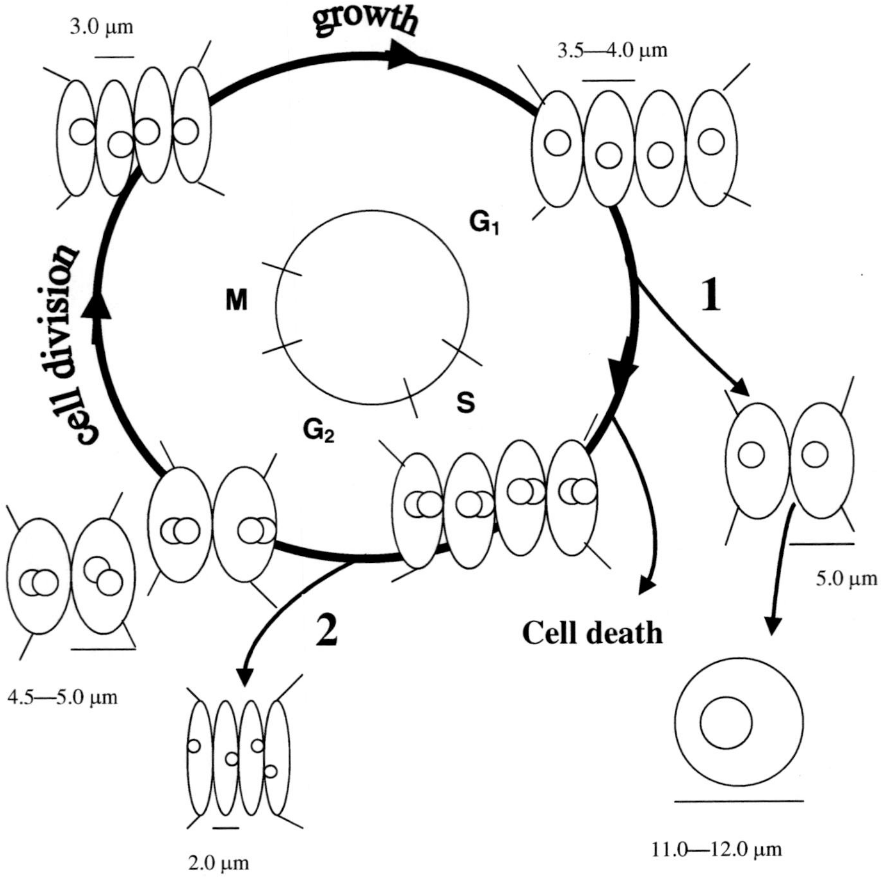

Figure 8. *S. quadricauda* cell cycle in control culture and after toxic treatment.
The average cell sizes are shown. M – mitosis, S – synthetic period, G_1 and G_2 – pre- and postsinthetic periods. The cell cycle changes in the presence of toxicants are marked as arrows. 1 — cell division inhibition in the presence 0.001 and 1.0 mg/L imazalil sulfate and 0.001 mg/L chromium; 2 – division of immature cells and cell death in the presence of lethal toxicant concentrations.

The algal population proved to be a convinient model for investigating this problem. Using this model, we attempted to answer the question as to why the inhibitory effect of low concentrations of the toxicants dissappears with an ancrease in its concentrations.

First, we found that the growth delay of the algal culture in the presense of low toxicant concentrations is due to a long-term cell division arrest in a fraction of the cell population rather than to cell death or deceleration of cell division. Therefore, at low concentrations, cell heterogeneity with respect to their tolerance to toxic influence is a primary importance. It seems likely, that during the first day, the cells whose division was stimulated by the toxicants were damaged. The toxicants probably activated cell proliferation with a subsequent impairment of the cell cycle. In addition, low concentrations seem to be unsufficient for triggering reparatory processes, which may explain the fact that cells did not resume their division for a long period of time.

The absence of the inhibitory effect and even a small positive action of moderate-strength treatment is called a "dead zone" on the concentration-response curve. The most common explanation of this phenomenon is based on the assumption that such an amount (threshold) of the harmful agent activates protective and reparative responses in cells. These responses compensate for the injuries, which may also lead to a hypercompensation effect. The later is known as hormesis.

As seen from characteristics of the photosynthetic apparatus, cell tolerance increased (thermal stability increased by 1.5-2 ^{0}C) even within first hours after treatment with moderate concentrations, and cell division was arrested for two days. We suppose that this unspecific cell response is a cooperative transition of cells to a new quasi-steady state, i. e. stress. While being in this state, cells have time to repair damage and initiate and complete genome-dependent processes that modify cell structure to adjust it to the new conditions.

The cells overcame stress on the third day, resuming their division at the same time. They retained an elevated thermal stability. In the presence of toxicants, the population resumed growth at an even higher rate. It can be said that cell sensitivity to the toxicants declined after adaptation by a factor of 1000 (both moderate and sublethal concentrations reduced cell number to the same extent).

In other words, the new state of cells adapted to growth at the elevated toxicant concentrations can be called hormesis by definition. Hence, hormesis is the active strategy of survival under altered conditions (or pollution impact). Our data show that there is also passive method to survive which was used by cells at low and sublethal concentrations, i. e. transition to a resting state and survival with the formation of giant cells (long-term growth without division). Such a state of the algae was reversible. Giant cells rapidly resumed their division after being transferred to a toxicant-free medium.

2. Structural Changes and Adaptation of Algal Population under Different Regimens of Toxic Exposure.

2.1. Chromium contamination effect investigation.

We tried to develope an experimental model of toxic effect using constant toxicant dose per cell during the experiments.

The presented data show (Figure 9), that at presence of high chromium concentration (1.0 mg/L and more) the total cell number of *S. quadricauda* and *T. weisflogii* slightly varied or decreased, since the moment of the first chromium addition and down to the end of experiment in comparison with the initial cell number and drastically decreased in comparison which control without chromium. At toxic influence of such intensity, the dose of chromium per one cell remains practically constant during all term of experiment. Therefore with reference to high concentration of substances it is possible to speak about concurrence of concepts “concentration” and “dose” even if we add the toxicant one time at the beginning of the experiment.

At medium chromium concentration of 0.1 mg/L number of cells increased, but growth rate of culture has been slowed down in comparison with control one (without chromium). At low chromium concentration of 0.001 and 0.01 mg/L growth rate of *S. quadricauda* corresponded to the control parameters down to 10th day of experiment, then growth rate have decreased, however by the end of experiment number of cells at presence of these concentrations of chromium has appeared close to the control. Thus, the most sensitive stage at repeated additions of chromium in medium is, apparently, second half of logarithmic growth phase (10-14 day of experiment). As concentration of chromium of 0.001 and 0.01

mg/L are low enough, it is not likely, that they provoke selection of resistant cells. In this case chromium could cause so called "synchronization" (full or partial) of cultures seaweed by delay or arrest of cellular division at 7th-10th days of experiment. After that there was an acclimation of algal cells, and cellular division also was synchronously restored. Thus cultures have reached "control" levels of number of cells.

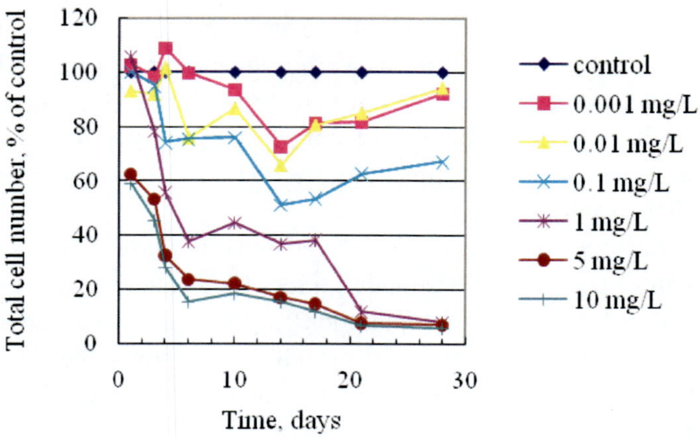

Figure. 9. Changes of the total cell number of *S. quadricauda* under chromium exposure (multiple chromium additions).

Thus, at low chromium concentrations of 0.001 and 0.01 mg/L during the experiments with the periodical additions growth rate of *S. quadricauda* was close to the control (without chromium) and to the conventional "control" (single chromium addition at the start of experiments, see detail description in "Materials and Methods"), although the total final concentrations were 3.3-3.4 times more than initial ones.

The final cell number of *T. weissflogii* was slightly decreased in the presence of 0.001 mg/L chromium and was reliably smaller in the presence of 0.01; 0.1 and 1 mg/L chromium during the multiple intoxication as compared with the single one (Figure 10).

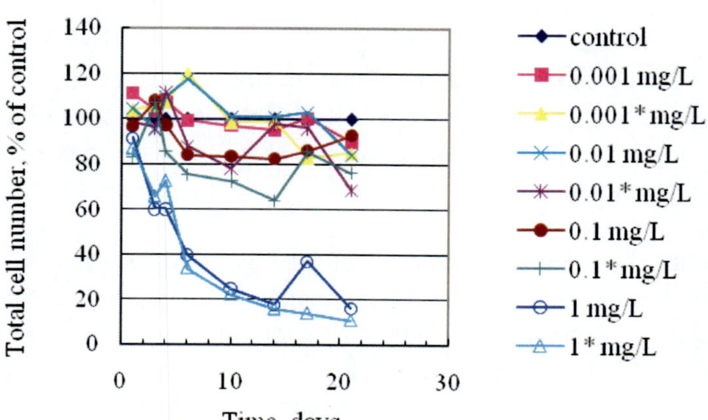

Figure. 10. Changes of the total cell number of *T. weissflogii* under chromium exposure: single addition at the start of experiment and multiple (*) additions at 0, 3, 6, 10 and 13 day of experiment.

The share of dead and dying cells was slightly higher at the multiple intoxication than at the single one during experiments with both species.

2.2. The number of the toxicant-resistant cells within S. quadricauda population

There are many experimental data about algal adaptation to heavy metals. The result of adaptation is increasing of resistance to toxicants during the time. In the case of chronic intoxication this process can develop by selection of already existent forms in genetically heterogeneous population (genetic adaptation) or by forming of resistant cells of algae within population (biochemical or phenotypic adaptation). It is important to know the limits of algal population resistance to long-term high intensive toxic effects for hydrosphere monitoring.

Our results have demonstrated that living cells were remained in the cultures treated by the toxicants at lethal concentrations. Data are available about size spectrum (as an example see Figure 6) and photosynthetic characteristics of these cells. It was interesting to estimate the resistant cell quantity in the heterogenous algal population.

In present work we estimated resistance of laboratory population of green chlorococcal alga *Scenedesmus quadricauda* (Turp.) Breb. to chromium (as potassium dichromate, $K_2Cr_2O_7$) as a model toxicant.

We worked out a program of "step by step" experiment (duration of every step was approximately 30 days), which has been carried out to develop Cr-tolerant cells of algae through previous exposure at various concentrations of chromium 0.1; 1.0; 3.0; 10.0 mg/L. Then the alga was re-inoculated twice in medium with 10.0 mg/L chromium or in the medium without toxicant. The re-inoculation was made by following manner: after intoxication during 30 days the algae were infiltrated via membrane filters NN 4 and 5, washed by distilled water and transferred to the Uspenskii medium with or without toxicant. The three experiments were conducted according to this scheme. After step II before re-inoculation the control cultures were diluted by Uspenskii medium to the initial cell number $2x10^5$ cells/mL. At the end of step III of experiment the algae were re-inoculated in the Uspenskii medium without chromium adding (step IV) for estimation of population restore possibility. In spring we made an additional experiment with chromium. After 30-day exposure with 10.0 mg/L the algae were we re-inoculated twice in Uspenskii medium with 10.0 mg/L chromium. Then, the algae were transferred in the medium without toxicant.

The scheme of the experiment (chromium concentrations, mg/L, which the algae were inoculated in consecutively are indicated) is shown in the table.

The cultures were pre-adapted to the chromium action because of growing with various concentrations of the toxicant. Then the algae were transferred to the Uspenskii medium with 10 mg/L chromium (step I).

In the end of step II pre-adaptation has led to the following results. The number of living algal cells was different: the more the initial chromium concentration was, the less the cell number was. The maximal cell number was 73 000 cells/mL in the culture previously exposed in the presence of 0.1 mg/L chromium (seemingly inactive concentration, "dead zone" on the dose-response curve). We suggested that the increasing of algal response to the toxic action is a result of initial exposition at this concentration.

Table 1.

Steps and terms their carrying out (excluding variant 5)	Variants of the experiment (Cr, mg/L)					
	Control	1	2	3	4	5
I	0	0.1	1	3	10	10
II	↓ 0	↓ 10	↓ 10	↓ 10	↓ 10	↓ 10
III	↓ 0	↓ 10	↓ 10	↓ 10	↓ 10	↓ 10
IV	↓ 0	↓ 0	↓ 0	↓ 0	-	↓ 0

Note: "0" – culture without toxicant;
"-' – algae were not re-inoculated.

After the re-inoculation in 10.0 mg/L chromium we revealed that the cell number was 6000-8000 cells/mL in all samples (step III). In sample, pre-adapted with 10 mg/L chromium, living cells were not found in winter, but in spring the cell number was 5000 cells/mL (variant 5). It means that metal-resistance changes in the course of year. During the experiments efficiency of photosynthesis decreased accordingly to chromium concentrations changes: the higher concentration was, the lower efficiency of photosynthesis was.

Thus, in spite of the long-term exposition with toxicant some algal cells remained alive. Their number was 5-7 % of initial cell number.

We analyzed the size-age population structure and photosynthetic activity in control cultures and after treatment. It was demonstrated that cell size spectrum is rather the same as control one (as it can be seen from comparison of figure 2 and figure 11). It indicates that after toxic exposure the normal algal cells remain in population. The photosynthetic activity of these cells was the same than control one, too. The number of these cells (5-7 %) corresponds with frequency of mutation for unicellular algae, fungi and bacteria in nature.

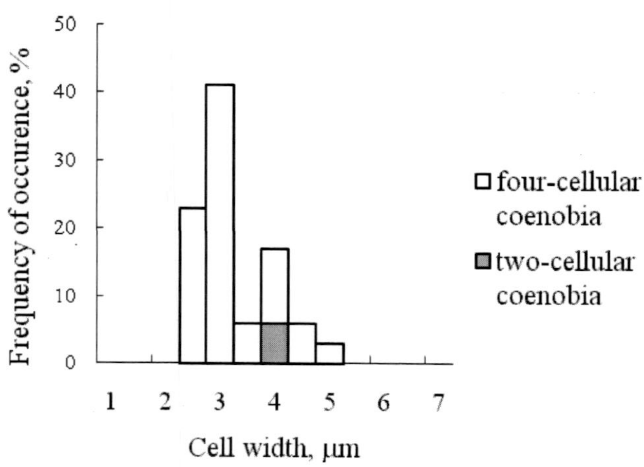

Figure 11. *S. quadricauda* cell width distribution after the triple intoxication of 10.0 mg/L chromium.

The resistant cells cause quick population restoration after the intoxication arrest. For example, the growth rate of the cells, which were pre-adapted with 3.0 mg/L chromium and re-inoculated twice to the medium with 10.0 mg/L chromium, was ten times as many as that of the control.

The presence of resistant cells can be related to their constant presence in population or is the result of selection. It is need of special research for clarification of this phenomenon.

2.3. Analysis of transformation from chromium sensitivity to chromium resistance. Mutation rate evaluation

In the present study we have analyzed the spontaneous occurrence of chromium-resistant cells in cultures of chromium-sensitive (wild-tipe) cells of *S. quadricauda* and *T. weissflogii*. For this purpose, a modified fluctuation analysis was carried out, using algae as experimental organisms.

Fluctuation analysis [Luria & Delbrück, 1943; Cairns et al., 1988; Tlsty et al., 1989] was used to distinguish between resistant cells arising by rare spontaneous pre-adaptive mutations occurring randomly during replication of organisms prior to the incorporation of chromium and chromium-resistant cells arising through physiological or specifically acquired post-selective adaptation in response to chromium and, subsequently, to estimate the rate of occurrence of resistant cells.

On the base of hypothesis that adaptation to chromium occurs by selection of spontaneous mutations, the controls should have had a low variance-to-mean ratio consistent with the error in sampling resistants from one large culture, whereas the fluctuation test cultures should have had a high variance-to-mean ratio. Thus, spontaneous mutation predicts a high variance-to-mean ratio in the number of resistant cells among cultures, whereas resistance acquired in response to exposure predicts a variance-to-mean ratio that is approximately equal to 1, as expected from the Poisson distribution.

When algal cultures were exposed to 2.5 mg/L (*S. quadricauda*) and 1.5 mg/L (*T. weissflogii*) chromium, growth of the algae were inhibited. Chromium killed the wild-type sensitive cells but allowed the growth of resistant cells. The culture survived due to the growth of variants that were resistant to chromium.

Every experimental culture of both sets 1 and 2 apparently collapsed following chromium exposure. In set 1, only some cultures recovered after 14 day of chromium exposure, apparently due to the growth of chromium resistant cells (recovered cultures increased their cell number compared to the control level). A high fluctuation in set 1 (in contrast with the scant variation in set 2) was found in both species (tables 2 and 3), which indicated that the high variance found in set 1 cultures should be due to processes other than sampling error.

The data from a fluctuation test were used to calculate a spontaneous mutation rate per cell division using the proportion of cell cultures that exhibit no mutants at all [Luria & Delbrück, 1943]. The estimated mutation rates (μ) using the P_0 estimator were $5.2{\cdot}10^{-6}$ and $3.1{\cdot}10^{-6}$ mutants per cell division in *S. quadricauda* and *T. weissflogii*, respectively.

Table 2. Fluctuation analysis of resistant variants in *Scenedesmus quadricauda*.

	Set 1	Set 2
No. of replicate cultures	52	30
No. of cultures containing the following no. of resistant cells/mL:		
0	45	0
0-2x10^4	2	0
2x10^4-10^5	5	30
>10^5	0	0
Variance/mean (of the no. of resistant cells per replicate)	61.5	3.2
μ (mutants per cell division)	5.2 x 10^{-6}	

Table 3. Fluctuation analysis of resistant variants in *Thalassiosira weissflogii*.

	Set 1	Set 2
No. of replicate cultures	49	30
No. of cultures containing the following no. of resistant cells/mL:		
0	36	0
1-1300	4	0
1300-5000	9	30
>5000	0	0
Variance/mean (of the no. of resistant cells per replicate)	16.8	0.95
μ (mutants per cell division)	3.1 x 10^{-6}	

The data of this study correspond to the results of other work carried out on understanding algal adaptation to anthropogenic chemical water pollutants, such as antibiotics, herbicides, substances of military use and others. The rate of mutation from $3.1 \cdot 10^{-6}$ to $5.2 \cdot 10^{-6}$ mutants per cell per generation was the same order (or one order lower or higher) of magnitude found for the resistance to several pollutants in other cyanobacterial and microalgal species [Costas et al., 2001; López-Rodas et al., 2001; Baos et al., 2002; García-Villada et al., 2002, 2004; Flores-Moya et al., 2005]. The presence of resistant cells in the populations of algae is regulated by the recurrent appearance of mutants and their elimination by selection, yielding an equilibrium frequency of 3-5 resistant cells per 10^6 cell divisions. This fraction of resistant mutants is presumably enough to assure the adaptation of algal populations to catastrophic water contamination, since the algal natural populations are composed of countless cells. Nevertheless, mutations usually imply an energetic cost that may affect the survival of adapting populations [Coustau et al., 2000], as was demonstrated by a growth rate in resistant cells only one-sixth of that in sensitive ones, in the absence of the herbicide [López-Rodas et al., 2007]. (Isolated resistant mutants growing in the absence of the selective agent, i.e., without herbicide in the culture medium, showed growth rates only one-sixth of those found in sensitive cells [López-Rodas 2007].) Flores-Moya [Flores-Moya et al., 2005] observed that resistant cells grew approximately 23% more slowly than sensitive cells in permissive medium: there is a cost associated with resistance. Thus, resistant cells could develop in freshwater ecosystems in the presence of pollutants, but their contribution to primary production will be significantly lower than that occurring in pristine ecosystems with sensitive cells.

3. Algostatic Effect of Silver

One of the main characteristics of hydrospheric pollution is the level of heavy metals, which is estimated on the base of biological and chemical analysis. According to literature data, silver and its compounds are toxic enough and the less investigated, simultaneously [Silver..., 2002]. That is why there is necessity of their monitoring in the environment and studying the effects of silver for water organisms.

Algae are used to evaluate the risk of new chemicals via laboratory research and these organisms are used for bioassays to measure the toxicity of waste water streams. The toxic effect of silver depends on algal species, growth medium, population density, etc. The aim of our research was the investigation of silver action (as a component part of silver sulfate, Ag_2SO_4) on the laboratory population of unicell algae: green chlorococcal *Scenedesmus quadricauda* (Turp.) Breb. and diatom *Thalassiosira weissflogii* (Grunow) Fryxell et Hastle. It is important to indicate that the maximum permissible concentrations of silver are not standardized by now [Silver..., 2002].

At low silver concentrations 0.0001; 0.001 and 0.01 mg/L we observed insignificant slowdown population growth as compared to the control culture starting from 3d – 4th days of the experiments. Such effect was more strongly marked in the marine medium (culture of the *T. weissflogii*). In the freshwater medium we observed the slight growth inhibition in the presence of the lowest concentration 0.0001 mg/L and stimulation of algal growth at moderate concentrations 0.001 and 0.01 mg/L.

Analysis of cell size distribution showed the appearance of enlarged cells both freshwater, and marine medium (110-120 % of control values) at the low toxicant concentrations. It was seemingly caused by cell division inhibition. Thus, the reason of population growth delay was the arrest of proliferation of some cells rather than deceleration of cell cycle in all cells. Toxicant had not strong effect on the photosynthetic activity as compared to the control level. The share of alive cells was around 85-90 % (the share of alive cells in the control culture was 95 % at the end of experiment).

The statistically and biologically significant responses (hormesis and paradoxical, three-phase curves) frequently occur below the NOAEL [Ewijk & Hoekstra, 1993; Calabrese & Balwin, 2001; Christofi et al., 2002]. It supports the non-random nature of such responses and need to transform the phenomena to an accepted for risk assessment. Low-dose effects deal with homeostasis disruptions that are mediated by agonist concentration gradients with different affinities for stimulatory and inhibitory regulatory pathways. The response of toxicological systems to low levels of exposure has been challenged especially for the hormesis and large implication for the safety standards for health and environment have been indicated [Calabrese & Balwin, 2003]. We have shown earlier that nonlinear concentration response curve of cell survival reflects of hierarchy of cell responses to increasing concentration of imazalil sulfate and chromium: cell division inhibition in low doses, stress and adaptive tolerance increasing in moderate doses and immature cell division and cell death in high doses (see above) [Prokhotskaya et al., 2000; 2003].

At high silver concentrations 0.02, 0.05, 0.1, 0.2 and 0.5 mg/L we observe algostatic effect, e. g. the total number of cells preserved on the constant level close to initial values. We suppose that such effect is related with inhibition of the dead cells bacterial lysis. Accordingly to the literature data the bacteria are the most sensitive organisms to silver action [Silver..., 2002]. It was obviously that in this case the cell number decreasing was caused by their death, but during the first day of cultivation the cell number did not change. The very small cells appeared within population. Therefore, toxicant first initiated cell division in all cells, including those that had not attained the mature cell size. Since the total cell number did not change, it is clear that a certain part of cells died. Therefore, the analysis of size-age population structure can find out the lethal effect earlier than counting of cell number.

The number of dead cells in the cultures increased only at high toxicant concentrations 0.1 and 0.5 mg/L (98-99 % of the total cell number). We were shown earlier that the lack of effect at the moderate toxicant concentrations ("dead zone") was caused by renewal of cell division after temporary inhibition [Prokhotskaya et al., 2000]. At these concentrations the toxicant initiated cell transfer to the state of nonspecific resistance (stress) and the cell reparative mechanisms were activated. In the presence of silver at moderate concentration we observed toxic (sublethal) effect. That implies absence of algal cells adaptation in this case.

After 1-day incubation at high concentrations of silver the photosynthetic activity of the *S. quadricauda* culture was reduced to a double as compared to the control level. It implies that cell damage was irreversible. The number of cells did not attain the control values even after the washing and transferring of silver-treated cells in the toxicant-free medium. It was supposed that the irreversible injuries were caused by silver uptake.

The number of silver-resistant cells. With the aim to estimate the share of silver-resistant cells within the heterogeneous algal population we carried out experiment with double silver intoxication during 60 days. In the course of this experiment we transferred the *S. quadricauda* cells previously treated (during 30 days) with 0.001 and 0.01 mg/L silver in the medium with 0.05 mg/L silver. In spite of the long-term exposition with toxicant some algal cells remained alive. Their number was 3-5 % of initial cell number. We analyzed the size-age population structure and photosynthetic activity in control cultures and after treatment. The cell size spectrum in the presence of silver was rather the same as control one. It indicates that after toxic exposure the normal algal cells remain in population. The photosynthetic activity of these cells was the same as control one, too. The number of these cells (3-5 %) corresponds with frequency of mutation for unicellular algae, fungi and bacteria in nature. The presence of resistant cells can be related to their constant presence in population or is the result of selection. It is need of special research for clarification of this phenomenon.

The resistant cells cause quick population restoration after the intoxication. For example, the growth rate of the cells, which were pre-adapted with 0.001 and 0.01 mg/L silver and re-inoculated to the medium with 0.5 mg/L toxicant, was two times as many as that of the control. The maximal resistance of the algae to the toxicant was revealed in spring-summer, the minimal resistance – in winter.

CONCLUSION

The concentration-response curve of cell survival reflects a hierarchy of cell responses to increasing concentration of the toxicants. On the base of structural and functional population characteristics analysis we suggest to appropriate the following types of population reaction to the toxicant action: at low toxicant concentrations (0.001 mg/L), the decreasing of cell number is the result of cell division arrest; at moderate (0.01-0.1 mg/L), the absence of effect is caused by renewal of cell division after temporary arrest; at sublethal concentrations (1.0-3.0 mg/L), we can observe long-term cell division inhibition and giant cells forming; at lethal concentration (10.0 mg/L), the cell division is stimulated and the small immature cells predominated at the beginning of intoxication. We offer using described types of reaction to the toxic action for risk assessment and biotesting.

Our data demonstrated that the informational value of DF characteristics is most appropriate for recording the responses of algal cultures to lethal concentrations of toxic agents. At low concentrations, DF characteristics are more due to the proportion of various cell types in the population [Prokhotskaya et al., 2006].

There is a vast information about chemical waste effects on plants, including algal adaptation to toxicant action [Ahner et al., 1994, Hall, 2002, Lasat, 2002]. The limits of algal cells resistance to long-term high intensive toxic effects determine survival of population as a whole. In the present research we demonstrated the method of proportion of resistant cells estimation in the heterogeneous algal population. Our experiments with algal cultures *Scenedesmus quadricauda* (Turp.) Breb. and *Thalassiosira weissflogii* (Grunow) Fryxell et Hastle grown in the presence of toxicants showed the increasing resistance of pre-adapted cultures by means of the total cell number and share of alive cells growth. The morphological characteristics of the resistant cells were differed from the control ones by the predominance of small cell fraction as a possible result of changes in their growth rates. The population heterogeneity ensured the cell number restoration after the removing of toxic pressure due to the minimal amount of the most resistant cells (3-6 % of the initial cell number).

The present study is a simple model of algal adaptation to stressful environments. Our results suggest that rare pre-selective mutants can be sufficient to ensure the adaptation of eukaryotic algae to extreme natural habitats. These values are low ($\sim 10^{-6}$ mutants per cell division). Such mutation rate coupled with rapid growth rates, are presumably enough to ensure the adaptation of microalgae to water contamination. The resistant cells arise randomly by rare spontaneous mutation during replication of cells prior to the addition of the contaminant. The pre-selective mutations are able to survival of microalgae in contaminated environments. Resistant mutants are maintained in the absence of contaminants as the result of balance between new resistant cells arising from spontaneous mutation and resistant cells eliminated by natural selection, so that about 3-5 chromium-resistant mutants per million cells are present in the absence of chromium. Within limits microalgal species should survive in polluted environments as a result of physiological adaptation. With increasing concentrations of contaminants, however, physiological adaptation is not enough, but the genetic variability of natural populations could assure the survival of at least some genotypes [Mettler et al., 1988]. New alleles arising by rare spontaneous mutations during replication of organisms under nonselective conditions could play the principal role in the survival of microalgae in polluted environments. Mutation is the fundamental source of genetic variability, because only mutation is able to generate new adaptive alleles. Genetic variability in natural populations is the most important guarantee of surviving most environmental changes [Lewontin, 1974; Mettler et al., 1988]. Some populations are being exposed to new xenobiotics for the first time. Sudden toxic spills of residual materials can be lethal to microalgae. Rare spontaneous pre-adaptive mutations are enough to ensure the survival of microalgal populations in contaminated environments when the population size is large enough. Adaptation of algal populations to modern pollution-derived environmental hazards seems to be the result of a rare instantaneous events and the result of resistant cells selection within heterogeneous population.

During the long-term toxic exposure the resistant communities have been forming in the environment. The increasing of algal resistance to acting factor under the chronic toxic pressure can be result of selection in the heterogenous population (genotypic adaptation) or can be related with the initial presence of the resistant cells (phenotypic adaptation). All the populations always have the different potential reactions on the stress factors. That is why the one of the tasks of the toxic effect ecological description is to give an idea of duration of response and degree of population resistance. In the present research we demonstrated the method of proportion of resistant cells estimation in the heterogeneous algal population.

Our experiments with algal cultures *Scenedesmus quadricauda* (Turp.) Breb. and *Thalassiosira weissflogii* (Grunow) Fryxell et Hastle grown in the presence of silver showed the increasing resistance of pre-adapted cultures by means of the total cell number and share of alive cells growth. The morphological characteristics of the resistant cells were differed from the control ones by the predominance of small cell fraction as a possible result of changes in their growth rates. The population heterogeneity ensured the cell number restoration after the removing of toxic pressure due to the minimal amount of the most resistant cells (3-5 % of the initial cell number). At silver concentration of 0.1 and 0.5 mg/L the total cell number changed insignificantly, so, we observed the algostatic effect.

Thus, in the long-term intoxication of algal populations experiments we can see the common rules of adaptive and compensation reaction, e. g. elimination of the most sensitive cells and reconstruction the population as a whole system already in the new conditions. Changes of the population structural and functional characteristics can be special way of survival in unfavourable conditions.

Data on the cell number, their photosynthetic characteristics, population structure and share of alive and dead cells will be appropriate for use to predict the most sensitive ecosystem responses and indicate the permissible amount of toxicants in the environment.

REFERENCES

[1] Ahner, B. A., Price, N. M. & Francois, M. M. M. (1994). Phytochelatin production by marine phytoplankton at low free metal ion concentrations: laboratory studies and field data from Massachusetts Bay. *Proc. Natl. Acad. Sci. USA*, *91*, 8433-8436.

[2] Baos, R., Garcia-Villada, L., Agrelo, M., López-Rodas, V., Hiraldo, F. & Costas, E. (2002). Short-term adaptation of microalgae in highly stressful environments: an experimental model analysing the resistance of *Scenedesmus intermedius*

(Chlorophyceae) to the heavy metals mixture from the Aznalcóllar mine spill. *Eur. J. Phycol.*, *37*, 593-600.

[3] Belfiore, N. M. & Anderson, S. L. (2001). Effects of contaminants on genetic patterns in aquatic organisms: a review. *Mutat. Res.*, *489*, 97-122.

[4] Cairns, J., Overbaugh, J. & Miller, S. (1988). The origin of mutants. *Nature*, *335*, 142-145.

[5] Calabrese, E. J. & Balwin, L. A. (2001). Hormesis: U-shaped dose responses and their centrality in toxicology. *Trends Pharmacol Sci*, *22*, 291.

[6] Calabrese, E. J. & Balwin, L. A. (2003). Toxicology rethinks its central belief. *Nature. 421*. 691-692.

[7] Christofi, N., Hoffman, C. & Tosh, L. (2002). Hormesis response of free and immobilized light-emitting bacteria. *Ecotoxicol Environ Saf*, *52*, 227-231

[8] Costas, E., Carrillo, E., Ferrero, L. M., Agrelo, M., García-Villada, L., Juste, J. & López-Rodas, V. (2001). Mutation of algae from sensitivity to resistance against environmental selective agents: the ecological genetics of *Dictyosphaerium chlorelloides* (Chlorophyceae) under lethal doses of 3-(3,4-dichlorophenyl)-1,1-dimethylurea herbicide. *Phycologia*, *40*, 391-398.

[9] Coustau, C., Chevillon, C. & Ffrench-Constant, R. (2000). Resistance to xenobiotics and parasites: can we count the cost? *Trends Ecol. Evol.*, *15*, 378-383.

[10] Ewijk, van P. H. & Hoekstra, J. A. (1993). Calculation of the EC50 and its confidence interval when subtoxic stimulus is present. *Ecotoxicol Environ Saf*, *25*, 25-32.

[11] Flores-Moya, A., Costas, E., Bañares-España, E., García-Villada, L., Altamirano, M. & López-Rodas, V. (2005). Adaptation of *Spirogyra insignis* (Chlorophyta) to an extreme natural environment (sulphureous waters) through preselective mutations. *New Phytol.*, *166*, 655-661.

[12] García-Villada, L., López-Rodas, V., Bañares-España, E., Flores-Moya, A., Agrelo, M., Martín-Otero, L. & Costas, E. (2002). Evolution of microalgae in highly stressing environments: an experimental model analyzing the rapid adaptation of *Dictyosphaerium chlorelloides* (Chlorophyceae) from sensitivity to resistance against 2,4,6-trinitrotoluene by rare preselective mutations. *J. Phycol*, *38*, 1074-1081.

[13] García-Villada, L., Rico, M., Altamirano, M., Sánchez-Martín, L., López-Rodas, V. & Costas, E. (2004). Occurrence of copper resistant mutants in the toxic cyanobacterium *Microcystis aeruginosa:* characterization and future implications in the use of copper sulphate as an algaecide. *Water Res.*, *38*, 2207-2213.

[14] Hall, J. L. (2002). Cellular mechanisms for heavy metal detoxification and tolerance. *J. Exp. Bot.*, *53*, 1-11.

[15] Hoffmann, A. A. & Parsons, P. A. (1991). *Evolutionary Genetics and Environmental Stress.* : Oxford University Press Inc.

[16] Holzhutter, H.-G. & Quedenau, J. (1995). Mathematical modeling of cellular responses to external signals. *J Biol Systems*, *3*, 127-138.

[17] Ivorra, N., Barranguet, C., Jonker, M., Kraak, M.H.S. & Admiraal, W. (2002). Metal-induced tolerance in the freshwater microbenthic diatom *Gomphonema parvulum. Environ. Pollu*, *116*, 147-157.

[18] Knauer, K., Behra, R. & Hemond, H. (1999). Toxicity of inorganic and methylated arsenic to algal communities from lakes along an arsenic contamination gradient. *Aquat. Toxicol.*, *46*, 221-230.

[19] Lasat, M. M. (2002). Phytoextraction of toxic metals: A review of biological mechanisms. *J. Environ. Qualit.*, *31*, 109-120.

[20] Lewontin, R. C. (1974). *The genetic basis of evolutionary change.* New York: Columbia University Press.

[21] López-Rodas, V., Agrelo, M., Carrillo, E., Ferrero, L. M, Larrauri, A., Martín-Otero, L. & Costas, E. (2001). Resistance of microalgae to modern water contaminants as the result of rare spontaneous mutations. *Eur. J. Phycol.*, *36*, 179-190.

[22] López-Rodas, V., Flores-Moya, A., Maneiro, E., Perdigones, N., Marva, F., García, M. E. & Costas, E. (2007). Resistance to glyphosate in the cyanobacterium *Microcystis aeruginosa* as result of pre-selective mutations. *Evol. Ecol.*, *21*, 535-547.

[23] Luria, S. E. & Delbrück, M. (1943). Mutations of bacteria from virus sensitivity to virus resistance. *Genetics*, *28*, 491-511.

[24] Mettler, L. E., Gregg, T. & Schaffer, H. E. (1988). *Population Genetics and Evolution.* New York: Prentice-Hall, Englewood Cliffs.

[25] Nyström, B., Björnsater, B. & Blanck, H. (1999). Effects of sulfonylurea herbicides on non-target aquatic micro-organisms: growth inhibition of microalgae and short-term inhibition of adenine and thymidine incorporation in periphyton communities. *Aquat. Toxicol.*, *47*, 9-22.

[26] Prokhotskaya, V. Yu., Ipatova V. I. & Dmitrieva, A. G. (2006). Intrapopulation Changes of Algae under Toxic Exposure. *Proc. Int. Conf. on Complex Systems 2006*, http://necsi.org/events/iccs6/viewpaper.php?id=50.

[27] Prokhotskaya, V. Yu., Veselova, T.V., Veselovskii, V.A., Dmitrieva, A.G. & Artyukhova (Ipatova), V.I. (2003). The dimensional-age structure of a laboratory population of *Scenedesmus quadricauda* (Turp.) Breb. in the presence of imazalyl sulfate. *Intern. J. Algae.*, *5*, 82-91.

[28] Prokhotskaya, V. Yu., Veselovskii, V. A., Veselova, T. V., Dmitrieva, A. G. & Artyukhova (Ipatova), V. I. (2000). On the nature of the three-phase response of *Scenedesmus quadricuda* populations to the action of imazalil sulfate. *Russian J Plant Physiol*, *6*. 772-778.

[29] Santos, M. M., Moreno-Garrido, I., Goncalves, F., Soares, A. & Ribeiro, R. (2002). An *in situ* bioassay for estuarine environments using microalga *Phaeodactilum tricornutum. Envirom Toxicol Chem*, *21*. 567-574.

[30] Senger, H. & Krupinska, K. (1986). Changes in molecular organization of thylakoid membranes during the cell cycle of *Scenedesmus obliquus. Plant Cell Physiol.*, *27*, 1127-1139.

[31] Silver and silver compounds: environmental aspects. (2002). Geneva: World Health Organization.

[32] Tamiya, H. (1966). Synchronous cultures of algae. *Ann. Rev. Plant Physiol.*, *17*, 1-26.

[33] Tamiya, H., Iwamura, T., Shibata, K., Hase, E. & Nihei, T. (1953). Correlation between photosynthesis and light-independent metabolism in the growth of *Chlorella. Biochim Biophys Acta*, *12*. 23-40.

[34] Tlsty, T. D., Margolin, B. H. & Lum K. (1989). Differences in the rate of gene amplification in nontumorigenic and tumorigenic cell lines as measured by Luria-Delbrück fluctuation analysis. *Proc. Natl. Acad. Sci. USA*, *86*, 9441-9445.

[35] Toxicological profile for silver. (1990). Agency for toxic substances and disease registry Department of health and human service. USA.

[36] Wang, W. (1997). Chromate ion as a reference toxicant for aquatic phytotoxicity tests. *Environ. Toxicol. Chem.*, *6*, 953-960.

In: Cell Division: Theory, Variants and Degradation
Editors: Y. N. Golitsin, M. C. Krylov, pp. 59-79
ISBN: 978-1-60876-986-5

Chapter 3

CELL DIVISION AND CELL ELONGATION OF *CORYNEBACTERIUM GLUTAMICUM*, A ROD-SHAPED BACTERIUM THAT LACKS ACTIN-LIKE HOMOLOGUES

Michal Letek, María Fiuza, Efrén Ordóñez, Almudena F. Villadangos, Luís M. Mateos and José A. Gil*
Departamento de Biología Molecular, Área de Microbiología, Facultad de Biología, Universidad de León, León, 24071, Spain.

ABSTRACT

Homologues to actin are ubiquitous in nature, and actin-based cellular skeletons are crucial for the maintenance of prokaryotic and eukaryotic cellular morphology. Regarding the prokaryotes, MreB actin-homologues sustain the peptidoglycan (PG) synthesis along the lateral cell wall of most rod-shaped bacteria; FtsA actin-homologues are essential for cell division in *Escherichia coli* or *Bacillus subtilis*. However, the rod-shaped actinomycete *Corynebacterium glutamicum* has lost during evolution any homologues to actin found in most of other bacteria. Instead, this bacterium elongates in a mycelium fashion, synthesizing PG at the cell poles sustained by internal structures made of a coiled-coil rich protein called DivIVA. This protein interacts with the molecular machinery involved in polar PG synthesis, mainly comprised by RodA, a transporter of PG-precursors, and the class A penicillin-binding proteins. The cell division of *C. glutamicum* is also accomplished by the absence of any actin-homologue. In fact, the cell division machinery of this bacterium is a minimalist version of other septum molecular structures described in most bacteria. Despite of the minimalism exhibited in such crucial processes, the coordination of cell growth, cell division and DNA partition of *C. glutamicum* have been elusive to researchers for a long period of time. This coordination must be tightly controlled since *C. glutamicum* is able to change its cellular morphology to a coco-bacillus shape depending on the environmental

* Corresponding autor: Tel. 34-987-291503, Fax. 34-987-291479. E-mail: jagils@unileon.es.

conditions. Nevertheless, recent reports have characterized some of the molecular factors involved in the spatio-temporal regulation of cell division and cell growth in this bacterium. This regulation implicates protein phosphorylation, which is also exceptional in bacterial cell-shape acquisition. In summary, *Corynebacterium glutamicum* is able to generate a rod-shaped cell by using in a different way the molecular mechanisms that are generally accepted as involved in bacterial morphogenesis.

Keywords: *Corynebacterium*; cell division; cell growth; FtsZ; DivIVA; FtsI; HMW-PBP; PknA; PknB; cell wall.

INTRODUCTION

Corynebacterium glutamicum, a soil-borne microorganism, was firstly identified during a screening for natural producers of amino acids in the late 1950s [69]. Since then, this bacterium has been broadly used in the industrial production of the taste enhancer L-glutamic acid or the essential amino acid for animal nutrition L-lysine, among other applications [52]. Nowadays, the production of these two amino acids by Corynebacteria is estimated to be more than 1 million tons per year [52]. Because of the huge economical interest, the study of the metabolism of *C. glutamicum* and its manipulation has been the main focus of numerous research initiatives worldwide. This has led to the genome sequencing of three different strains of *C. glutamicum* and the closely related *Corynebacterium efficiens* by four independent laboratories [61,66,80,126]. The availability of these genome sequences has been accompanied with the development and application of a wide range of molecular biology tools: from efficient transformation methods [96], unmarked deletion systems [64,105], numerous cloning vectors for gene complementation or overexpression [11,12,97], to genome-wide proteomics and transcriptomics [7,53,89]. The use of all of these technologies has permitted ultimately the genetic engineering of the *C. glutamicum* metabolism [5,13,56,60,84,100], seeking for a rapid amino acid production increase.

The genus *Corynebacterium* has also medical interest, firstly because of its close relatedness to the pandemic man-killer *Mycobacterium tuberculosis* [43], but in addition, the *Corynebacterium* genus itself comprises several human pathogenic species which genomes have been rapidly sequenced in the last few years. The most prominent member of the pathogenic Corynebacteria is the causative agent of diphtheria, *Corynebacterium diphtheriae* [14], however, there has been a substantial increase in the interest for the study of several emergent pathogens such as *Corynebacterium jeikeium* [109], *Corynebacterium urealyticum* [34] or *Corynebacterium amycolatum* [73]. These pathogens are frequently multi-drug resistant and cause nosocomial infections in immunosupressed patients. At the moment of writing this chapter, 26 genomes from 17 different *Corynebacterium* species have being sequenced or are in the process of being sequenced (source: http://www.genomesonline.org/); 15 of these sequenced species are considered pathogenic, which could be illustrative of the medical importance of the genus *Corynebacterium.*

However, Corynebacteria are not only interesting from a biotechnological or medical point of view. These rod-shaped bacteria are fascinating in the molecular strategies used to achieve their cellular shape. They share molecular determinants involved in cell division and cell elongation with other bacterial models like *Escherichia coli*, *Bacillus subtilis* or

Caulobacter crescentus, although they differ profoundly in the way that they use these factors. Because of this, the objective of this chapter is to revise the knowledge accumulated to date regarding the molecular biology of Corynebacterial cell morphogenesis. Apart from the study of fundamental and evolutionary related concepts, the analysis of bacterial cell division and cell-shape acquisition could have also crucial applications for the human kind. Essentially, this knowledge could allow the rational design of new compounds to fight bacterial infections, since most of the proteins involved in these processes are essential for bacteria but absent in humans, and thus may serve as targets of new antimicrobial agents or new antibiotics [59,63,83,104,113,118,120,123,127]. This is of uttermost importance, since the rate at which new antibiotics are being discovered by traditional approaches is much slower than the rate at which bacteria are becoming resistant to currently available antibiotics [19]. In addition, from the financial side of things, the manipulation of the cellular growth rate or the properties of the bacterial cell envelope could be also beneficial to improve the biotechnological production derived from Corynebacteria [54,91].

Morphological Eccentricities of Corynebacteria: Club Shape, Outer Membrane, Pleomorphism, and Snapping Division

The name *Corynebacterium* comes from the Greek words corunë (club) and bacterion (rod). This refers to the peculiar morphology of this bacterium, since the cell poles of cultured *Corynebacterium* are frequently engrossed, which confers a "club" shape to the cells [20]. This could be due to intracellular polyphosphate accumulations called volutin granules, which have been recurrently observed at the cellular poles [82] and could constitute 18–37% of the total cell volume.

Corynebacteria are high GC-content gram-positive actinomycetes that belong to the group of mycolata, which also includes the genera *Gordonia, Mycobacterium, Nocardia* or *Rhodococcus*. The mycolata are characterized by a lipid-rich cell envelope surrounding the cell wall, which has been described as an outer membrane of gram-positive bacteria and is thought to act as a permeability barrier [27,55,128]. In *Mycobacterium*, this outer membrane is considered a virulence factor (the so-called *cord factor*), since it confers to this pathogen resistance to antimicrobials and different stress conditions during intracellular growth [107]. In *Corynebacterium*, this lipid domain is composed of corynemycolic acids, which contain 30–36 carbon atoms and a non-reduced β-keto group [18,90]. In addition of this mycolic acid membrane, several species of Corynebacteria possess an extensive S-layer [16,49,85].

The Corynebacteria can exhibit a certain rod-to-coccoid pleomorphism during cell growth, which is influenced by the culture conditions [20]. This type of rod-to-coccoid morphological change has been observed in many different bacteria when the stationary phase of the growth curve is reached [44,65,77]. It has been postulated that these coccoid cells are the product of an arrested cell elongation event during several and consecutive cell division rounds [65]. This type of pleomorphism usually appears in response to nutrient deprivation or other stress conditions. It has been postulated that in these conditions, the bacteria tend to produce a larger number of cells with a smaller cellular size in order to distribute on a higher number of individuals a certain stress factor, increasing the probabilities of survival of at least a few of these individuals [65]. In *E. coli* the rod-to-coccoid pleomorphism is transcriptionally controled by *bolA* which represses the expression of different morphogenes such as *dacA*, *dacC*, *ampC* or the *mreBCD* cluster [42,99]. *bolA* expression is in turn modulated by the sigma factor *rpoS* in response to stress conditions [1,2,41,70,98]. The Corynebacterial genomes do not contain any orthologues to *bolA*, thus the molecular mechanism by which *Corynebacterium* controls its pleomorphism is still unknown. However, *divIVA*, a gene that is essential to maintain the rod-shape in *C. glutamicum* (see below and [75]), would be the perfect target for gene regulation by a *bolA*-like repressor in this bacterium.

After cell elongation, the Corynebacteria undergo a very quick and drastic "snapping" cell division event (Fig. 1) [72]. The cell constriction is apparently accomplished faster in one half of the septum than in the other, generating what is called a post-fission movement, which leads to two daughter cells that remain joined together forming a characteristic V-shape [20,72]. After a new cell elongation step, the cells can often lie in clusters resembling Chinese letters or palisades (Fig. 1).

Cell Elongation At The Cell Poles

The Corynebacterial genomes lack any *mreB* actin-like orthologues, which have been proved to be essential for the cell elongation of *E. coli* [26], *Bacillus subtilis* [35], or *Caulobacter crescentus* [36], among others. It seems that Corynebacteria and Mycobacteria have been evolved to generate rod-shaped cells using an *mreB*-independent mechanism of cell elongation [68,75]. In high contrast, *S. coelicolor* has a cluster of *mreBCD* genes (Table 1), although these genes are apparently involved in the sporulation process [78]. It is possible to speculate that the actin-like bacterial *mreB* homologues have been lost long ago in the actinomycete genomes, now having just a role in the sporulation of some genera. In contradiction to this hypothesis, some *Rhodococcus* species, which similarly to *Corynebacterium* are also not-sporulated mycolata, share a rhodococcal-specific *mreB* gene adjacently located to a *rodA/pbp* fusion gene (RHA1_ro00247-8 and ROP_03780-90), which strongly suggests a role of this *mreB* homologue in cell shape acquisition. In any case, the cell wall elongation of *Corynebacterium*, *Mycobacterium* or *Streptomyces* is accomplished in a mycelial fashion, i.e. polarly, and this is dependent on the presence of the coiled-coil protein DivIVA [39,68,75,93,121]. Therefore, the possible role of *mreB* in the cell shape acquisition of some Actinobacteria must differ to what it has been described in other models.

All studied models of Actinobacteria synthesize new peptidoglycan, and consequently elongate, at the cellular poles [21,112]. In the recent years, the fluorescent vancomycin staining clearly confirmed this polar model of growth, previously proposed for *C. diphtheriae* [115]. In *C. diphtheriae*, cell elongation was found to resemble the growth pattern of fungal or *Streptomyces* hyphae and was therefore called apical growth [40,115]. Similar patterns of cell elongation were recently recognized in *C. glutamicum* and *M. tuberculosis* by staining of newly synthesized peptidoglycan with Vancomycin-FL [21,112]. Because of these evidences, Actinobacteria were proposed to employ a strategy for cell elongation radically different from the ones used by representative gram-positive bacteria such as *B. subtilis,* which elongates at the lateral cell wall using an *mreB*-based PG synthesis machinery, and *Staphylococcus aureus*, which cellular growth is derived from the divisome [21,87].

In all studied models of Actinobacteria, this polar cell wall synthesis requires *divIVA*, a gene located downstream from the *dcw* cluster of most gram-positives [72] (Fig. 2). DivIVA has a conserved, short N-terminal domain, which is essential for the localization of this protein in *de novo* formed cellular poles [71,121]. In addition, DivIVA has at least two coiled-coil regions by which the protein oligomerizes and probably interacts with the PG synthesis machinery [71,79,103,121]. The *divIVA* genes show poor DNA-sequence conservation [73] and their protein products exhibit a broad diversity of functions in gram-positive bacteria. In *B. subtilis* DivIVA sequesters the MinCD complex to the poles, thus participating in the spatial regulation of cell division and in chromosome segregation during sporulation [6,15,29]. DivIVA is also present in a variety of gram-positive cocci that lack the MinCD system, such as *Enterococcus faecalis, Streptococcus pneumoniae*, and *Staphylococcus aureus*. In *E. faecalis* and *S. pneumoniae*, DivIVA is required for nucleoid segregation, cell division, and cell growth [31,92], whereas in *S. aureus* the protein is not essential for growth, viability, or nucleoid segregation but localizes at the septum [88]. In *C. glutamicum*, DivIVA also localizes at the septum, but only when the nucleoids are already segregated [75]. Thus, it may have additional functions related to a final stage in cell division or cell-pole maturation, as suggested for *S. pneumoniae* DivIVA [32].

However, the main function of DivIVA in *C. glutamicum* is the maintenance of cell elongation [75,93] as in *Streptomyces* or *Mycobacterium* [39,68]. When the protein is overexpressed, the accumulated excess of DivIVA localizes mainly at one cell pole, which in turn becomes a very active site of PG synthesis [75,93]. Low-level expression of DivIVA in *C. glutamicum* results in a total lack of polar PG synthesis, and a consequent loss of the rod-shaped cellular morphology, yielding coccoid cells [75]. DivIVA interacts with PBP1a, a high-molecular-weight penicillin-binding protein (HMW-PBP), involved in polar cell-wall synthesis in *C. glutamicum* (see below and [116]). Moreover, DivIVA assembles into higher-order structures in the absence of any cofactors thanks to its coiled-coil domains [121]. Due to all these observations, it has been postulated that DivIVA oligomerizes at the cell poles creating an internal scaffold required for the maintenance of membrane integrity during PG synthesis [39,75,93]. It is clear that this protein is essential for the morphogenesis of Actinobacteria, thus, it is reasonable to affirm that DivIVA is another member of the family of cytoeskeletal proteins, and perhaps, a bacterial homologue of eukaryotic intermediate filaments (IF) [3]. Up to now, two bacterial homologues to IF proteins have been described in *C. crescentum* [3] and *S. coelicolor* A3(2) [4].

PENICILLIN-BINDING PROTEINS

The penicillin-binding proteins (PBPs) are essential for the last steps of bacterial cell-wall biosynthesis [116]. As the name suggests, PBPs are often the targets of β-lactam antibiotics and, probably because of this, the bacteria have shielded themselves against these antimicrobials by having multiple copies of *pbp* genes, which in many cases are now functionally redundant [47,101].

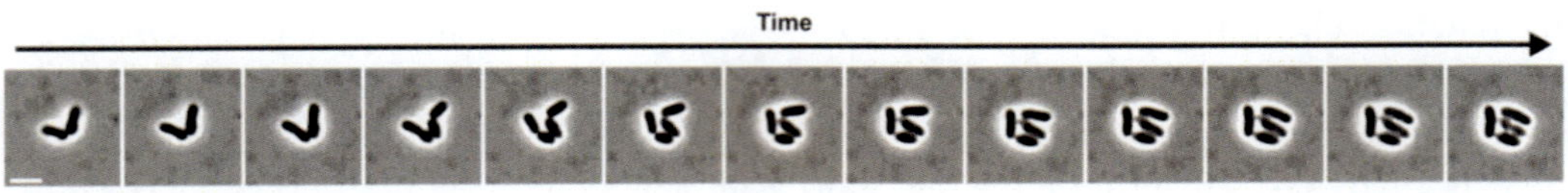

Fig. 1. Timelapse of *C. glutamicum* growing on complex medium at room temperature. The pictures were taken every 20 minutes during 12 hours. Scale bar represents 1 µm.

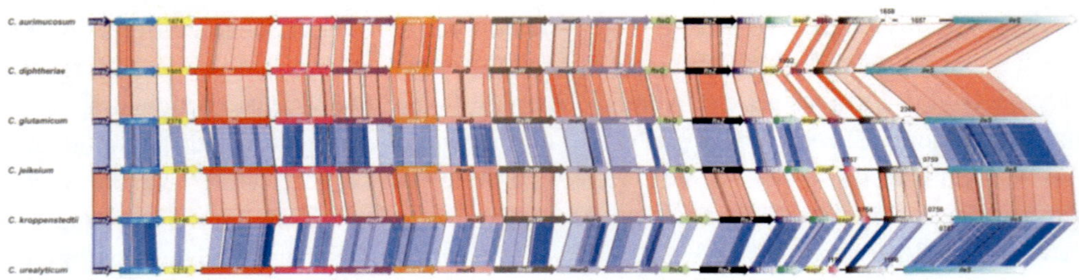

Fig. 2. Genetic organization and ACT pairwise comparisons of the *dcw* cluster in different corynebacteria. Genes are represented by thick arrows indicating direction of transcription and homologous genes are shown in the same colour; genes not related to cell division or peptidoglycan biosynthesis are colourless. Regions with significant similarity (tBLASTx) are connected by coloured lines (red, sequences in direct orientation; blue, sequences in reverse orientation). The intensity of the colour indicates the strength of the sequence homology (pink/light blue, lowest; red/deep blue, highest). Note that in the genomes of *Corynebacterium jeikeium* and *Corynebacterium kroppenstedtii* the *dcw* clusters are inverted in the chromosome when compared to the remaining genomes.

In *C. glutamicum*, from the nine proteins identified as putative penicillin-binding transpeptidases, five of them are High Molecular Weight-PBPs (HMW-PBPs) [116] and thus, they are directly involved in PG synthesis. Of these five, two are class A HMW-PBPs (PBP1a and PBP1b) with transglycosylase and transpeptidase domains, and three are class B HMW-PBPs (FtsI, PBP2a and PBP2b) with only the transpeptidase domain characteristic of this family of proteins. Except for FtsI, which is the only essential HMW-PBP and it is found just at the septum [117], all HMW-PBPs are present at both cell poles and at the septum, suggesting a role in both cell elongation and cell division. However, *C. glutamicum* cells lose their rod shape only when they are deprived of both class A HMW-PBPs, which demonstrates that PBP1a and PBP1b are essential for cell-wall synthesis at the poles [116]. Whereas class B HMW-PBPs are closely associated with septal PG synthesis during cell division and their disruption or partial depletion leads to filamentation. In support to this hypothesis, class B HMW-PBPs interact more prominently with cell-division proteins, such as FtsZ or FtsW, whereas class A HMW-PBPs are associated with the cell elongation effectors DivIVA and RodA [116]. The latter protein is required for the control of rod shape in *E. coli* and *B. subtilis* [51,62] and it is also essential for cell elongation in *C. glutamicum* (Maria Fiuza, unpublished observations), presumably by transporting PG precursors through the membrane at the cell poles.

All of the HMW-PBPs in *C. glutamicum* show a certain level of interaction between them [116], suggesting that they are part of the same machinery of PG synthesis. Thus, depending on the stage of the cell cycle, the HMW-PBPs complex could synthesize PG at the septum (cell division) or at the cell poles (cell elongation). The orchestration of these events may well be carried out by *pknAB*, as discussed below. On the other hand, when the transpeptidase domain of the PBPs is blocked by a specific β-lactam treatment, these proteins lose their localization in the cell [116], indicating that HMW-PBP localization could be dependent upon substrate recognition. Nevertheless, the spatio-temporal regulation of cell growth and cell division is probably a complex interaction network of positive and negative molecular effectors of cell division or cell growth, their activation or inactivation and their presence or absence at certain cell locations during specific steps of the bacterial cytokinesis. Therefore, it shall be nearly impossible to unravel the complexity of this process without a systems biology approach.

Genes Involved in Corynebacterial Cell Division and Its Regulation

Most of the genes required for the entire process of cell division in bacteria are located in the conserved *dcw* (division cell wall) gene cluster (Fig. 2). Despite of its high level of conservation, the different arrangements of the *dcw* clusters clearly separate the rod-shaped model actinomycetes *M. tuberculosis, S. coelicolor* and *C. diphtheriae* from other bacteria [108]. In *C. glutamicum*, many of the *dcw* genes have been extensively studied, such as *ftsZ* [57,58,74,95], *ftsI* [117,124], *murE* [124], *murD, murC*, and *ftsQ* [37,57,94,119], or *divIVA* [71,75,93]. In comparison with other well-studied *dcw* clusters, there is a number of cell-division genes not present in Corynebacteria or Mycobacteria (*ftsA, ftsN* or *ftsL*, Table 1) but essential to the process in other well-studied bacterial models. This clearly indicates that cell division of *Corynebacterium* or *Mycobacterium* must differ from other bacteria. However, there is an increasing amount of evidence supporting the notion that there is a functional redundancy in some of the *fts*-encoded proteins [8,45]. Therefore, *Corynebacterium* and *Mycobacterium* may have just the minimal version of a more sophisticated divisome of other bacteria in which some proteins have overlapping functions.

Furthermore, the well-known positive or negative regulators of cell division are missing from the *dcw* clusters and genomes of Corynebacteria [72,74]. In addition, and similarly to other Actinobacteria like *M. tuberculosis* or *S. coelicolor* (Table 1), in the Corynebacterial genomes there are neither homologues to positive regulators involved in FtsZ polymerization e.g., *zipA* or *zapA*, nor to negative regulators, e.g., *ezrA*, *noc*, *slmA*, *sulA*, and *minCD* [72,74].

It is believed that *ftsA*, *zipA* or *zapA* are involved in the stabilization of Z-ring polymerization in *E. coli* [76,86]. Similarly to *M. tuberculosis* [23], in *C. glutamicum* this role could be fulfilled by FtsW which interacts directly with FtsZ [116]. The *C. glutamicum sepF* homologue *cg2363* could also have a role in the Z-ring stabilization, as described in *B. subtilis* [48]. However, the *cg2363* gene is apparently not essential for either the growth or the cell viability of Corynebacteria [57].

In addition, the actinomycetes have a unique cluster of seven genes closely located to their chromosomal origin of replication (Fig. 3). This conserved cluster usually includes two transmembrane serine/threonine protein kinases (STPKs), named *pknA* and *pknB*, and a phosphatase that antagonize them [10,17,22]. These two STPKs are involved in the regulation of cell growth and cell division, at least in *Corynebacterium* and *Mycobacterium* [38,67].

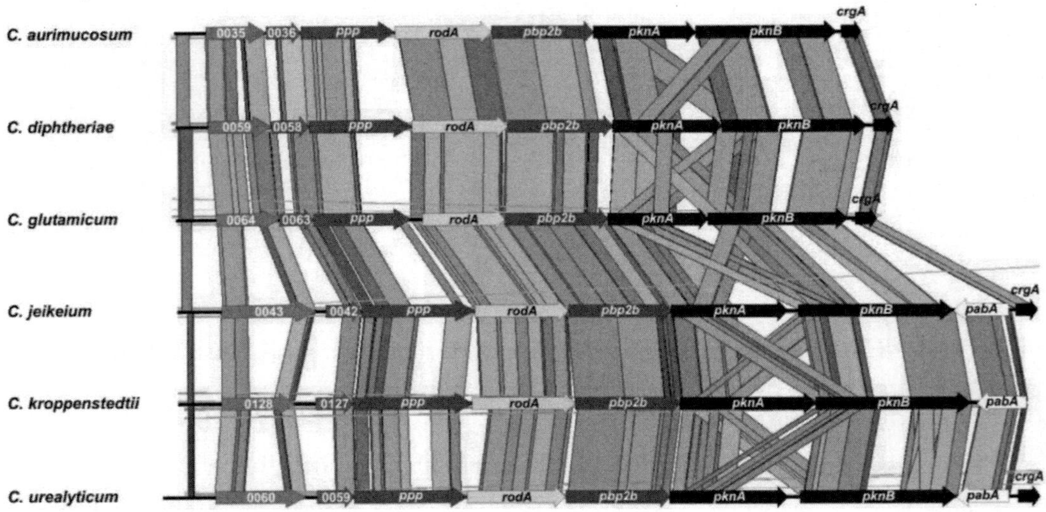

Fig. 3. Genetic organization and ACT pairwise comparisons of the *pknAB* cluster in different corynebacteria. The first two genes of this cluster are always conserved, strongly suggesting a possible implication in cell growth and/or cell division despite their function is still unknown. The gene *crgA* is present in the chromosome of *Corynebacterium kroppenstedtii* but it is not located in the *pknAB* cluster.

Both kinases are essential for *C. glutamicum*, in contrast with the other two STPKs present in the genome [38]. The partial depletion of *pknAB* generates elongated cells and alters cell growth and cell viability. Their overexpression also alters cell growth but it produces chains of coccoid cells, which in some cases are devoid of nucleoids [38]. These coccoid cells show a total lack of polar peptidoglycan synthesis, resembling a partial depletion of DivIVA [75]. In addition, they usually remain attached, suggesting a disruption in the final stages of cell division or in cell-pole maturation. However, none of the four *C. glutamicum* STPKs phosphorylate DivIVA *in vitro* [38], in high contrast with *M. tuberculosis* where it is phosphorylated by either PknA or PknB [67] or with *S. coelicolor* A3(2) where DivIVA is phosphorylated by the protein kinase AfsK (Klas Flardh, personal communication). This illustrates that signal transduction signals could be different between these closely related Actinobacteria.

It is known that PknA phosphorylates the essential peptydoglycan ligase MurC in *C. glutamicum*, which negatively modulates its ligase activity [37]. This indicates that a partial depletion of PknA should maintain active MurC and therefore the synthesis of peptidoglycan. However, the phenotype observed by *pknAB* partial depletion or overexpression suggests that there is/are other substrate/s or their phosphorylation that should be implicated in the final stages of cell growth or cell division processes. Since neither PknA nor PknB regulate DivIVA, it is possible to speculate that the target of these STPKs should be a penicillin-binding protein, like the *pbp2b* gene that lies adjacently to *pknAB* genes in the same cluster (Figure 3). In agreement with this hypothesis, the disruption of *pbp2b* or the inhibition of PBP2b by the beta-lactam antibiotic mecillinam generates a strikingly similar phenotype to *pknA* or *pknB* partial depletion [38,116], and the *pbp2b* orthologue of *M. tuberculosis* is phosphorylated by PknB [22]. Finally, PBP1A/1B are required for the correct synthesis of PG

Table 1. Genes related to cell division and cell growth present in different bacterial genomes. The functions of the codified proteins were recently reviewed [30,46].

Gene name	*E. coli*	*B. subtilis*	*C. glutamicum*	*M. tuberculosis*	*S. coelicolor*
amiC	b2817	BSU35620	cg3424	Rv3915	SCO2345
crgA	-	-	cg0055	Rv0011c	SCO3854
divIVA	-	BSU15420	cg2361	Rv2145c	SCO2077
ezrA	-	BSU29610	-	-	-
ftsA	b0094	BSU15280	-	-	-
ftsB	b2748	-	cg1112	Rv1024	SCO3095 (*divIC*)
ftsE	b3463	BSU35260	cg0914	Rv3102c	SCO2969
ftsI	b0084	BSU15170	cg2375	Rv2163c	SCO2090
ftsK	b0890	BSU29800 (*ytpT*) BSU16800 (*spoIIIE*)	cg2158	Rv2748c	SCO3934 SCO4508 SCO5750
ftsL	b0083	BSU15150	-	-	-
ftsN	b3933	-	-	-	-
ftsQ	b0093	-	cg2367	Rv2151c	SCO2083
ftsW	b0089	BSU14850 (*ftsW*) BSU15210 (*spoVE*)	cg2370	Rv2154c	SCO2085 (*ftsW*) SCO2607 (*sfr*)
ftsX	b3462	BSU35250	cg0915	Rv3101c	SCO2968
ftsZ	b0095	BSU15290	cg2366	Rv2150c	SCO2082
minC	b1176	BSU28000	-	-	-
minD	b1175	BSU27990	-	-	-
minE	b1174	-	-	-	-
mreB	b3251	BSU14470 (*mreBH*) BSU28030 (*mreB*) BSU36410 (*mbl*)	-	-	SCO2611
mreC	b3250	BSU28020	-	-	SCO2610
mreD	b3249	BSU28010	-	-	SCO2609
noc	-	BSU40990	-	-	-
pknA	-	-	cg0059	Rv0015c	SCO3848
pknB	-	-	cg0057	Rv0014c	-
rodA	b0634	BSU38120	cg0061	Rv0017c	SCO3846
sepF	-	BSU15390	cg2363	RV2147c	SCO2079
smlA	b3641	-	-	-	-
sulA	b0958	-	-	-	-
zapA	b2910	-	-	-	-
zipA	b2412	-	-	-	-

at the cell poles in *C. glutamicum*. A disruption of both *pbp1A/1B* genes or their inhibition by a cefsulodin treatment [116], generate chains of coccoid cells, similarly to the phenotype observed by the overexpression of either *pknA* or *pknB*. This suggests that the phosphorylation mediated by the PknA/B STPKs could modulate either positively or negatively many different proteins required for various stages of the cell division and cell elongation processes of *C. glutamicum*, similarly to *M. tuberculosis* where the list of identified PknA/B substrates includes FtsZ, Wag31 (DivIVA), MurD and PbpA among others

[22,67,110,111]. It is worth to mention that *pknAB* have been identified as very attractive substrates for the screening of potential anti-tuberculosis drugs [28,33,50,106,122].

In *E. coli* or *B. subtilis* two different FtsZ-polymerization inhibitors accomplish the spatio-temporal regulation of cytokinesis: the nucleoid occlusion and the *min* system. The Z-ring can assemble in *C. glutamicum* even before nucleoids are completely segregated [95], suggesting that the inhibition of cell division by the presence of DNA at the midcell reported in *E. coli* or *B. subtilis* [9,125] does not take place in Corynebacteria, similarly to other actinomycetes [102]. The lack of any nucleoid occlusion effectors in *C. glutamicum*, such as *noc* [125] and *slmA* [9], strengthen the hypothesis that the regulation of the Z-ring assembly is independent of the chromosomal replication timing in these bacteria. The *minCD* system is also absent in all Corynebacterial genomes, as well as the topological effector MinE from *E. coli* [24]. In *B. subtilis*, the function of *minE* is overtaken by *divIVA* [15], which, as previously discussed, has a radically different function in Actinobacteria [39,68,75]. Thus, the question that is still unanswered is how Corynebacteria coordinate its cell division and cell elongation. It is very likely that the *pknAB* cluster is controlling this process in Actinobacteria. In addition to the proposed function of these protein kinases, it has been demonstrated that *crgA*, a gene located downstream from the *pknAB* cluster in many Actinobacteria (Fig. 3), is a cell division inhibitor in *S. coelicolor* [25]. However, the role as a Z-ring antagonist of this integral membrane protein in the cytokinesis of other Actinobacteria still remains to be verified. It is clear that Corynebacteria, and in general Actinobacteria, coordinate its cell division and cell growth events very differently than any other bacteria and therefore it is very likely that in the next few years of research there are going to be identified new positive and negative effectors of the different stages of cytokinesis that will be *Corynebacterium*-specific. This has been the case of several recent reports that described novel Corynebacterial proteins involved in such diverse processes as maturation of the cellular poles or DNA-damage induced cell division arrest [81,114].

CONCLUSION

The sequencing of the genomes of different *Corynebacterium* species and comparison of the sequences to those of other well-known model bacteria (Table 1), together with the application of new molecular biology and microscopy techniques, have provided a major impulse to our understanding of the cell-cycle in these bacteria.

Most rod-shaped cells require MreB, which assembles into wire-like structures that run between the poles of the cell and distributes various components of PG metabolism along the cell's length. When the cell has acquired the appropriate length, it enters into the cell-division process. The divisome is responsible for the formation of two symmetrical daughter cells after constriction of the Z-ring and synthesis of the cell envelope.

C. glutamicum lacks MreB and thus represents a model of cell elongation/division distinct from that of typical rod-shaped bacteria such as *E. coli* or *B. subtilis*, which express MreB. During cell elongation, the polar PG-synthesis protein complex is mainly formed by DivIVA, RodA, and class A HMW-PBPs (PBP1a and PBP1b) (Fig. 4), whereas the core of the cell-division machinery (divisome) comprises FtsZ, FtsEX, FtsK, FtsQ, FtsB, FtsW, and three class B HMW-PBPs (FtsI, PBP2a, and PBP2b) (Fig. 4).

How the cell "decides" between synthesizing PG at mid-cell vs. at the cell poles is still unknown, but these two pathways might be regulated by phosphorylation, as in the case of *M. tuberculosis*, in which the protein kinases PknA and PknB regulate cell growth and cell division [67,110]. Therefore, future efforts should focus on the characterization and identification of these cell-cycle regulators as well as other proteins involved in cell-shape acquisition by *C. glutamicum*. All these proteins are known to orchestrate the localization of cell-wall synthetic complexes, resulting in co-ordinated and efficient PG synthetic activity at the septum (cell division) or at the cell poles (cell elongation). However, to date, the details of these processes remain poorly understood in Actinobacteria.

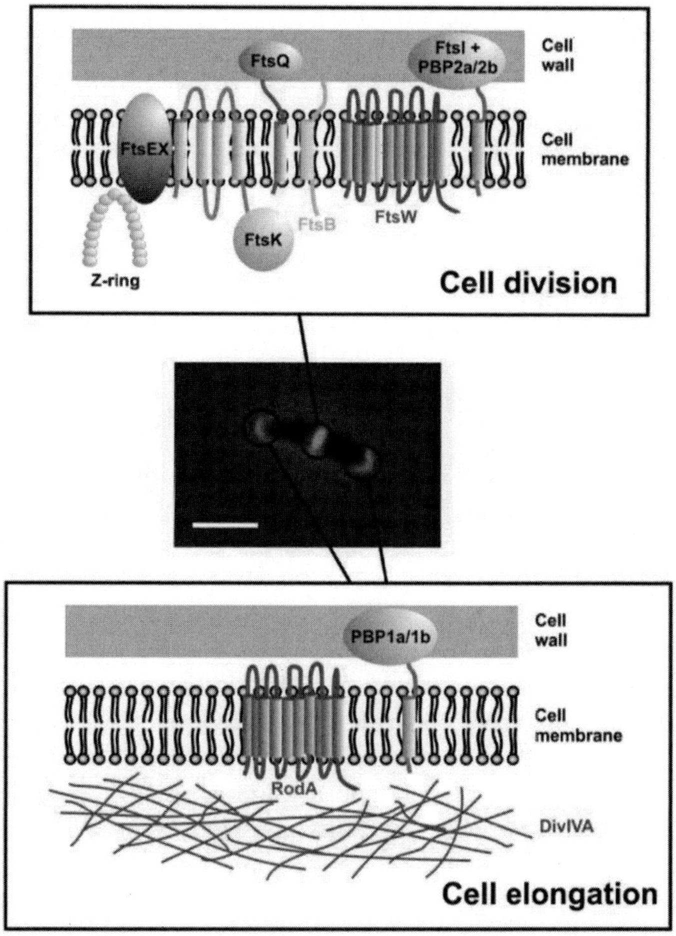

Fig. 4. Vancomycin-FL staining of *C. glutamicum* (central figure, scale bar represents 1 μm) and comparison of the division and elongation machineries. The wild-type strain synthesizes peptidoglycan at the cell poles; when the correct size is reached the cells begin to synthesize peptidoglycan at the septum. The key component of the divisome (cell-division machinery) is FtsZ. This protein polymerizes to form a Z-ring that acts as a scaffold of the multi-protein complex comprising the divisome. The hierarchy for assembly of the remaining proteins (FtsEX, FtsK, FtsQ, FtsW, FtsI, Pbp2a, and PBP2b) is still unclear, but FtsZ is known to interact with FtsW, and FtsZ/FtsW with FtsI and PBP2a/2b. The essential component of the cell-elongation machinery is DivIVA, which polymerizes at the cell poles and permits the cell-wall synthesis carried out by RodA, PPB1a, and PBP1b.

Acknowledgments

M. Letek and M. Fiuza were beneficiaries of fellowships from the Ministerio de Educación y Ciencia (Spain); E. Ordóñez and A. F. Villadangos from the Junta de Castilla y León. This work was funded by grants from the Junta de Castilla y León (Ref. LE040A07), University of León (ULE 2001-08B), and Ministerio de Ciencia y Tecnología (BIO2005-02723 and BIO2008-00519).

References

[1] Aldea, M., Garrido, T., Hernandez-Chico, C., Vicente, M. & Kushner, S. R. (1989). Induction of a growth-phase-dependent promoter triggers transcription of *bolA*, an *Escherichia coli,* morphogene. *EMBO J., 8*, 3923-3931.

[2] Aldea, M., Hernandez-Chico C., de la Campa, A. G., Kushner, S. R. & Vicente, M. (1988). Identification, cloning, and expression of *bolA*, an *ftsZ*-dependent morphogene of *Escherichia coli.*, *J. Bacteriol.*, *170*, 5169-5176.

[3] Ausmees, N., Kuhn J. R. & Jacobs-Wagner, C. (2003). The bacterial cytoskeleton: an intermediate filament-like function in cell shape. *Cell.*, *115*, 705-713.

[4] Bagchi, S., Tomenius, H., Belova, L. M. & Ausmees, N. (2008). Intermediate filament-like proteins in bacteria and a cytoskeletal function in *Streptomyces. Mol. Microbiol.*, *70*, 1037-1050.

[5] Becker, J., Klopprogge, C., Herold, A., Zelder, O., Bolten, C. J. & Wittmann, C. (2007). Metabolic flux engineering of L-lysine production in *Corynebacterium glutamicum*-- over expression and modification of G6P dehydrogenase. *J. Biotechnol.*, *132*, 99-109.

[6] Ben-Yehuda, S., Rudner, D. Z. & Losick, R. (2003). RacA, a bacterial protein that anchors chromosomes to the cell poles. *Science.*, *299*, 532-536.

[7] Bendt, A. K., Burkovski, A., Schaffer, S., Bott, M., Farwick, M. & Hermann, T. (2003). Towards a phosphoproteome map of *Corynebacterium glutamicum. Proteomics.*, *3*, 1637-1646.

[8] Bernard, C. S., Sadasivam, M., Shiomi, D. & Margolin, W. (2007). An altered FtsA can compensate for the loss of essential cell division protein FtsN in *Escherichia coli. Mol. Microbiol.*, *64*, 1289-1305.

[9] Bernhardt, T. G. & de Boer, P. A. (2005). SlmA, a nucleoid-associated, FtsZ binding protein required for blocking septal ring assembly over chromosomes in *E. coli. Mol. Cell.*, *18*, 555-564.

[10] Boitel, B., Ortiz-Lombardia, M., Duran, R., Pompeo, F., Cole, S. T., Cervenansky, C. & Alzari, P. M. (2003). PknB kinase activity is regulated by phosphorylation in two Thr residues and dephosphorylation by PstP, the cognate phospho-Ser/Thr phosphatase, in *Mycobacterium tuberculosis. Mol. Microbiol.*, *49*, 1493-1508.

[11] Cadenas, R. F., Fernández-González, C., Martín, J. F. & Gil, J. A. (1996). Construction of new cloning vectors for *Brevibacterium lactofermentum. FEMS Microbiol. Lett.*, *137*, 63-68.

[12] Cadenas, R. F., Martín, J. F. & Gil, J. A. (1991). Construction and characterization of promoter-probe vectors for Corynebacteria using the kanamycin-resistance reporter gene. *Gene*. *98*, 117-121.

[13] Carpinelli, J., Kramer, R. & Agosin, E. (2006). Metabolic engineering of *Corynebacterium glutamicum* for trehalose overproduction: role of the TreYZ trehalose biosynthetic pathway. *Appl. Environ. Microbiol.*, *72*, 1949-1955.

[14] Cerdeño-Tarraga, A. M., Efstratiou, A., Dover, L. G., Holden, M. T., Pallen, M., Bentley, S. D., Besra, G. S., Churcher, C., James, K. D., De, Z. A., Chillingworth, T., Cronin, A., Dowd, L., Feltwell, T., Hamlin, N., Holroyd, S., Jagels, K., Moule, S., Quail, M. A., Rabbinowitsch, E., Rutherford, K. M., Thomson, N. R., Unwin, L., Whitehead, S., Barrell, B. G. & Parkhill, J. (2003). The complete genome sequence and analysis of *Corynebacterium diphtheriae* NCTC13129. *Nucleic Acids Res.*, *31*, 6516-6523.

[15] Cha, J. H. & Stewart, G. C. (1997). The *divIVA* minicell locus of *Bacillus subtilis*. *J. Bacteriol.*, *179*, 1671-1683.

[16] Chami, M., Bayan, N., Dedieu, J., Leblon, G., Shechter, E. & Gulik-Krzywicki, T. (1995). Organization of the outer layers of the cell envelope of *Corynebacterium glutamicum*: a combined freeze-etch electron microscopy and biochemical study. *Biol. Cell.*, *83*, 219-229.

[17] Chopra, P., Singh, B., Singh, R., Vohra, R., Koul, A., Meena, L. S., Koduri, H., Ghildiyal, M., Deol, P., Das, T. K., Tyagi, A. K. & Singh, Y. (2003). Phosphoprotein phosphatase of *Mycobacterium tuberculosis* dephosphorylates serine-threonine kinases PknA and PknB. *Biochem. Biophys. Res. Commun.*, *311*, 112-120.

[18] Collins, M. D., Goodfellow, M. & Minnikin, D. E. (1982). Fatty acid composition of some mycolic acid-containing coryneform bacteria. *J. Gen. Microbiol.*, *128* (Pt 11): 2503-2509.

[19] Courvalin, P. & Davies, J. (2003). Antimicrobials: time to act! *Curr. Opin. Microbiol.*, 6, 425-529.

[20] Cure, G. L. & Keddie, R. M. (1973). Methods for the morphological examination of aerobic coryneform bacteria.: 123-135.

[21] Daniel, R. A. & Errington, J. (2003). Control of cell morphogenesis in bacteria: two distinct ways to make a rod-shaped cell. *Cell.*, *113*, 767-776.

[22] Dasgupta, A., Datta, P., Kundu, M. & Basu, J. (2006). The serine/threonine kinase PknB of *Mycobacterium tuberculosis* phosphorylates PBPA, a Penicillin-Binding Protein required for cell division. *Microbiology.*, *152*, 493-504.

[23] Datta, P., Dasgupta, A., Bhakta, S. & Basu, J. (2002). Interaction between FtsZ and FtsW of *Mycobacterium tuberculosis*. *J. Biol. Chem.*, *277*, 24983-24987.

[24] de Boer, P. A., Crossley, R. E. & Rothfield, L. I. (1989). A division inhibitor and a topological specificity factor coded for by the minicell locus determine proper placement of the division septum in *E. coli*. *Cell.*, *56*, 641-649.

[25] del, Sol. R., Pitman, A., Herron, P. & Dyson, P. (2003). The product of a developmental gene, *crgA*, that coordinates reproductive growth in *Streptomyces* belongs to a novel family of small actinomycete-specific proteins. *J. Bacteriol.*, *185*, 6678-6685.

[26] Doi, M., Wachi, M., Ishino, F., Tomioka, S., Ito M., Sakagami, Y., Suzuki, A. & Matsuhashi, M. (1988). Determinations of the DNA sequence of the *mreB* gene and of

the gene products of the *mre* region that function in formation of the rod shape of *Escherichia coli* cells. *J. Bacteriol.*, *170*, 4619-4624.

[27] Dover, L. G., Cerdeño-Tarraga, A. M., Pallen, M. J., Parkhill, J. & Besra, G. S. (2004). Comparative cell wall core biosynthesis in the mycolated pathogens, *Mycobacterium tuberculosis* and *Corynebacterium diphtheriae*. *FEMS Microbiol. Rev.*, *28*, 225-250.

[28] Drews, S. J., Hung, F. & Av-Gay, Y. (2001). A protein kinase inhibitor as an antimycobacterial agent. *FEMS Microbiol. Lett.*, *205*, 369-374.

[29] Edwards, D. H. & Errington, J. (1997). The *Bacillus subtilis* DivIVA protein targets to the division septum and controls the site specificity of cell division. *Mol. Microbiol.*, *24*, 905-915.

[30] Errington, J., Daniel, R. A. & Scheffers, D. J. (2003). Cytokinesis in bacteria. *Microbiol. Mol. Biol. Rev.*, *67*, 52-65.

[31] Fadda, D., Pischedda, C., Caldara, F., Whalen, M. B., Anderluzzi, D., Domenici, E. & Massidda, O. (2003). Characterization of *divIVA* and other genes located in the chromosomal region downstream of the dcw cluster in *Streptococcus pneumoniae*. *J. Bacteriol.*, *185*, 6209-6214.

[32] Fadda, D., Santona, A., D'Ulisse, V., Ghelardini, P., Ennas, M. G., Whalen, M. B. & Massidda, O. (2007). *Streptococcus pneumoniae* DivIVA: localization and interactions in a MinCD-Free context. *J Bacteriol.*, *189*, 1288-1298.

[33] Fernandez, P., Saint-Joanis, B., Barilone, N., Jackson, M., Gicquel, B., Cole, S. T. & Alzari, P. M. (2006). The Ser/Thr protein kinase PknB is essential for sustaining mycobacterial growth. *J. Bacteriol.*, *188*, 7778-7784.

[34] Fernández-Natal, I., Guerra, J., Alcoba, M., Cachón, F. & Soriano, F. (2001). Bacteremia caused by multiply resistant *Corynebacterium urealyticum*: six case reports and review. *Eur. J. Clin. Microbiol. Infect. Dis.*, *20*, 514-517.

[35] feu Soufo, H. J. & Graumann, P. L. (2005). *Bacillus subtilis* actin-like protein MreB influences the positioning of the replication machinery and requires membrane proteins MreC/D and other actin-like proteins for proper localization. *BMC. Cell Biol.*, *6*, 10.

[36] Figge, R. M., Divakaruni, A. V. & Gober, J. W. (2004). MreB, the cell shape-determining bacterial actin homologue, co-ordinates cell wall morphogenesis in *Caulobacter crescentus*. *Mol. Microbiol.*, *51*, 1321-1332.

[37] Fiuza, M., Canova, M. J., Patin, D., Letek, M., Zanella-Cleon, I., Becchi, M., Mateos, L. M., Mengin-Lecreulx, D., Molle, V. & Gil, J. A. (2008). The MurC ligase essential for peptidoglycan biosynthesis is regulated by the serine/threonine protein kinase PknA in *Corynebacterium glutamicum*. *J. Biol. Chem.*, *283*, 36553-36563.

[38] Fiuza, M., Canova, M. J., Zanella-Cleon, I., Becchi, M., Cozzone, A. J., Mateos, L. M., Kremer, L., Gil, J. A. & Molle, V. (2008). From the characterization of the four serine/threonine protein kinases (PknA/B/G/L) of *Corynebacterium glutamicum* toward the role of PknA and PknB in cell division. *J. Biol. Chem.*, *283*, 18099-18112.

[39] Flärdh, K. (2003). Essential role of DivIVA in polar growth and morphogenesis in *Streptomyces coelicolor* A3(2). *Mol. Microbiol.*, *49*, 1523-1536.

[40] Flärdh, K. (2003). Growth polarity and cell division in *Streptomyces*. *Curr. Opin. Microbiol.*, *6*, 564-571.

[41] Freire, P., Amaral, J. D., Santos, J. M. & Arraiano C. M. (2006). Adaptation to carbon starvation: RNase III ensures normal expression levels of *bolA1p* mRNA and sigma(S). *Biochimie.*, *88*, 341-346.

[42] Freire, P., Moreira, R. N. & Arraiano, C. M. (2009). BolA inhibits cell elongation and regulates MreB expression levels. *J. Mol. Biol., 385*, 1345-1351.

[43] Frieden, T. R., Sterling, T. R., Munsiff, S. S., Watt, C. J. & Dye, C. (2003). Tuberculosis. *Lancet., 362*, 887-899.

[44] Fuhrmann, C., Soedarmanto, I. & Lammler, C. (1997). Studies on the rod-coccus life cycle of *Rhodococcus equi. Zentralbl. Veterinarmed. B., 44*, 287-294.

[45] Geissler, B. & Margolin, W. (2005). Evidence for functional overlap among multiple bacterial cell division proteins: compensating for the loss of FtsK. *Mol. Microbiol., 58*, 596-612.

[46] Goehring, N. W. & Beckwith, J. (2005). Diverse paths to midcell: assembly of the bacterial cell division machinery. *Curr. Biol., 15*, R514-R526.

[47] Goffin, C. & Ghuysen, J. M. (1998). Multimodular Penicillin-Binding Proteins: an enigmatic family of orthologs and paralogs. *Microbiol. Mol. Biol. Rev., 62*, 1079-1093.

[48] Hamoen, L. W., Meile, J. C., de, J. W., Noirot, P. & Errington, J. (2006). SepF, a novel FtsZ-interacting protein required for a late step in cell division. *Mol. Microbiol., 59*, 989-999.

[49] Hansmeier, N., Bartels, F. W., Ros, R., Anselmetti, D., Tauch, A., Puhler, A. & Kalinowski, J. (2004). Classification of hyper-variable *Corynebacterium glutamicum* surface-layer proteins by sequence analyses & atomic force microscopy. *J. Biotechnol. 112*, 177-193.

[50] Hegymegi-Barakonyi, B., Szekely, R., Varga, Z., Kiss, R., Borbely, G., Nemeth, G., Banhegyi, P., Pato, J., Greff, Z., Horvath, Z., Meszaros, G., Marosfalvi, J., Eros, D., Szantai-Kis, C., Breza, N., Garavaglia, S., Perozzi, S., Rizzi, M., Hafenbradl, D., Ko, M., Av-Gay, Y., Klebl, B. M., Orfi, L. & Keri, G. (2008). Signalling inhibitors against *Mycobacterium tuberculosis*--early days of a new therapeutic concept in tuberculosis. *Curr. Med. Chem., 15*, 2760-2770.

[51] Henriques, A. O., Glaser, P., Piggot, P. J. & Moran, C. P., Jr. (1998). Control of cell shape and elongation by the *rodA* gene in *Bacillus subtilis. Mol. Microbiol., 28*, 235-247.

[52] Hermann, T. (2003). Industrial production of amino acids by coryneform bacteria. *J. Biotechnol., 104*, 155-172.

[53] Hermann, T., Pfefferle, W., Baumann, C., Busker, E., Schaffer, S., Bott, M., Sahm, H., Dusch, N., Kalinowski, J., Puhler, A., Bendt, A. K., Kramer, R. & Burkovski, A. (2001). Proteome analysis of *Corynebacterium glutamicum. Electrophoresis., 22*, 1712-1723.

[54] Hirasawa, T., Wachi, M. & Nagai, K. (2000). A mutation in the *Corynebacterium glutamicum ltsA* gene causes susceptibility to lysozyme, temperature-sensitive growth, and L-glutamate production. *J. Bacteriol., 182*, 2696-2701.

[55] Hoffmann, C., Leis, A., Niederweis, M., Plitzko, J. M. & Engelhardt, H. (2008). Disclosure of the mycobacterial outer membrane: cryo-electron tomography and vitreous sections reveal the lipid bilayer structure. *Proc. Natl. Acad. Sci. U.S.A., 105*, 3963-3967.

[56] Holatko, J., Elisakova, V., Prouza, M., Sobotka, M., Nesvera, J. & Patek, M. (2009). Metabolic engineering of the L-valine biosynthesis pathway in *Corynebacterium glutamicum* using promoter activity modulation. *J. Biotechnol., 139*, 203-210.

[57] Honrubia, M. P., Ramos, A. & Gil, J. A. (2001). The cell division genes *ftsQ* and *ftsZ*, but not the three downstream open reading frames YFIH, ORF5 and ORF6, are essential for growth and viability in *Brevibacterium lactofermentum* ATCC 13869. *Mol. Genet. Genomics.*, *265*, 1022-1030.

[58] Honrubia-Marcos, M. P., Ramos, A. & Gil, J. A. (2005). Overexpression of the ftsZ gene from Corynebacterium glutamicum (Brevibacterium lactofermentum) in Escherichia coli. Can. J Microbiol., 51, 85-89.

[59] Huang, Q., Tonge, P. J., Slayden, R. A., Kirikae, T. & Ojima, I. (2007). FtsZ: a novel target for tuberculosis drug discovery. *Curr. Top. Med. Chem.*, *7*, 527-543.

[60] Ikeda, M., Mitsuhashi, S., Tanaka, K. & Hayashi, M. (2009). Reengineering of a *Corynebacterium glutamicum* L-arginine and L-citrulline producer. *Appl. Environ. Microbiol.*, *75*, 1635-1641.

[61] Ikeda, M. & Nakagawa, S. (2003). The *Corynebacterium glutamicum* genome: features and impacts on biotechnological processes. *Appl. Microbiol. Biotechnol.*, *62*, 99-109.

[62] Ikeda, M., Sato, T., Wachi, M., Jung, H. K., Ishino, F., Kobayashi, Y. & Matsuhashi, M. (1989). Structural similarity among *Escherichia coli* FtsW and RodA proteins and *Bacillus subtilis* SpoVE protein, which function in cell division, cell elongation, and spore formation, respectively. *J. Bacteriol.*, *171*, 6375-6378.

[63] Iwai, N., Nagai, K. & Wachi, M. (2002). Novel S-benzylisothiourea compound that induces spherical cells in *Escherichia coli* probably by acting on a rod-shape-determining protein(s) other than penicillin-binding protein 2. *Biosci. Biotechnol. Biochem.*, *66*, 2658-2662.

[64] Jäger, W., Schäfer, A., Pühler, A., Labes, G. & Wohlleben, W. (1992). Expression of the *Bacillus subtilis sacB* gene leads to sucrose sensitivity in the gram-positive bacterium *Corynebacterium glutamicum* but not in *Streptomyces lividans*. *J. Bacteriol.*, *174*, 5462-5465.

[65] James, G. A., Korber, D. R., Caldwell, D. E. & Costerton, J. W. (1995). Digital image analysis of growth and starvation responses of a surface-colonizing *Acinetobacter* sp. *J Bacteriol.*, *177*, 907-915.

[66] Kalinowski, J., Bathe, B., Bartels, D., Bischoff, N., Bott, M., Burkovski, A., Dusch N., Eggeling, L., Eikmanns, B. J., Gaigalat, L., Goesmann, A., Hartmann, M., Huthmacher, K., Kramer, R., Linke, B., McHardy, A. C., Meyer, F., Mockel, B., Pfefferle, W., Puhler, A., Rey, D. A., Ruckert, C., Rupp, O., Sahm, H., Wendisch, V. F., Wiegrabe, I. & Tauch, A. (2003). The complete *Corynebacterium glutamicum* ATCC 13032 genome sequence and its impact on the production of L-aspartate-derived amino acids and vitamins. *J. Biotechnol.*, *104*, 5-25.

[67] Kang, C. M., Abbott, D. W., Park, S. T., Dascher, C. C., Cantley, L. C. & Husson, R. N. (2005). The *Mycobacterium tuberculosis* serine/threonine kinases PknA and PknB: substrate identification and regulation of cell shape. *Genes Dev.*, *19*, 1692-1704.

[68] Kang, C. M., Nyayapathy, S., Lee, J. Y., Suh, J. W. & Husson, R. N. (2008). Wag31, a homologue of the cell division protein DivIVA, regulates growth, morphology and polar cell wall synthesis in mycobacteria. *Microbiology.*, *154*, 725-735.

[69] Kinoshita, S., Udaka, S. & Shimono, S. (1957). Studies on the aminoacid fermentation. Part I. Production of L-glutamic acid by various microorganisms. *J. Gen. Appl. Microbiol.*, *3*, 193-205.

[70] Lange, R. & Hengge-Aronis, R. (1991). Growth phase-regulated expression of *bolA* and morphology of stationary-phase *Escherichia coli* cells are controlled by the novel sigma factor sigma S. *J. Bacteriol.*, *173*, 4474-4481.

[71] Letek, M., Fiuza, M., Ordoñez, E., Villadangos, A. F., Flardh, K., Mateos, L. M. & Gil, J. A. (2009). DivIVA uses an N-terminal conserved region and two coiled-coil domains to localize and sustain the polar growth in *Corynebacterium glutamicum. FEMS Microbiol. Lett.*, *297*, 110-116.

[72] Letek, M., Fiuza, M., Ordoñez, E., Villadangos, A. F., Ramos, A., Mateos, L. M. & Gil, J. A. (2008). Cell growth and cell division in the rod-shaped actinomycete *Corynebacterium glutamicum. Antonie Van Leeuwenhoek.*, *94*, 99-109.

[73] Letek, M., Ordoñez, E., Fernandez-Natal, I., Gil, J. A. & Mateos, L. M. (2006). Identification of the emerging skin pathogen *Corynebacterium amycolatum* using PCR-amplification of the essential *divIVA* gene as a target. *FEMS Microbiol Lett.*, *265*, 256-263.

[74] Letek, M., Ordoñez, E., Fiuza, M., Honrubia-Marcos, P., Vaquera, J., Gil, J. A. & Mateos, L. M. (2007). Characterization of the promoter region of *ftsZ* from *Corynebacterium glutamicum* and controlled overexpression of FtsZ. *Int. Microbiol.*, *10*, 271-282.

[75] Letek, M., Ordoñez, E., Vaquera, J., Margolin, W., Flardh, K., Mateos, L. M. & Gil, J. A. (2008). DivIVA is required for polar growth in the MreB-lacking rod-shaped actinomycete *Corynebacterium glutamicum. J. Bacteriol.*, *190*, 3283-3292.

[76] Low, H. H., Moncrieffe, M. C. & Lowe, J. (2004). The crystal structure of ZapA and its modulation of FtsZ polymerisation. *J. Mol. Biol.*, *341*, 839-852.

[77] Luscombe, B. & Gray, T. (1974). Characteristics of *Arthrobacter* grown in continuous culture. *J Gen Microbiol.*, *82*, 213-222.

[78] Mazza, P., Noens, E. E., Schirner, K., Grantcharova, N., Mommaas, A. M., Koerten, H. K., Muth, G., Flardh, K., van Wezel, G. P. & Wohlleben, W. (2006). MreB of *Streptomyces coelicolor* is not essential for vegetative growth but is required for the integrity of aerial hyphae and spores. *Mol. Microbiol.*, *60*, 838-852.

[79] Muchova, K., Kutejova, E., Scott, D. J., Brannigan, J. A., Lewis, R. J., Wilkinson A. J. & Barak, I. (2002). Oligomerization of the *Bacillus subtilis* division protein DivIVA. *Microbiology.*, *148*, 807-813.

[80] Nishio, Y., Nakamura, Y., Kawarabayasi, Y., Usuda, Y., Kimura, E., Sugimoto, S., Matsui, K., Yamagishi, A., Kikuchi, H., Ikeo, K. & Gojobori, T. (2003). Comparative complete genome sequence analysis of the amino acid replacements responsible for the thermostability of *Corynebacterium efficiens. Genome Res.*, *13*, 1572-1579.

[81] Ogino, H., Teramoto, H., Inui, M. & Yukawa, H. (2008). DivS, a novel SOS-inducible cell-division suppressor in *Corynebacterium glutamicum. Mol. Microbiol.*, *67*, 597-608.

[82] Pallerla, S. R., Knebel, S., Polen, T., Klauth, P., Hollender, J., Wendisch, V. F. & Schoberth, S. M. (2005). Formation of volutin granules in *Corynebacterium glutamicum. FEMS Microbiol. Lett.*, *243*, 133-140.

[83] Paradis-Bleau, C., Sanschagrin, F. & Levesque, R. C. (2004). Identification of *Pseudomonas aeruginosa* FtsZ peptide inhibitors as a tool for development of novel antimicrobials. *J. Antimicrob. Chemother.*, *54*, 278-280.

[84] Peters-Wendisch, P., Stolz, M., Etterich, H., Kennerknecht, N., Sahm, H. & Eggeling L. (2005). Metabolic engineering of *Corynebacterium glutamicum* for L-serine production. *Appl. Environ. Microbiol.*, *71*, 7139-7144.

[85] Peyret, J. L., Bayan, N., Joliff, G., Gulik-Krzywicki, T., Mathieu, L., Schechter, E. & Leblon, G. (1993). Characterization of the *cspB* gene encoding PS2, an ordered surface-layer protein in *Corynebacterium glutamicum. Mol. Microbiol.*, *9*, 97-109.

[86] Pichoff, S. & Lutkenhaus, J. (2005). Tethering the Z ring to the membrane through a conserved membrane targeting sequence in FtsA. *Mol. Microbiol.*, *55*, 1722-1734.

[87] Pinho, M. G. & Errington, J. (2003). Dispersed mode of *Staphylococcus aureus* cell wall synthesis in the absence of the division machinery. *Mol. Microbiol.*, *50*, 871-881.

[88] Pinho, M. G. & Errington, J. (2004). A *divIVA* null mutant of *Staphylococcus aureus* undergoes normal cell division. *FEMS Microbiol Lett.*, *240*, 145-149.

[89] Polen, T. & Wendisch, V. F. (2004). Genomewide expression analysis in amino acid-producing bacteria using DNA microarrays. *Appl. Biochem. Biotechnol.*, *118*, 215-232.

[90] Puech, V., Chami, M., Lemassu, A., Laneelle M. A., Schiffler, B., Gounon, P., Bayan, N., Benz, R. & Daffe, M. (2001). Structure of the cell envelope of corynebacteria: importance of the non-covalently bound lipids in the formation of the cell wall permeability barrier and fracture plane. *Microbiology*. *147*, 1365-1382.

[91] Radmacher, E., Alderwick, L. J., Besra, G. S., Brown, A. K., Gibson, K. J., Sahm H. & Eggeling, L. (2005). Two functional FAS-I type fatty acid synthases in *Corynebacterium glutamicum. Microbiology*. *151*, 2421-2427.

[92] Ramírez-Arcos, S., Liao, M., Marthaler, S., Rigden, M. & Dillon, J. A. (2005). *Enterococcus faecalis divIVA*: an essential gene involved in cell division, cell growth and chromosome segregation. *Microbiology.*, *151*, 1381-1393.

[93] Ramos, A., Honrubia, M. P., Valbuena, N., Vaquera, J., Mateos, L. M. & Gil, J. A. (2003). Involvement of DivIVA in the morphology of the rod-shaped actinomycete *Brevibacterium lactofermentum. Microbiology.*, *149*, 3531-3542.

[94] Ramos, A., Honrubia, M. P., Vega, D., Ayala, J. A., Bouhss, A., Mengin-Lecreulx, D. & Gil, J. A. (2004). Characterization and chromosomal organization of the *murD-murC-ftsQ* region of *Corynebacterium glutamicum* ATCC 13869. *Res. Microbiol.*, 155, 174-184.

[95] Ramos, A., Letek, M., Campelo, A. B., Vaquera J., Mateos, L. M. & Gil, J. A. (2005). Altered morphology produced by *ftsZ* expression in *Corynebacterium glutamicum* ATCC 13869. *Microbiology.*, *151*, 2563-2572.

[96] Santamaria, R. I., Gil, J. A. & Martin, J. F. (1985). High-frequency transformation of *Brevibacterium lactofermentum* protoplasts by plasmid DNA. *J. Bacteriol. 162*, 463-467.

[97] Santamaria, R. I., Martin, J. F. & Gil, J. A. (1987). Identification of a promoter sequence in the plasmid pUL340 of *Brevibacterium lactofermentum* and construction of new cloning vectors for corynebacteria containing two selectable markers. *Gene.*, *56*, 199-208.

[98] Santos, J. M., Freire, P., Vicente, M. & Arraiano, C. M. (1999). The stationary-phase morphogene *bolA* from *Escherichia coli* is induced by stress during early stages of growth. *Mol. Microbiol.*, *32*, 789-798.

[99] Santos, J. M., Lobo, M., Matos, A. P., de Pedro, M. A. & Arraiano, C. M. (2002). The gene *bolA* regulates *dacA* (PBP5), *dacC* (PBP6) and *ampC* (AmpC), promoting normal morphology in *Escherichia coli. Mol. Microbiol. 45*, 1729-1740.

[100] Sasaki, M., Jojima, T., Kawaguchi, H., Inui, M. & Yukawa, H. (2009). Engineering of pentose transport in *Corynebacterium glutamicum* to improve simultaneous utilization of mixed sugars. *Appl. Microbiol. Biotechnol.*

[101] Scheffers, D. J. (2005). Dynamic localization of Penicillin-Binding Proteins during spore development in *Bacillus subtilis. Microbiology., 151*, 999-1012.

[102] Schwedock, J., McCormick, J. R., Angert, E. R., Nodwell, J. R. & Losick, R. (1997). Assembly of the cell division protein FtsZ into ladder-like structures in the aerial hyphae of *Streptomyces coelicolor. Mol. Microbiol., 25*, 847-858.

[103] Stahlberg, H., Kutejova, E., Muchova, K., Gregorini, M., Lustig, A., Muller, S. A., Olivieri, V., Engel, A., Wilkinson, A. J. & Barak, I. (2004). Oligomeric structure of the *Bacillus subtilis* cell division protein DivIVA determined by transmission electron microscopy. *Mol. Microbiol., 52*, 1281-1290.

[104] Stokes, N. R., Sievers, J., Barker, S., Bennett, J. M., Brown, D. R., Collins, I., Errington, V. M., Foulger, D., Hall, M., Halsey, R., Johnson, H., Rose, V., Thomaides, H. B., Haydon, D. J., Czaplewski, L. G. & Errington, J. (2005). Novel inhibitors of bacterial cytokinesis identified by a cell-based antibiotic screening assay. *J Biol Chem., 280*, 39709-39715.

[105] Suzuki, N., Nonaka, H., Tsuge, Y., Inui, M. & Yukawa, H. (2005). New multiple-deletion method for the *Corynebacterium glutamicum* genome, using a mutant *lox* sequence. *Appl. Environ. Microbiol., 71*, 8472-8480.

[106] Szekely, R., Waczek, F., Szabadkai, I., Nemeth, G., Hegymegi-Barakonyi, B., Eros, D., Szokol, B., Pato, J., Hafenbradl, D., Satchell, J., Saint-Joanis, B., Cole, S. T., Orfi, L., Klebl, B. M. & Keri, G. (2008). A novel drug discovery concept for tuberculosis: inhibition of bacterial and host cell signalling. *Immunol. Lett., 116*, 225-231.

[107] Takayama, K., Wang, C. & Besra, G. S. (2005). Pathway to synthesis and processing of mycolic acids in *Mycobacterium tuberculosis. Clin. Microbiol. Rev., 18*, 81-101.

[108] Tamames, J., González-Moreno, M., Mingorance, J., Valencia, A. & Vicente, M. (2001). Bringing gene order into bacterial shape. *Trends Genet., 17*, 124-126.

[109] Tauch, A., Kaiser, O., Hain, T., Goesmann, A., Weisshaar, B., Albersmeier, A., Bekel, T., Bischoff, N., Brune, I., Chakraborty, T., Kalinowski, J., Meyer, F., Rupp, O., Schneiker, S., Viehoever, P. & Pühler, A. (2005). Complete genome sequence and analysis of the multiresistant nosocomial pathogen *Corynebacterium jeikeium* K411, a lipid-requiring bacterium of the human skin flora. *J Bacteriol., 187*, 4671-4682.

[110] Thakur, M. & Chakraborti, P. K. (2006). GTPase activity of mycobacterial FtsZ is impaired due to its transphosphorylation by the eukaryotic-type Ser/Thr kinase, PknA. *J. Biol. Chem., 281*, 40107-40113.

[111] Thakur, M. & Chakraborti, P. K. (2008). Ability of PknA, a mycobacterial eukaryotic-type serine/threonine kinase, to transphosphorylate MurD, a ligase involved in the process of peptidoglycan biosynthesis. *Biochem. J., 415*, 27-33.

[112] Thanky, N. R., Young, D. B. & Robertson, B. D. (2007). Unusual features of the cell cycle in mycobacteria: polar-restricted growth and the snapping-model of cell division. *Tuberculosis. (Edinb.)., 87*, 231-236.

[113] Tsao, D. H., Sutherland, A. G., Jennings, L. D., Li, Y., Rush, T. S., III, Alvarez, J. C., Ding, W., Dushin, E. G., Dushin, R. G., Haney, S. A., Kenny, C. H., Malakian, A. K., Nilakantan R. & Mosyak L. (2006). Discovery of novel inhibitors of the ZipA/FtsZ complex by NMR fragment screening coupled with structure-based design. Bioorg.Med.Chem. 14: 7953-7961.

[114] Tsuge, Y., Ogino, H., Teramoto, H., Inui, M. & Yukawa, H. (2008). Deletion of *cgR_1596* and *cgR_2070*, encoding NlpC/P60 proteins, causes a defect in cell separation in *Corynebacterium glutamicum* R. *J. Bacteriol.*, *190*, 8204-8214.

[115] Umeda, A. & Amako, K. (1983). Growth of the surface of Corynebacterium diphtheriae. Microbiol. Immunol., 27, 663-671.

[116] Valbuena, N., Letek, M., Ordoñez, E., Ayala, J., Daniel, R. A., Gil, J. A. & Mateos L. M. (2007). Characterization of HMW-PBPs from the rod-shaped actinomycete *Corynebacterium glutamicum*: peptidoglycan synthesis in cells lacking actin-like cytoskeletal structures. *Mol. Microbiol.*, *66*, 643-657.

[117] Valbuena, N., Letek, M., Ramos, A., Ayala, J., Nakunst, D., Kalinowski, J., Mateos, L. M. & Gil, J. A. (2006). Morphological changes and proteome response of *Corynebacterium glutamicum* to a partial depletion of FtsI. *Microbiology.*, *152*, 2491-2503.

[118] Vicente, M., Hodgson, J., Massidda, O., Tonjum, T., Henriques-Normark, B. & Ron, E. Z. (2006). The fallacies of hope: will we discover new antibiotics to combat pathogenic bacteria in time? *FEMS Microbiol Rev.*, *30*, 841-852.

[119] Wachi, M., Wijayarathna, C. D., Teraoka, H. & Nagai, K. (1999). A *murC* gene from coryneform bacteria. *Appl. Microbiol. Biotechnol.*, *51*, 223-228.

[120] Wang, J., Galgoci, A., Kodali, S., Herath, K. B., Jayasuriya, H., Dorso, K., Vicente, F., Gonzalez, A., Cully, D., Bramhill, D. & Singh, S. (2003). Discovery of a small molecule that inhibits cell division by blocking FtsZ, a novel therapeutic target of antibiotics. *J. Biol. Chem.* *278*, 44424-44428.

[121] Wang, S. B., Cantlay, S., Nordberg, N., Letek, M., Gil, J. A. & Flardh, K. (2009). Domains involved in the in vivo function and oligomerization of apical growth determinant DivIVA in *Streptomyces coelicolor*. *FEMS Microbiol. Lett.*

[122] Wehenkel, A., Fernandez, P., Bellinzoni, M., Catherinot, V., Barilone, N., Labesse, G., Jackson, M. & Alzari, P. M. (2006). The structure of PknB in complex with mitoxantrone, an ATP-competitive inhibitor, suggests a mode of protein kinase regulation in mycobacteria. *FEBS Lett.*, *580*, 3018-3022.

[123] White, E. L., Suling, W. J., Ross, L. J., Seitz, L. E. & Reynolds, R. C. (2002). 2-Alkoxycarbonylaminopyridines: inhibitors of *Mycobacterium tuberculosis* FtsZ. *J. Antimicrob. Chemother.*, *50*, 111-114.

[124] Wijayarathna, C. D., Wachi, M. & Nagai, K. (2001). Isolation of *ftsI* and *murE* genes involved in peptidoglycan synthesis from *Corynebacterium glutamicum*. *Appl. Microbiol. Biotechnol.*, *55*, 466-470.

[125] Wu, L. J. & Errington, J. (2004). Coordination of cell division and chromosome segregation by a nucleoid occlusion protein in *Bacillus subtilis*. *Cell.*, *117*, 915-925.

[126] Yukawa, H., Omumasaba, C. A., Nonaka, H., Kos, P., Okai, N., Suzuki, N., Suda, M., Tsuge, Y., Watanabe, J., Ikeda, Y., Vertes, A. A. & Inui, M. (2007). Comparative analysis of the *Corynebacterium glutamicum* group and complete genome sequence of strain R. *Microbiology.*, *153*, 1042-1058.

[127] Zervosen, A., Lu W. P., Chen, Z., White, R. E., Demuth, T. P., Jr. & Frere, J. M. (2004). Interactions between penicillin-binding proteins (PBPs) and two novel classes of PBP inhibitors, arylalkylidene rhodanines and arylalkylidene iminothiazolidin-4-ones. *Antimicrob. Agents Chemother.*, *48*, 961-969.

[128] Zuber, B., Chami, M., Houssin, C., Dubochet, J., Griffiths, G. & Daffe, M. (2008). Direct visualization of the outer membrane of mycobacteria and corynebacteria in their native state. *J. Bacteriol.*, *190*, 5672-5680.

In: Cell Division: Theory, Variants and Degradation
Editors: Y. N. Golitsin, M. C. Krylov, pp. 81-93
ISBN: 978-1-60876-986-5

Chapter 4

THE IMPACT OF CELL CYCLE REGULATION ON THE TUMORIGENESIS PROCESS

Odair Aguiar Jr., Glaucia Monteiro de Castro and Daniel Araki Ribeiro*

Department of Biosciences, Federal University of São Paulo, UNIFESP, SP, Brazil

ABSTRACT

Cell division is a highly coordinated process by which living organisms grow, develop and reproduce. It starts in the zygote, is essential during embryogenesis and lasts for the entire life as a source of new cells for repairing purposes. The molecular mechanisms underlying mitotic cell division is under intense investigation due to their key role in the discovery of potential molecular targets for cell therapy. For cell cycle entry and commitment to completion, the exposure to growth factors is required. After receptor activation, signals transmit by phosphorylating substrates leading to the trigger of a number of early signaling cascades, including activation of tyrosine kinases (Tyr K), Ras, and phospholipase C, among others. These proteins subsequently activate secondary effectors that regulate transcription factors such as c-Myc. Cell cycle orchestration is guided by molecular mechanisms that govern crucial irreversible transitions assuring that steps take place in the right order. Progress has been made toward the understanding of cell cycle regulation through better characterization of the cyclin role, the promoting anaphase complex (APC), and the functions of cyclin kinases. Disruptions in such mechanisms can trigger cell transformations and contribute to tumorigenesis. Cell cycle checkpoint deficiencies have also been proposed as events whereby cells lose their ability to avoid division until the optimal conditions are reached. Humans are exposed to a large range of disruptors, from their own physiology to environmental substances which are constantly challenging their cells and potentially inciting disturbances in the cell cycle and division mainly by virtue of a series of DNA injuries.

Key words: cell divison, cell cycle control, tumorigenesis, neoplastic conversion

---

* Corresponding author: Phone 55 13 32218058, Fax 55 13 32232592, E-mails daribeiro@unifesp.br, daribeiro@pesquisador.cnpq.br

Cell Division: Life Guardian or Death Promoter

Whenever a cell divides, the organisms are growing, repairing tissues, producing gametes, responding to external or internal signals or even becoming committed to die. The evolution culminates with multicellularity where high complex cell networks are under functional interdependence and collaboration. When some cells of such a network become unable to properly control division, they can allow genetic errors and trigger the tumorigenesis process, which will compromise the homeostasis of the remaining cells and the organism's survival.

The mitotic division cycle of eukaryotic cells comprises four periods or phases: the S phase, marked by the DNA replication process; the M phase in which the genetic material is segregated into two identical daughter cells; and two gap phases (G), one preceding S (G1 phase) and one preceding M (G2 phase), both characterized by cell growth (Quereda and Malumbres, 2009). To ensure the correct progression over the cycle, cells use specific points whereby they check the fidelity of the events. These so-called checkpoints were proposed by Chen et al. (1989) and have been crucial to the understanding of the cell cycle control mechanisms (Malumbres and Barbacid, 2009). They verify whether the processes at each phase of the cycle have been accurately completed before progression into the next phase (Malumbres and Barbacid, 2009).

The key molecules of the cell cycle control are the cyclins, proteins discovered during studies with sea urchin eggs (Evans et al., 1983) and later characterized as the essential element of the heterodimeric enzymatic complexes containing a cyclin subunit and a kinase protein known as "cyclin-dependent kinase (CDK)" (Hochegger et al., 2008). Progression of a cell through the cycle is promoted by a number of CDKs which, when complexed with their specific cyclins, drive the cell forward through the cell cycle phases. The expression pattern of the cyclins is time-specific and defines the relative position of the cell within the cycle (Schwartz and Shah, 2005).

The kinase activities of the complex CDK-cyclin are responsible for triggering the events leading the cells enter mitosis (DNA replication, chromosome condensation and nuclear envelope disassembly) and finish division (chromosome decondensation and nuclear envelope restructuration). Without the cyclin partner, the kinase is inactive. Besides the physical union between CDK/cyclin, the full activation of the complex is only achieved when the CDK is phosphorylated at a key threonine residue on the polypeptide chain (Hochegger et al., 2008).

When mammalian cells receive a stimulus to division, which is usually effected by mitogens (e.g., growth factors), they progress through G1 and the initiation of the DNA synthesis phase (S) is cooperatively regulated by several cyclins and their associated CDKs, which integrate the flow of information from outside the cell, including multiple environmental signs such as the availability of nutrients and hormone stimulation (Nacusi and Sheaff, 2007; Lapenna and Giordano, 2009).

To pass through the interphase (G1, S and G2) and enter the M phase, cells activate various cyclin-CDK complexes. By mitogenic stimulus, D-type cyclins (D1, D2 and D3), known as G1 cyclins, accumulate during the G1 phase in association with CDK4 or CDK6 and facilitate the cell's entry into S, so that overexpression of D-type cyclins shortens the G1 phase and allows rapid entry into S (Das, 2009). Retinoblastoma protein (pRB) negatively controls the D-type cyclins by inactivating the gene regulatory proteins of the E2F family, which promotes the gene expression of G1/S cyclins. To antagonize its transcriptional repressor role, a series of phosphorylation events regulate the RB function in relation to the cell cycle phase and in response to mitogenic stimulation. Under such stimulus, RB becomes progressively phosphorylated by the activity of some G1 CDK-cyclins and loses its affinity to E2F, allowing the expression of its target genes and cell progression through G1 (Knudsen and Knudsen, 2006).

Additionally, cyclin A-CDK2 complex is required during the progression in the S phase, whereas binding of cyclin A or B to CDK1 is essential for the G2-M phase transition. Active CDK1-cyclin phosphorylates more than 70 substrates and triggers fundamental processes such as centrosome separation, Golgi and microtubule dynamics, nuclear envelope breakdown and chromatin compactation to form mitotic chromosomes (Das, 2009; Lapenna and Giordano, 2009).

The action of CDKs is constrained by the CKIs (CDK inhibitor proteins) which accumulate in quiescent cells (those in a phase known as G_0) and are repressed with the onset of proliferation. Thus, the cell's permission to divide results from the balance between the positive and the negative cell cycle regulators (Das, 2009). In early mitosis, cyclin A is degraded and another complex (cyclin B-CDK1) is required for M phase progression. Finally, to the completion of mitosis, CDK1 activity is switched off by proteolytic destruction of its associated cyclin B (Lapenna and Giordano, 2009). Such destruction is effected by a protein complex known as Anaphase-Promoting Complex (APC), which is a highly regulated ubiquitin ligase. Ubiquitylation processes mark the proteins to be degraded in the cytosolic proteasomes (Alberts et al., 2007).

Concluding the cell division, the sister-chromatid separation, which characterizes the mitotic anaphase, requires accurate preceding events in order to form two genetically equal daughter cells. The signal that triggers the anaphase is the tension force resulting from the pulling of sister chromatids to opposite cell poles through their kinetochore-microtubule attachment (Alberts et al., 2007). Only when all kinetochores are attached to the spindle microtubules, the protein known as Cdc20 activates the APC and the anaphase starts. Until the attachment is in progress, Cdc20 is confined to the kinetochores and is not able to exert its function. When the attachment is completed, Cdc20 activates the APC which degrades the proteins securin and the cyclin B. With the degradation of securin, separase is free to cleave the cohesins which hold the cohesion between the sister chromatids, resulting in their separation to the opposite cell poles (Kares, 2005; Li and Zhang, 2009). The fidelity of such processes is crucial to the correct distribution of the genetic material into the newly formed nuclei.

A successful cell division ensures genomic stability and therefore a series of mechanisms have evolved to overcome possible undesired events. As mentioned above, the checkpoints are the guardians of the cell cycle as they operate by mechanisms which temporarily stop the division, providing enough time to fixing events. They are not essential for cell cycle progression, but are critical for the cellular responses to stress, including abnormal mitogenic stimuli and DNA damage (Satyanarayana et al., 2008).

Cells use checkpoints to enter the cycle, in the transitions between the phases G1-S, G2-M, and also to complete the chromosome segregation and cytoplasmic division. In each G1phase, decisions are made whether to enter the new cell cycle if the conditions are favorable or, alternatively, to enter a quiescent phase (G_0) and even regarding which division (mitosis or meiosis) proceed (Tvgard et al., 2007). The G1-S checkpoint (also known as "DNA damage checkpoint") is primarily responsible for preventing damaged DNA from being replicated. It results in the activation of the tumor suppressor protein p53, which induces the transcription of the gene to p21. The protein p21, which is a CDK-inhibitor (CKI), binds to and inhibits CDK2-cyclin E complexes, thereby arresting cells at G1-S transition (Satyanarayana et al., 2008). If the damage is not successfully corrected, p53 activates the proapoptotic protein BAX, which promotes the release of cytochrome c from the mitochondria and trigger the apoptotic death program (Ho et al., 2006). Dysregulation of the control mechanisms at the G1-S transition may lead to mutations, chromosomal fragmentation, and genetic instability, which are events known to promote cancer development (Tvgard et al., 2007).

To the G2-M transition, a checkpoint is activated by DNA damage and also by incompletely replicated DNA (DNA replication checkpoint or S-M checkpoint) also providing a break to correct the defects (Zheng et al., 2005).

When cells progress through the M phase they reach a critical point where they have to check whether the conditions are propitious to segregate the sister chromatids and divide the cytoplasm. Therefore, they activate the "spindle assembly checkpoint" which monitors the proper attachment of the chromosomes to the mitotic spindle before the onset of the anaphase. To prevent premature separation of the sister-chromatids, the formation of the APC/Cdc20 complex is inhibited by the sequestering Cdc20 at the kinetochore in association with the proteins Mad2 and BubR1. Only when the sister chromatids are aligned at the metaphase plate and have established bivalent spindle attachment can the inhibition of Cdc20 be released and activates the APC to promote the anaphase (Li and Zhang, 2009).

All this molecular orchestration have ensured for billions of years the progressive construction of the life's complexity. However, such machinery is prone to fail more than it is supposed to do. Degeneration of the cell division process can be caused by internal mechanisms or by influence of external (environmental) factors. Such misadjustments can lead to chromosome segregation errors and mainly to the appearance of uncontrolled rapidly proliferating cells—tumors or cancers—which work independently and can lead to the organism's death. Such mechanisms will be discussed below.

The Cell Proliferation Stimuli

Competency for proliferation and cell-cycle progression require the stringent execution of regulatory cascades that are governed by the temporal/spatial integration of physiological signals that modulate the activation and suppression of genes that control these processes (Stein et al., 2006).

In this way, growth factors, hormones, neurotransmitters and extracellular matrix bind to and activate receptor tyrosine kinases, G-protein-coupled receptors and integrins, respectively, triggering a series of cytoplasmatic signal transduction cascades that transmit signals from the cell surface to the nucleus (Roovers and Assoian, 2000). These extracellular stimuli induce sequential activation of the Ras/extracellular-signal–regulated kinase (ERK) pathway. In this pathway, the induction of kinase activity is achieved by a conserved signaling cascade in which the levels are designated MAP4K, MAP3K, MAP2K and MAPK

(Mitogen-Activated Protein Kinase) sequentially from kinase to substrate. Multiple signals can sometimes activate multiple MAPKs and there is considerable cross-talk between these pathways. The specificity of the pathways has, therefore, been evolutionarily refined by multiple mechanisms: different tissues express different patterns; there are distinct hierarchal concentration-dependent substrate specificities between kinases and their substrates provided by specific docking sites; the localization of these kinases can be regulated and scaffolding organization of these pathways modulate local concentrations of selected kinases and substrates (MacCorkle and Tan, 2005; Torii et al., 2006).

The four distinct MAPK cascades are named according to the subgroup of their MAPK components: extracellular signal-regulated kinase 1 and 2 (ERKs); c-Jun N-terminal kinase (JNK), also know as stress-activated protein kinase 1 (SAPK1); and P38 α-δ and ERK5, also known as Big MAPK. Thus, distinct MAPK cascades seem to differ in their physiological activities (Rubinfeld and Seger, 2005).

After extracellular signals activate the tyrosine kinase receptors, this leads to phosphorylation of tyrosine residues, the signal is transmitted through the adaptors protein such as growth-factor-receptor-bound-2 (GRN2), and it is followed by recruitment and activation of Ras proteins. The Ras proteins are small GTPases that cycle between inactive guanosine diphosphate (GDP)-bound and guanosine triphosphate-bound conformations (Ras-GDP and Ras-GTP, respectively). Guanine-nucleotide-exchange factors (GEFs), named SOS (Son of Sevenless), catalyze the transition from GDP-bound, inactive Ras to GTP-bound, active Ras. Then, active Ras-GTP binds to the effector protein Raf and subsequently recruits Raf to the cell membrane, where this protein is activated. Once active, Raf phosphorylates MEK-ERK kinases cascade (Schubbert et al., 2007; Karreth and Tuveson, 2009).

Raf activates MEK-1 and MEK-2 (Mitogen-Activated Protein Kinase Kinase) by phosphorylation on two serine residues. In this turn, MEK phosphorylates ERK-1 and ERK-2 (Extracellular signal-regulated kinase). In addition, scaffold proteins have an important role in the regulation of this pathway, stabilizing and coordinating interactions between the individual components, which increase the efficiency of signaling and maintains fidelity by restricting interactions between closely related components (Wellbrock et al., 2004).

To extracellularly signal the trigger of the cell-cycle progression, ERK activation must be sustained until approximately two or three hours before the onset of the S phase, which is a key factor ensuring G1 phase progression. Sustained ERK activation also induces sustained phosphorylation of immediate early genes products, leading to they stabilization and activation, resulting in gene expression of proteins that promote the cell cycle progression (MacCorkle and Tan, 2005; Torii et al., 2006).

There are many substrates of ERK in the cytosol, cytoskeleton, and a group of substrates that resides in the nucleus, as the nuclear transcription factor Elk1, which induces the expression of the immediate early genes c-Fos and c-Jun. In the nucleus, ELK1 regulates the transcription through its interaction with the serum response factor (SRF) and c-Fos promoter enhancer at the serum response element (SRE). The products of early immediate genes have been implicated in regulating subsequent induction of delayed early genes, including a first class of G1 cyclins, cyclin D. The cyclin D upregulation results in the expression of the D-CDK4/6 complex, which are the regulatory subunits for the cyclin-dependent kinase 4 and 6 (CDK4 and CDK6) catalytic subunits. The activation of cyclin D-CDK4/6 complex kinase activity phosphorylate and inactivate Rb protein (retinoblastoma tumor suppressor), leading to activation of transcription factor E2F, and upregulation of genes necessary to transition toward S phase (Torii et al., 2006).

At early G1, hypophosphorylated Rb binds to E2F and inhibits its activity. During mid-G1, Rb is sequentially phosphorylate by CDKs and finally releases E2F, which initiates transcription genes required for G1/S transition such as cyclin D, cyclin E cyclin A, *c-myc, c-myb* and DNA polymerase (Matsumura et al., 2003).

The MEK-ERK typically controls G1 phase progression by regulating the expression of cyclin D1 and/or downregulating the cdk-inhibitory proteins such as $p21^{CIP1}$ and $p27^{KIP1}$. In CDK inhibitors (CKIs) activity, low levels of activated Raf-1 cause cell cycle progression, whereas high levels cause cell cycle arrest and $p21^{Waf/Cip1}$ induction in a p53-independent manner (Rubinfeld and Seger, 2005).

In addition to receptor tyrosine kinases, MAPK pathway can also be regulated by G-protein-coupled receptors (GPCRs). These receptors can be activated by different external stimuli such as growth factors, hormones and neurotransmitters. GPCRs consist of seven hydrophobic transmembrane helixes with a large hydrophobic tail at the C-terminus which interacts with heterotrimeric G protein, composed by alpha subunit and beta/gamma dimmer. Upon binding of GPCRs to ligands, the G protein is activated, leading to conversion from the inactive GDP-bound state into the active GTP-bound state. Once activated, G proteins can activate several effector enzymes, such as phospholipase C (PLC) species or adenylate cyclases. Activation of adenylate cyclases leads to the generation of cyclic AMP (cAMP) from ATP, which can subsequently activate protein kinases A (PKAs). Besides, most GPCRs activate MAPK via Ras-dependent signaling pathways or through PLC or protein kinases C (PKC), which can directly phosphorylate Raf-1 (Helleman and Boonstra, 2001).

Cell-surface receptors also promote cell-cycle progression through the phosphatidylinositol 3-kinase (PI3-K) pathway. PI3-Ks contribute to cyclin D1 mRNA induction as well as to regulate the translation and stability of cyclin D1 protein. Phosphotyrosine residues can bind with high affinity to the one or both of the SH2 domains in regulatory subunits of the PI3Ks, leading to their recruitment into receptor signaling complex. An important element governing the activity of PI3Ks in this signaling complex is the direct association of Ras with an RBD (Ras-binding domain) motif in the p110 catalytic subunit of PI3K, which translocates to the cell membrane and interact with tyrosine kinases or Ras. The PI3K thus activated produces the second messenger polyphosphoinositides PI-3,4-P_2 and PI-3,4,5-P_3, which in turn activate a number of phosphoinositide-dependent kinases (PDKs). Akt or protein kinase B (PKB) is the first direct downstream effector of PI3K. The substrates phosphorylate by the Akt include glycogen synthase kinase 3 (GSK3) and the pro-apoptotic members of *bcl2* family protein. (Takuma and Takuma, 2001; Hawkins et al., 2006).

Cancer arises when the molecular network connecting proliferation and tumor suppression become uncoupled. Many studies point to the importance of MAPK pathway mutations, which result in abnormal cellular signaling, proliferation, survival and responses to growth factors. Receptor tyrosine kinases could suffer mutations that abnormally activate Ras and downstream substrates (Karreth and Tuveson, 2009; Zhang and Yang, 2009). The RAS-ERK pathway has long been associated with human cancers because, mutations in RAS occurs ~15% of cancers and ERK is hyperactivated in ~30% of cancers. The most common substitutions are gain-of-function mutations that render the kinase constitutively active, conferring to this cell a greater chance of progressing all the way to a cancerous state. This somatic missence Ras mutations found in cancer cells introduce amino-acid substitutions that impair the intrinsic GTPase activity and confer resistance to GAPs (GTPase activating proteins) (Wellbrock et al., 2004; Schubbert et al., 2007).

The Role of Cell Cycle Control in Oncogenesis

Cancer cells are characteristically independent of growth stimulus due to mutations of intracellular signal pathways (Foster, 2008). Within the human genome, ~300 genes have been found to be mutated in cancer and many others exhibit altered levels or patterns of expression. Such changes contribute to deregulation of cell cycle kinases, which is often associated with unscheduled proliferation of cancer cells (Lapenna and Giordano, 2009). As examples, dysregulations of CDK4 and CDK6 activities have been implicated in a wide variety of tumors, and CDK4 is altered in a set of melanoma patients by a miscoding mutation (Arg24Cys). Also, E-type cyclins are often overexpressed in human tumors, and the expression of the CKIs p21 and p27 is frequently silenced during tumor development (Malumbres and Barbacid, 2009).

Nowadays, the proportion of cells committed to the cycle may be easily assessed by Ki-67 or MIB-1 antibodies, which identify an antigen expressed in G1, S and G2 phases of cycling cells (Cattoretti et al., 1992). In addition, PCNA is a DNA polymerase delta auxiliary protein of 36KDa, which is closely related to the replication of DNA and is indispensable to cell proliferation. PCNA level increases rapidly in mid-G1, remains elevated throughout the S phase, and then decreases from G2/M to G1 (Linden et al., 1992). PCNA-positive cells can be regarded as cells involved in the proliferating process. A decrease in the PCNA-positive cells reflects a decrease in S phase and, thus, a reduced proliferative activity. Detection of PCNA antigen is considered a reliable marker of cell proliferation (Tanaka et al., 2002). Previous studies conducted by our group have revealed that PCNA positive nuclei were higher either in oral dysplasia or in squamous cell carcinomas when compared to ordinary oral mucosa (Silva et al., 2007). These results suggest that the expression of PCNA is closely involved during neoplastic conversion.

Retinoblastoma (Rb) and p16 gene products are part of the retinoblastoma pathway that negatively controls the cell cycle. The Rb gene is located on the long arm of chromosome 13. The retinoblastoma protein is a nuclear phosphoprotein that is expressed in most normal cells. Rb functions during the G1–S transition within the cell cycle (Muirhead et al., 2006). The hypophosphorylated form of the retinoblastoma protein mediates G1 arrest (Muirhead et al., 2006). Rb and p16 genes inactivation have been reported in many cancers (Nemes et al., 2006). Cyclin-dependent kinase inhibitors (CDKIs), such as p21 exert a direct control on the cell cycle. p21 is a negative regulators of cyclin-dependent kinases and in this function they are negative check-point regulators of the cell cycle. Some studies have suggested that p21 in carcinoma of oral cavity seems to be predictive parameter in regulation and prognosis of squamous cell carcinomas (Goto et al., 2005). Cellular DNA damage leads via p53-activation to an up-regulation of p21 to cause cell-cycle arrest in the G1 phase with the cellular possibility for DNA-repair or the induction of apoptosis (Hill et al., 2008). In addition, p21 can be regulated independent of p53 by cellular growth factors (Ciccarelli et al., 2005). IN particular, our results have demonstrated no significant statistically differences ($p>0.05$) in expression of all tumor suppressor genes along medium-term oral carcinogenesis assay (Ribeiro et al., 2007).

Dysregulation of the cell cycle in cancer cells can also be due to inactivation of critical CKIs or to overexpression of cyclins. For example, the inhibition of the CKI p16, generally by hypermethylation of its promoters, leads to loss of function and has been associated with various malignancies such as melanoma, lung, breast and colorectal tumors (Schwartz and Shah, 2005). Therefore, the goal in cancer therapy was the development artificial CKI targeted to CDKs. Such agents are pan-cyclin-dependent kinase (CDK) inhibitors (e.g., Flavopiridol) resulting in cell cycle arrest, with consequent arrest of the uncontrolled growth and induction of apoptotic cell death by inhibition of antiapoptotic molecules including bcl-2 (Schwartz and Shah, 2005). This is because no mutations in the p16CDKN2A exon 2 were found in any experimental periods evaluated that corresponded to normal oral mucosa, hyperplasia, dysplasia and squamous cell carcinomas following oral carcinogenesis induced by 4NQO (Minicucci et al., 2009a). However, the levels of Rb were increased ($p<0.05$) in pre-neoplastic lesions at 12 weeks following carcinogen exposure. In well-differentiated squamous cell carcinoma induced after 20 weeks of treatment with carcinogen, p16 and Rb were expressed in some tumor cells (Ribeiro et al., 2007). Taken together, our results support the notion that expression of Rb is closely event related to malignant transformation and conversion of the oral mucosa, being reliable biomarker linked to oral cancer pathogenesis.

The gene of the tumor suppressor protein (p53) mentioned above has been regarded as the “guardian of the genome” since it protects against the proliferation of mutated cells (Foster, 2008). Loss of p53 function as well as Rb protein may result from mutation, deletion of the gene, or binding with other proteins. Absence of a functional p53 allows accumulation of oncogenic DNA lesions since its pro-apoptotic regulation, through the DNA damage checkpoint, has been removed. Tumor promoters act as survival factors, preventing apoptosis, and so increasing the proportion of damaged cells likely to survive (Foster, 2008). The p53 gene encodes a protein, p53, which has a molecular weight of 53 kDa (Whyte et al., 2002). The protein product of the *Tp53* gene restrains cellular proliferation by binding to specific regions of DNA, where it can regulate the expression of other genes. It also suppresses cell growth by controlling entry into the S phase of the cell cycle.

It has been proposed that in many tumors the G1 phase is a frequent primary target, since most, if not all, human cancers show a dysregulated control of G1 progression where the major targets are exactly the Rb and p53 pathways, which contain several targets (Rb, p53, CDKs, cyclins) often altered (Dela Val and Birnbaun, 2007). Treating such tumors by trying to kill these mutated cells with DNA-damaging agents such as ionizing radiation and DNA-targeting drugs results in cell checkpoint-mediated arrest at S or G2. Such remaining checkpoints can be used by the tumor cells to protect themselves from radiation or cytotoxic agents. The situation may be tackled by associating the ionizing radiation or DNA-damaging drugs with inhibitors of S or G2 checkpoints, forcing the cancer cells carrying DNA lesions to enter mitosis, prompting a mitotic catastrophe and associated cell death. So, abrogation of DNA-damage checkpoint in S or G2 is a strategy for selectively targeting G1-checkpoint defective cancer cells (Lapenna and Giordano, 2009). Normally, wild-type p53 has a very short half-life on the order of 6–20 min, and therefore it cannot be detected by standard immunohistochemical methods. Therefore, positive staining for p53 has been proposed as an indicator of mutations within the *Tp53* gene (Okazaki et al., 2002). In addition, regulatory defects of the *Tp53* gene may, in some cases, result in the over-expression or stabilization of the wild-type p53 protein (Sjodren et al., 1996). In an earlier study performed by our research group, an increased number of faintly or densely stained p53-positive cells, which were either wild-type and/or mutant, were found in the epithelium of dysplastic lesions and squamous cell carcinoma when compared to ordinary oral mucosa (Minicucci et al., 2009b).

Bcl-2 and bax are also two important effector genes responsible for arresting cell cycle as a result of triggering the apoptosis process. The bcl-2 proto-oncogene was originally discovered by analysis of the t(14;18) chromosomal translocation associated with human follicular B-cell lymphoma (Tsujimoto et al., 1985). The bcl-2 gene encodes a protein located in the nuclear membrane, on the inner surface of mitochondria, and the endoplasmic reticulum (Akao et al. 1994). It is the most important gene of the bcl-2 family and has been shown to be an inhibitor of apoptosis (Lu et al., 1996). Immunohistochemical overexpression of bcl-2 has been observed in carcinomas of the nasopharynx, lung, urinary bladder, colon, prostate, breast, thyroid and oral cavity (Singh et al., 1998). Bax, another member of the bcl-2 family, is considered to be a major effector of apoptosis (Oltvai et al., 1993). In normal and tumour tissues, the distribution of bax is inversely related to that of bcl-2 (Krajewski et al. 1994). Thus, the bcl-2/bax ratio controls the relative susceptibility of cells to lethal stimuli (Korsmeyer et al., 1993). Our data pointed to an overexpression of bcl-2 and bax ($p < 0.01$) in all layers of rat oral "normal" epithelium exposed to chemical carcinogen during four weeks (Ribeiro et al., 2005). The expression levels were the same in all layers of epithelium for both antibodies used (bcl-2 or bax). In dysplastic lesions at 12 weeks following carcinogen administration, the levels of bcl-2 and bax expression did not increase when compared to negative control with the immunoreactivity for bcl-2 being restricted to the superficial layer of epithelium (Ribeiro et al., 2005). In well-differentiated squamous cell carcinoma induced after 20 weeks of treatment with neoplasm inducer, bcl-2 was expressed in some cells of tumour islands. On the other hand, immunostaining for bax was widely observed at the tumour nests. The labeling index for bcl-2 and bax showed an increase ($P < 0.05$) after only four weeks (Ribeiro et al., 2005). In conclusion, our results suggest that abnormalities in the apoptosis pathways are associated with the development of persistent clones of mutated epithelial cells in the oral mucosa. Bcl-2 and bax expression appears to be associated with a risk factor in the progression of oral cancer.

In mammals, apoptosis is mainly modulated by two protein families, the bcl-2 and inhibitor of apoptosis (IAP) proteins (Altieri, 2003). Among IAP proteins, interest has been addressed to survivin, a multifunctional protein that suppresses apoptosis by association with caspases and Smac/DIABLO and regulates mitosis by interacting with other chromosomal passenger proteins (Altieri, 2004). Unlike other IAP proteins broadly expressed in adult cells, survivin is expressed during embryonic development, and is not detectable in most differentiated normal adult tissues (Altieri, 2003; Altieri, 2004). Survivin is expressed in a wide variety of human malignancies (Miyachi et al., 2003), apparently as a requirement for cancer-cell immortalization and/or malignant progression (Altieri, 2003; 2004). Although no histopathological abnormalities were induced in the oral epithelium of Wistar rats after four weeks of carcinogen exposure, survivin was expressed in some cells of the "normal" oral epithelium (Ribeiro et al., 2007). In pre-neoplastic lesions at 12 weeks following carcinogen exposure, the levels of survivin were increased ($p < 0.05$) when compared to negative control. In well-differentiated squamous cell carcinoma induced after 20 weeks of treatment with chemical carcinogen, survivin was expressed in some tumor cells (Ribeiro et al., 2007). Lack of immunoreactivity for both markers was observed in the negative control group. Taken together, it seems that expression of survivin is considered an early event during malignant transformation and conversion of the oral mucosa.

The start point of cell division degeneration is multifactorial in nature. It can arise from the natural aging process, from high levels of reactive oxygen species (ROS), and can also be induced by environmental agents (e.g., solar radiation), pollutants, chemicals and a series of other processes. The possible relationship between aging and oncogenesis is of special interest due to the global incremental rise in life expectancy. Such a correlation has been, however, converversial and no definitive answer has been achieved. The aging process is caused mainly by the cellular senescence, the process by which cells lose the telomeres by a progressive shortening in the absence of the enzyme telomerase, normally absent in most somatic tissues (Kim et al., 2002). Considerable telomere loss has been associated with chromosomal instability (CIN), being both a physiological and pathologically accelerated telomere loss, and is therefore considered as having clinico-oncologic significance (Tallen et al., 2007). However, contrary to tumor cells, senescent cells accumulate active p53 and p16/Rb suppressor tumors, which can protect against a defective division through the induction of an irreversible growth arrest (Tallen et al., 2007). Cellular senescence and death, then, can be considered tumor suppressive. On the other hand, somatic mutations, some of which can inactivate genes required for such senescence response, accumulate throughout life (Kim et al., 2002).

Cancer research is a constantly expanding area. Whatever the oncogenic nature, knowledge of the molecular basis summarized here underlying such misadjusted cell physiology provides tools for tracking and predicting tumorigenic candidates.

REFERENCES

Akao, Y; Otsuki, Y; Kataoka, S; Ito, Y; Tsujimoto, Y. Multiple subcellular localization of bcl-2: detection in nuclear outer membrane, endoplasmic reticulum membrane, and mitochondrial membranes. *Cancer Res*, 1994, 54, 2468-2471.

Alberts, B; Johnson, A; Lewis, J; Raff, M; Roberts, K; Walter, P. Molecular Biology of the Cell. *Garland Sciences,* (5th Edition), 1600, 2007.

Altieri, DC; Survivin. versatile modulation of cell division and apoptosis in cancer, Oncogene 2003, 22, 8581-8589.

Altieri, DC. Molecular circuits of apoptosis regulation and cell division control, the survivin paradigm, *J Cell Biochem*, 2004, 92, 656-663.

Catoretti, G; Becker, MHG; Key, G. Monoclonal antibodies agains recombinant parts of the Ki-67 antigen (MIB-1 and MIB-3) detect proliferating cells in microwave-processed formalin-fixed paraffin sections *J Pathol,* 1992, 168, 357-363.

Chen, PL; Scully, P; Shew, JY; Wang, JY; Lee, WH. Phosphorylation of the retinoblastoma gene product is modulated during the cell cycle and cellular differentiation. *Cell,* 1989, 58, 1193-1198.

Ciccarelli, C; Marampon, F; Scoglio, A; Mauro, A; Giacinti, C; De Cesaris, P; Zani, BM. p21WAF1 expression induced by MEK/ERK pathway activation or inhibition correlates with growth arrest, myogenic differentiation and onco-phenotype reversal in rhabdomyosarcoma cells Mol Cancer 2005, 4, 41-46.

Das SK. Cell cycle regulatory control for uterine stromal cell decidualization in implantation. *Reproduction,* 2009, 137, 889-899.

Dela Val, B; Birnbaun, D. A cell cycle hypothesis of cooperative oncogenesis. *International Journal Of Oncology*, 2007, 30, 1051-1058.

Evans, T; Rosenthal, ET; Youngblom, J; Distel, D; Hunt, T. Cyclin: a protein specified by maternal mRNA in sea urchin eggs that is destroyed at each cleavage division. *Cell,* 1983, 33, 389-396.

Foster, I. Cancer: A cell cycle defect. *Radiography*, 2008, 14, 144-149.

Goto, M; Tsukamoto, T; Inada, K; Mizoshita, T; Ogawa, T; Terada, A; Hyodo, I; Shimozato, K; Hasegawa, Y; Tatematsu, M. Loss of p21WAF1/CIP1 expression in invasive fronts of oral tongue squamous cell carcinomas is correlated with tumor progression and poor prognosis. *Oncol Rep,* 2005, 14, 837-846.

Hawkins, PT; Anderson, KE; Davidson, K; Stephens, LR. Signalling through class I PI3Ks in mammalian cells. *Biochem Soc Trans,* 2006, 34, 647-662.

Helleman, E; Boonstra, J. Regulation of G1 phase progression by growth factors and extracellular matrix. *Cell Mol Life Sci,* 2001, 58, 80-93.

Hill, R; Bodzak, E; Blough, MD; Lee, PW. p53 binding to the p21 promoter is dependent on the nature of DNA damage. *Cell Cycle*, 2008, 15, 2535-2543.

Ho, CC; Siu, WY; Lau, A; Chan, WM; Arooz, T; Poon, RYC. Stalled replication induces p53 accumulation through distinct mechanisms from DNA damage checkpoint pathways. *Cancer Res,* 2006, 66, 2233-2241.

Hochegger, H; Takeda, S. and Hunt T. Cyclin-dependent kinases and cell-cycle transitions: does one fit all? *Nature Reviews Molecular Cell Biology,* 2008, 9, 910-916.

Karess R. Rod-ZW10-Zwilch: a key player in the spindle checkpoint. *Trends Cell Biol,* 2005, 15, 386-92.

Karreth, FA; Tuveson, DA. Modelling oncogenic Ras/Raf signaling in the mouse. *Curr Op Gen Devlop.*, 2009, 19, 4-11.

Kim, S; Kaminker, P; Campis, J. Telomeres, aging and cancer: In search of a happy ending. *Oncogene,* 2002, 21, 503-511.

Knudsen, ES; Knudsen, KE. Retinoblastoma tumor suppressor: Where cancer meets the cell cycle. *Exp Biol Med,* 2006, 231, 1271-1281.

Korsmeyer, SJ; Shutter, JR; Veis, DJ; Merry, DE; Oltvai, ZN. Bcl-2/Bax: a rheostat that regulates an anti-oxidant pathway and cell death. *Cancer Biol*, 1993, 4, 327-332.

Krajewski, S; Krajewska, M; Shabaik, A; Miyashita, T; Wang, HG; Reed, JC. Immunohistochemical determination of in vivo distribution of Bax, a dominant inhibitor of Bcl-2 Am. *J Pathol,* 1994, 145, 1323-1336.

Lapenna, S. and Giordano, A. Cell cycle kinases as therapeutic targets for cancer. *Nature Reviews Drug Discovery*, 2009, 8, 547-566.

Li, M; Zhang, P. The function of APC/CCdh1 in cell cycle and beyond. *Cell Division*, 2009, 4, 2.

Linden, MD; Torrex, RX; Dubus, J; Zarbo, RJ. Clinical application of morphologic and immunocytochemical assessments of cell proliferation [editorial] Am. *J Clin Pathol,* 1992, 97, S4-13.

Lu, QL; Abel, P; FosterCS; Lalani, EN. Bcl-2: role in epithelial differentiation and oncogenesis. *Hum Pathol,* 1996, 27, 102-110.

MacCorkle, RA; Tan, TH. Mitogen-activated protein kinases in cell-cycle control. *Cell Biochem Biophys,* 2005, 43, 451-461.

Malumbres, M, Barbacid, M. Cell cycle, CDKs and cancer: a changing paradigm. *Nature Reviews Cancer,* 2009, 9, 153-166.

Matsumura, I; Tabaka, H; Kanakura, Y. E2F1 and C-Myc in cell growth and death. *Cell Cycle,* 2003, 2, 333-338.

Minicucci, EM; da Silva, GN; Ribeiro, DA; Favero Salvadori DM. No mutations found in exon 2 of gene p16CDKN2A during rat tongue carcinogenesis induced by 4-nitroquinoline-1-oxide. *J Mol Histol,* 2009, 40, 71-6a.

MInicucci, EM; Ribeiro, DA; Silva, GN; Pardini, ME; Mantovani, JC; Salvadori, DM. The role of TP53 gene during rat tongue carcinogenesis induced by 4-nitroquinoline 1-oxide, *Exp Toxicol Pathol,* 2009b, *in press.*

Miyachi, K; Sasaki, S; Onodera, T; Taguchi, M; Nagamachi, H; Kaneko M; Sunagawa, Correlation between survivin mRNA expression and lymph node metastasis in gastric cancer, *Gastric Cancer,* 2003, 6, 217-224.

Muirhead, DM; Hoffman, HT; Robinson, RA. Correlation of clinicopathological features with immunohistochemical expression of cell cycle regulatory proteins p16 and retinoblastoma: distinct association with keratinisation and differentiation in oral cavity squamous cell carcinoma *J Clin Pathol,* 2006, 59, 711-715.

Nacusi, LP; Sheaff, RJ. Deregulation of Cell Cycle Machinery in Pancreatic Cancer. *Pancreatology,* 2007, 7, 373-377.

Nemes, JA; Deli, L; Nemes, Z; Márton, IJ. Expression of p16(INK4A), p53, and Rb proteins are independent from the presence of human papillomavirus genes in oral squamous cell carcinoma *Oral Surg Oral Med Oral Pathol Oral Radiol Endod,* 2006, 102, 344-352.

Okazaki, Y; Tanaka, Y; Tonogi, M; Yamane, G. Investigation of environmental factors for diagnosing malignant potential in oral epithelial dysplasia *Oral Oncol,* 38, 562-573, 2002

Oltvai, ZN; Milliman, CL; Korsmeyer, SJ. Bcl-2 heterodimerizes in vivo with a conserved homolog, Bax, that accelerates programmed cell death *Cell,* 1993, 74, 609-619.

Quereda, V, Malumbres, M. Cell cycle control of pituitary development and disease. *J Mol Endocrinol,* 2009, 42, 75-86.

Ribeiro, DA; Kitakawa, D; Domingues, MA; Cabral, LA; Marques, ME; Salvadori, DM. Survivin and inducible nitric oxide synthase production during 4NQO-induced rat tongue carcinogenesis: a possible relationship *Exp Mol Pathol,* 2007, 83, 131-7.

Ribeiro, DA; Kitakawa, D; Domingues, MA; Cabral, LA; Marques, ME; Salvadori, DM. Survivin and inducible nitric oxide synthase production during 4NQO-induced rat tongue carcinogenesis: a possible relationship *Exp Mol Pathol,* 2007, 83, 131-7.

Ribeiro, DA; Salvadori, DM; Marques, ME. Abnormal expression of bcl-2 and bax in rat tongue mucosa during the development of squamous cell carcinoma induced by 4-nitroquinoline 1-oxide *Int J Exp Pathol,* 2005, 86, 375-81.

Roovers, K; Assoian, RK. Integrating the MAP kinase signal into the G1 phase cell cycle machinery. *BioEssays,* 2000, 22, 818-826.

Rubinfeld, R; Seger, R. The ERK cascade - A Prototype of MAPK signaling. *Mol Biotechnol,* 2005, 31, 151-174.

Satyanarayana, A; Hilton, MB; Kaldis, P. p21 inhibits Cdk1 in the absence of Cdk2 to maintain the G1/S phase DNA damage checkpoint. *Mol Biol Cell,* 2008, 19, 65-77.

Schubbert, S; Shannon, K; Bollag, G. Hyperactive Ras in developmental disorders and cancer. *Nature Rev Cancer*, 2007, 7, 295-308.

Schwartz, GK; Shah, MA. Targeting the Cell Cycle: A New Approach to Cancer Therapy. *J Clin Oncol*, 2005, 23, 9408-9421.

Silva, RN; Ribeiro, DA; Salvadori, DM; Marques, ME. Placental glutathione S-transferase correlates with cellular proliferation during rat tongue carcinogenesis induced by 4-nitroquinoline 1-oxide *Exp Toxicol Pathol*, 2007, 59, 61-8.

Singh, BB; Chandler, FW Jr; Whitaker, SB; Forbes-Nelson, AE. Immunohistochemical evaluation of bcl-2 oncoprotein in oral dysplasia and carcinoma *Oral Surg Oral Med Oral Pathol Oral Radiol Endod*, 1998, 85, 692-698.

Sjodren, S; Inganas, M; Norbert, T. The p53 gene in breast cancer: prognostic value of complementary DNA sequencing versus immunohistochemistry *J Natl Cancer Inst*, 1996, 88, 173-182.

Stein, GS; van Wijnen, AJ; Stein, JL; Lian, JB; Montecino, M; Zaidi, SK; Braastad, C. An architectural perspective of cell-cycle control at the G1/S phase cell-cycle transition. *J Cell Physiol.*, 2006, 209, 706-710.

Takuma, N; Takuma, Y. Reulation of cell cycle molecules by the Ras effector system. *Mol Cell Endocrinol.*, 2001, 177, 25-33.

Tallen, G; Soliman, MA; Riabowol, K. The cancer-aging interface and the significance of telomere dynamics in cancer therapy. *Rej Res,* 2007, 10, 387-395.

Tanaka, T; Kohno, H; Sakata, Y; Yamada, Y; Hirose, Y; Sugie, S; Mori, H. Modifying effects of dietary capsaicin and rotenone on 4-nitroquinoline 1-oxide-induced rat tongue carcinogenesis *Carcinogenesis,* 2002, 23, 1361-1367.

Torii, S; Yamamoto, T; Tsuchiya, Y; Nishida, E. ERK MAP kinase in G cell cycle progression and cancer. *Cancer Sci*, 2006, 97, 697-702.

Tsujimoto, Y; Jaffe, E; Cossman, J; Gorham, J; Nowell, PC; Croce, CM. Clustering of breakpoints on chromosome 11 in human B-cell neoplasms with the t(11;14) chromosome translocation *Nature,* 1985, 315, 340-343.

Tvegard, T; Soltani, H; Skjolberg, HC. A novel checkpoint mechanism regulating the G1/S transition. *Genes Dev,* 2007, 21, 649-654.

Van Diest, PJ; Burgal, G; Baak, JPA. Proliferation markers in tumors: interpretation and clinical value *J Clin Pathol*, 1998, 51, 716-724.

Wellbrock, C; Karasarides, M; Marais, R. The Raf proteins take centre stage. *Natrure Rev Mol Cell Biol*, 2004, 5, 875-885.

Whyte, DA; Brton, CE; Shillitoe, EJ. The unexplained survival of cells in oral cancer: what is the role of p53? *J Oral Pathol Med*, 31, 125-133, 2002.

Zhang, M; Yang, H. Negative growth regulators of the cell cycle machinery and cancer. 1: Pathophysiology, 2009. Available online DOI 10.1016/j.pathophys.2009.02.004.

Zheng, YL; Loffredo, CA; Alberg, AJ; Yu, Z; Jones, RT; Perlmutter, D; Enewold, L; Krasna, MJ; Yung, R; Shields, PG; Harris, CC. Less efficient G2-M checkpoint is associated with an increased risk of lung cancer in African Americans. *Cancer Res*, 2005, 65, 9566-9573.

In: Cell Division: Theory, Variants and Degradation ISBN: 978-1-60876-986-5
Editors: Y. N. Golitsin, M. C. Krylov, pp. 95-105

Chapter 5

ONE RING TO BIND THEM ALL AT THE CENTRE OF THE CELL

Angela Cadou and Xavier Le Goff*
CNRS UMR6061 Université de Rennes 1, Institut de Génétique et Développement de Rennes, IFR140, Université Européenne de Bretagne, Faculté de Médecine, 2 Av. du Prof. Léon Bernard, 35043 Rennes Cedex, France

ABSTRACT

In animal cells and fungi, cytokinesis is achieved by constriction of an actomyosin-based ring assembled during mitosis. The fission yeast *Schizosaccharomyces pombe* is an excellent model organism for unraveling cell division controls by combining molecular genetics with cell biology approaches. Once spatially defined, the ring assembly site is the place of sequential incorporation of a set of proteins during mitotic progression, most of which are evolutionarily conserved. Then, fission yeast divides medially to produce equally sized daughter cells. In the past years, several studies have explored mechanisms of division site determination. It has been demonstrated that positive signals for division plane positioning originate from the central region. Position of the predivided nucleus and the anilin-related protein Mid1 give spatial cues to establish the place of ring formation. In addition, negative signals controlled by the DYRK Pom1 kinase and emanating from the cell ends restrict ring formation in the central region. This dual system prevents illegitimate cell division outside the centre of the cell and subsequent polyploid cell formation. Recently, it has been shown that the mitotic regulator Cdr2 kinase is intrinsically involved in division plane specification by binding to Mid1 at the cell equator during interphase. Moreover, nuclear-to-cytoplasm shuttling of Mid1 is another independent crucial mechanism that couples nuclear position with the actomyosin ring assembly site late in the G2 phase. Kin1, another kinase that regulates morphogenesis and intracellular organization, shares an essential function with Pom1 in cytokinesis. Recent advances have also identified distinct pathways involved in completion of CAR formation. Therefore, multiple regulatory mechanisms act in parallel to accurately specify and build up the actomyosin ring at the centre of the cell.

* Corresponding author: Phone +33 2 23 23 45 27; Fax +33 2 23 23 44 78; E-mail xavier.le-goff@univ-rennes1.fr

Concomitant inhibition of these pathways dramatically affects cytokinesis and cell viability. Here we present these redundant pathways that contribute to faithful distribution of the genetic material into daughter cells.

INTRODUCTION

Specification of the division site is a crucial step in cell division control because it ensures that equal genetic material is spatially distributed into each daughter cell. An exciting question for cell biologists is how cells define the right position to separate. The cell division plane dictates the site of assembly of a rather conserved structure, called hereafter the contractile actomyosin ring (CAR), which is mostly composed of conserved proteins between fungi and animals. Many experiments, including nuclear manipulations, suggest that internal spatial cues exist which modulate the positioning of the division plane (for a review, see Burgess and Chang, 2005).

Simple unicellular eukaryotes such as yeasts are excellent model organisms for the study of cytokinesis because they are amenable to genetic screens and facilitate selection of cell division mutants. The fission yeast *Schizosaccharomyces pombe* exhibits a precise symmetric cell division pattern that uses a CAR assembled early in mitosis. Therefore, fission yeast has become a popular model organism for the study of cell division, especially because of its apparent proximity with animal cytokinesis. An important breakthrough came from the pioneer genetic studies with the isolation of cell division deficient cells, such as the multinucleate "cell plate formation" mutants in the original "*cdc*" collection of Nurse and colleagues (Nurse et al., 1976). Later, mutant alleles of *pom1*, *mid1* and *plo1*, which misplace and misorient the cell division plane, were isolated (Chang et al., 1996; Sohrmann et al., 1996; Bähler and Pringle, 1998; Bähler et al., 1998; Balasubramanian et al., 1998). These studies and molecular cloning of the corresponding genes provided evidence that numerous proteins participate in controlling different steps of cell division. Identification of synthetic lethal interactions suggested that non overlapping mechanisms operate. One of the early functions of these mechanisms is to provide the cell with a broad central cortical band, which is a reliable spatial cue for CAR component assembly.

At mitotic onset, Spindle Pole Bodies (SPB) are duplicated and the spindle is assembled within the nucleus. F-actin patches and cables disappear from the cell ends and the CAR, composed of F-actin and many other proteins, is formed at the geometric centre of the cell. CAR assembly is a step-by-step process (Wu et al., 2003; Wu et al., 2006; Hachet and Simanis, 2008). Later, at the end of anaphase, the spindle breaks down and a primary septum is centripetally synthesized from the cortex inside the cell together with CAR constriction and invagination of plasma membranes. Therefore, the CAR is used as a spatial landmark for specifying the septum synthesis area and thus the cell division site. The primary septum has a different polysaccharidic composition compared to the surrounding secondary septa and the lateral cell wall. This difference allows its specific degradation to trigger the release of daughter cells (for a review, see Sipiczki, 2007).

Crucial aspects of an appropriate CAR assembly site are narrowness and precise location at the geometric cell centre to ensure symmetry of cell division. Enlarging or mispositioning of this cortical region lead to cytokinesis failure.

1. Cell Division Site Determination

To produce equally sized daughter cells after cytokinesis, it is necessary that the CAR is assembled at the geometric centre and perpendicularly to the long axis of the cell. In animal cells, the contractile ring assembly site is defined by position of the spindle late in mitosis (Burgess and Chang, 2005). In contrast, CAR assembly and thus cell division site are defined in late G2/early mitosis in fission yeast. This area is dictated by the position of the predivided nucleus (Chang and Nurse, 1996; Paoletti and Chang, 2000; Tran et al., 2001; Daga and Chang, 2005; Tolic-Norrelykke et al., 2005). Maintenance of the interphase nucleus in the centre of the cell requires a dynamic microtubule network (Tran et al., 2001). Eccentric position of the nucleus can be obtained by cell centrifugation (Daga and Chang, 2005), by optical tweezers (Tolic-Norrelykke et al., 2005) or by mutations in a subset of genes affecting the cytoskeleton or intracellular organization (for instance, Morishita and Shimoda, 2000; La Carbona et al., 2004). In all cases, the division site is defined where the nucleus is misplaced.

Recent studies have revealed the existence of both positive signals emanating from the centre of the cell and negative signals inhibiting CAR assembly in the cell ends.

(a) Positive signals at the centre of the cell

During the G2 phase, the nucleus is maintained at the geometric centre of the cell by the combination of mechanisms involving the rod shape of cells and microtubule dependent pushing forces (Sipiczki and Bozsik, 2000; Tran et al., 2001; Daga et al., 2006). The position of the nucleus defines the area of actomyosin ring assembly through the distribution of the Mid1 protein (Chang et al., 1996; Sohrmann et al., 1996; Paoletti and Chang, 2000; Daga and Chang, 2005). Deletion or mutation of the *mid1* gene promotes mispositioned and misoriented CARs and septa into the cell even though the nucleus is properly centered (Chang et al., 1996; Sohrmann et al., 1996). Mid1 is a phosphoprotein containing a Pleckstrin homology domain and shows a weak sequence homology with the metazoan anilin protein. Mid1 exhibits both nuclear and cortical localizations. During the major part of interphase, the main pool of Mid1 is present in the nucleus. A small fraction of the protein is associated with the cell cortex at the vicinity of the nucleus (Paoletti and Chang, 2000; Celton-Morizur et al., 2004). At the end of the G2 phase and in early mitosis, Mid1 exits from the nucleus towards the plasma membrane and appears as a broad band in the cortical region overlying the nucleus (Paoletti and Chang, 2000). In addition, the nuclear export of Mid1 has been shown to be a key regulation of Mid1 function in CAR formation since a "Nuclear Export Signal" mutant of Mid1 exhibits a *mid1Δ* phenotype (see below, Paoletti and Chang, 2000). Mid1 shuttles from the nucleus to the cortex after its phosphorylation by the fission yeast polo kinase homolog Plo1 (Bähler et al., 1998). Plo1 is present in the SPB, in the metaphase spindle and in the CAR and plays several crucial functions in mitotic progression. Accordingly, loss-of-function alleles as well as Plo1 overexpression promote diverse mitotic and cytokinetic defects suggesting separate multiple functions during these cell cycle stages (Ohkura et al., 1995; Bähler et al., 1998; Tanaka et al., 2001). When Mid1 is localized at the cell cortex, it recruits CAR components at the centre of the cell to promote its assembly (Wu et al., 2003; Motegi et al., 2004).

(b) Negative signals from the cell ends

It has been reported that septa are never synthesized in the cell ends in a *mid1Δ* mutant. A negative regulatory mechanism preventing septum synthesis in the cell extremities and referred to as "Tip occlusion" has been proposed (Huang et al., 2007). This process involves the polarity factors Tea1, Tea4 and Pom1 that inhibit septum synthesis in these areas of the cell. Tip occlusion becomes essential if Mid1 function is compromised. Tea1 is a 'Kelch repeat' containing protein that marks the cortex at the cell ends to activate polarized cell growth (Mata and Nurse, 1997). Tea4 binds to Tea1 and links polarity with the stress-activated MAPK Spc1 pathway (Martin et al., 2005; Tatebe et al., 2005). *Tea1Δ* and *tea4Δ* mutants misplace the areas for growth and therefore cells are bent or T-shaped. They also exhibit a weak defect for placing the division site, even though the nucleus remains properly centered. Pom1 is a conserved protein kinase of the DYRK family that controls activation of polarized growth and CAR position and orientation (Bähler and Pringle, 1998; Bähler and Nurse, 2001; Tatebe et al., 2008). Recently, Pom1 has been identified as a key regulator of the cell size control that triggers mitotic onset in fission yeast (Martin and Berthelot-Grosjean, 2009; Moseley et al., 2009).

Since Tea1 and Tea4 are required for association of the Pom1 kinase with the cell end cortex (Bähler et al., 1998; Tatebe et al., 2005), it has been suggested that the three polarity factors act in the same functional pathway but the main tip occlusion function maybe carried out by Pom1. Tea1, Tea4 and Pom1 constitutes a sub-group with specific function(s) at cell ends since other tested polarity mutants (like *bud6Δ*, *tea3Δ* or *mod5Δ*; for a review, La Carbona et al., 2006) did not exhibit strong interactions with a *mid1* mutant (Huang et al., 2007) or a *kin1* mutant (see below, Cadou et al., 2009). However, the exact nature of Pom1, Tea1 and Tea4 association, whether they directly interact or not, remains to be determined as well as the existence of other binding partners.

In *pom1Δ* cells, the Mid1 protein is mislocalized on an entire hemi-cell, consistent with mispositioned and misoriented CARs observed in this mutant. It is thus surprizing that *tea1Δ* and *tea4Δ* only exhibit CAR mispositioning but not CAR misorientation defects, suggesting an additional Tea1- and Tea4-independent function of Pom1 in orientation of the CAR perpendicular to the long axis of cells. Other mutations, such as *par1Δ* (Le Goff et al., 2001) and *cdc15-gc1* (Huang et al., 2007), have been shown to rescue orientation but not position of septum in *mid1* mutants, suggesting that orientation and position of the CAR/septum could be uncoupled. However, evidence of direct phosphorylation of Mid1 by Pom1 failed, indicating the existence of components linking Pom1 and Mid1 functions like Cdr2 (see below, Almonacid et al., 2009). It has also been proposed that an as-yet-unidentified Pom1-independent mechanism would inhibit Mid1 spreading in the other hemi-cell cortex (Celton-Morizur et al., 2006; Padte et al., 2006).

The simultaneous loss of positive (*mid1-18*, *mid1Δ* mutations) and negative (*tea1Δ*, *tea4Δ* or *pom1Δ*) signals of cell division site specification is lethal due to septum synthesis in illegitimate cellular areas allowing formation of polyploid cell compartments (Huang et al., 2007). The Cdc15 protein is required for CAR maturation, plasma membrane organization during cytokinesis and septum synthesis (Fankhauser et al., 1995; Carnahan and Gould, 2003; Takeda et al., 2004; Wachtler et al., 2006). Huang and colleagues have proposed that Cdc15 acts antagonistically downstream of Tea1, Tea4 and Pom1 to regulate Tip occlusion, since the hypomorphic allele *cdc15-gc1* rescued tip occlusion deficiency (Huang et al., 2007). Unexpectedly, this allele did not rescue the viability of *mid1-18 tea1*Δ cells.

2. Novel Regulators Defining the Site for CAR Formation

Recently, two protein kinases have been shown to regulate CAR formation at different levels, suggesting that the picture is far from being complete.

(a) Cdr2, a novel regulator of cell division site specification

Membrane association of Mid1 with the central cortex remained unclear since two different modes of interaction were reported (Celton-Morizur et al., 2004). An amphipathic helix located in the C-terminus half of the protein targets this truncated Mid1 version to the cortex but this protein failed to complement a *mid1*Δ mutant. In addition, it was reported that an unkonwn mechanism promotes the localization of the N-terminus moiety of Mid1 with the central region of the cell (Celton-Morizur et al., 2004). Recently, Almonacid and colleagues have shown that the Cdr2 kinase controls the binding of Mid1 to the central cortex through the N-terminal part of the protein, identifying Cdr2 as a novel regulator of cell division plane positioning (Almonacid et al., 2009). Cdr2 was initially isolated as a mitotic inducer which links cell size and nutrient limitation with cell cycle progression through the negative Cdc2 regulator Wee1 (Breeding et al., 1998; Kanoh and Russell, 1998). Cdr2 is present at the centre of the cell during interphase (Morrell et al., 2004). Two recent reports independently showed that the Pom1 kinase regulates Cdr2 function at the cell middle linking cell polarity with mitotic onset (Martin and Berthelot-Grosjean, 2009; Moseley et al., 2009).

Moreover, Cdr2 localization does not depend on the position of the predivided nucleus but contributes to localize efficiently Mid1 at the central cortex during interphase (Almonacid et al., 2009). In late G2 phase, *cdr2*Δ cells still exhibit a central Mid1 broad band, indicating that a Cdr2-independent mechanism could operate to define the CAR assembly site if Mid1-Cdr2 interaction is compromised. Interestingly, it has been demonstrated that the late G2/early mitosis nuclear export of Mid1, through its phosphorylation by Plo1, leads to the accumulation of Mid1 protein at the central region of the cortex, independently of Cdr2. The conclusion from these data is that nuclear export of Mid1 links the position of the nucleus with the CAR assembly site. A version of Mid1 that is never present in the nucleus (Mid1^{nsm}) is properly localized and allows CAR formation in wild type cells. If the nucleus is artificially moved in these cells, CAR assembly remains central showing that a nuclear localization mutant of Mid1 uncouples nuclear and CAR assembly positions. Moreover, Almonacid et al. showed that Mid1^{nsm} is associated with the entire cell cortex in *cdr2*Δ cells, indicating a role for Cdr2 in restricting Mid1 at the centre of the cell. In this situation, CAR formation is severely compromised (Almonacid et al., 2009).

Therefore, two non overlapping mechanisms, Cdr2-dependent and nuclear export, target Mid1 to the middle cortex and act in parallel. Accordingly, concomitant mutations affecting both patways showed synthetic defects, resembling a *mid1*Δ mutant (Almonacid et al., 2009). As Pom1 regulates Cdr2 localization, the authors proposed that the Pom1-Cdr2 system controls Mid1 restiction to the cell middle (i.e. negative signals from the cell ends where Pom1 is more concentrated, see above). But it remains to be determined why only a hemi-cell and not the entire cell cortex is controlled by Pom1, especially if the gradient of Pom1 from the cell ends to the cell middle appears to be rather symmetric (Martin and Berthelot-Grosjean, 2009; Moseley et al., 2009)? Another puzzling question is whether mislocalized Mid1 can actually form functional "cortical nodes" (see below) at illegitimate locations on the cortex.

(b) Kin1, a regulator of internal cellular organization, interacts with Pom1

It has been shown that deletion of *kin1*, encoding a kinase related to animal PAR-1/MARK proteins, is synthetically lethal with the *pom1*Δ mutant. Double mutant cells were unable to undergo cytokinesis because of severe CAR formation defects (La Carbona and Le Goff, 2006). Additional negative genetic interactions affecting cytokinesis were reported between *kin1*Δ and both *tea1*Δ and *tea4*Δ mutants (La Carbona and Le Goff, 2006; Cadou et al., 2009), consistent with Pom1, Tea1 and Tea4 acting in the same pathway (Celton-Morizur et al., 2006; Padte et al., 2006; Huang et al., 2007) and in a parallel crucial cell division function with Kin1. Interestingly, other mutants with apparent similar polarity defects (*bud6*Δ, *tea3*Δ or *mod5*Δ) did not show a negative genetic interaction with *kin1*Δ, indicating a specific common function for Pom1, Tea1 and Tea4 (Cadou et al., 2009).

Kin1 does not regulate Mid1 localization or function but *kin1*Δ or Kin1 shut-off expression showed a role for this kinase in maintenance of the nucleus at the centre of interphase cells. Padte et al. reported that the nucleus was still signalling for CAR assembly in *pom1*Δ cells, even though Mid1 is misplaced in these cells (Padte et al., 2006). This might be due to a pool of nuclear Mid1 controlled by the nuclear export mechanism (Almonacid et al., 2009). Cadou et al. proposed that the *pom1*Δ-dependent Mid1 delocalization on the lateral cortex together with nuclear centering defects would severely compromise CAR formation. For instance, a slow rate of Mid1 diffusion at the cortex while the nucleus is not centered may be responsible for mispecification of CAR assembly site on a larger central region of the cell.

Consistently, other nuclear positioning defective cells showed aberrant CAR formation in both *pom1*Δ and *tea4*Δ backgrounds (Cadou et al., 2009). This would suggest again the existence of non overlapping control mechanisms that show strong synthetic defects for cytokinesis when they are concomitantly inhibited. Additional functions for Kin1 beside nuclear centering, such as interphase-to-mitosis repolarization of F-actin in *pom1*Δ and *tea4*Δ backgrounds may also contribute to its role in cytokinesis completion. In addition, the detection of Kin1 as a novel CAR component may suggest that Kin1 could act as a regulator of septation (Cadou et al., 2009).

3. Assembly of the CAR at the Cell Equator

Once spatially defined, assembly of the medial ring takes place through sequential steps. The ring is a dynamic structure composed of more than twenty proteins which join the ring in a precise order during mitosis (Wu et al., 2003). Two different models have been proposed to describe CAR assembly (Kamasaki et al., 2007; Vavylonis et al., 2008). The differences between these models reside essentially in the initial steps of CAR formation. However, these models appear to be complementary (see Roberts-Galbraith and Gould, 2008) and suggest that non overlapping mechanisms operate to carry out CAR assembly (Hachet and Simanis, 2008; Huang et al., 2008).

(a) The cortical node model

The first model proposes the existence of protein complexes named "cortical nodes" which form as a broad band at the centre of the cell. These nodes are composed of the Mid1 protein, the type II myosin heavy chain Myo2 and its light chains Rlc1 and Cdc4, the IQGAP Rng2 protein, profilin Cdc3 and formin Cdc12. The only essential component for node formation is Mid1 (Wu et al., 2006). It has been proposed that Cdc12 and Myo2 could stimulate the formation of a F-actin network between the nodes by a "capture" mechanism involving nucleation of F-actin cables (Wu et al., 2003; Wu and Pollard, 2005; Mishra and Oliferenko, 2008; Vavylonis et al., 2008). This F-actin network could eventually allow condensation of nodes and the formation of a ring structure. Later, this ring matures by the sequential incorporation of additional proteins such as tropomyosin Cdc8, alpha-actinin Ain1 and type II myosin heavy chain Myp2. However, the existence of a F-actin network between the nodes has not been clearly reported (Arai and Mabuchi, 2002; Kamasaki et al., 2007), nor the presence of the Myo2 activating protein Rng3 within the nodes of wild type cells (Lord and Pollard, 2004; Lord et al., 2008).

(b) The aster model

Studies of F-actin images using fluorescence microscopy and three-dimensional reconstitution of the medial ring with electron microscopy data led to another model for CAR assembly (Arai and Mabuchi, 2002; Kamasaki et al., 2007). In this model, F-actin cables which constitute the ring would be nucleated by Cdc12 from a single "leading cable" formed from a specific site called the aster at the centre of the cell (Chang, 1999; Arai and Mabuchi, 2002; Motegi et al., 2004; Kamasaki et al., 2007). Then, F-actin cables would progressively complete the cell equator and would serve as a scaffold structure to achieve formation of a mature ring. In contrast to the cortical node model, the aster model predicts that Cdc12 would function from a single site to promote actin nucleation and that the motor protein Myo2 is not involved in the initial steps of CAR formation.

(c) Role of the SIN singalling pathway in ring assembly

Initially, the Septum Initiation Network (SIN) signalling cascade was described for its role in maintenance and constriction of the CAR as well as in septum synthesis (for a review, see Krapp et al., 2004). It has also been proposed a direct role of the mitotic kinase Plo1 in regulating this pathway, suggesting a role for SIN components downstream of Plo1 function (Ohkura et al., 1995; Tanaka et al., 2001). Recently, Hachet and Simanis have unraveled a novel function of the SIN cascade in CAR assembly. These authors proposed distinct involvements of each model described above in ring formation (Hachet and Simanis, 2008). CAR assembly can be divided into three steps: (1) the formation of a cortical network of CAR proteins, (2) the lateral condensation of this network and (3) the maturation of the medial ring. The latter step, consisting of the incorporation of the Cdc15 protein into the CAR, depends on SIN function. Therefore, SIN mutants are unable to fully achieve CAR formation. In a heat sensitive *mid1-6* mutant unable to form cortical nodes, CAR formation is entirely under the control of the SIN signalling pathway and is carried out from an actomyosin filament rather than from a cortical protein network. This alternative mechanism may explain why such a pivotal gene product like Mid1 is not essential. Thus, the Mid1 protein and the SIN pathway regulate CAR assembly in parallel.

Conclusion

Accuracy of cytokinesis is essential for all living organisms in order to proliferate and maintain a high viability. Recent studies in the fission yeast *Schizosacharomyces pombe* have revealed the existence of multiple redundant mechanisms that prevent defects in specification or assembly of the contractile ring at mitosis. Thus, this single-celled organism has developed non overlapping mechanisms to preserve its cell division. Many aspects of the interplay between these pathways remain to be deciphered. Whether similar protective redundancy can be unraveled in other eukaryotes is an exciting perspective. A possible common theme may be the phosphoregulation of cytokinetic proteins mediated by conserved kinases.

References

Almonacid, M., Moseley, J. B., Janvore, J., Mayeux, A., Fraisier, V., Nurse, P., & Paoletti, A. (2009). Spatial control of cytokinesis by Cdr2 kinase and Mid1/anillin nuclear export. *Curr Biol, 19*, 961-966.

Arai, R., & Mabuchi, I. (2002). F-actin ring formation and the role of F-actin cables in the fission yeast Schizosaccharomyces pombe. *J Cell Sci, 115*, 887-898.

Bähler, J., & Nurse, P. (2001). Fission yeast Pom1p kinase activity is cell cycle regulated and essential for cellular symmetry during growth and division. *Embo J, 20*, 1064-1073.

Bähler, J., & Pringle, J. R. (1998). Pom1p, a fission yeast protein kinase that provides positional information for both polarized growth and cytokinesis. *Genes Dev, 12*, 1356-1370.

Bähler, J., Steever, A. B., Wheatley, S., Wang, Y., Pringle, J. R., Gould, K. L., & McCollum, D. (1998). Role of polo kinase and Mid1p in determining the site of cell division in fission yeast. *J Cell Biol, 143*, 1603-1616.

Balasubramanian, M. K., McCollum, D., Chang, L., Wong, K. C., Naqvi, N. I., He, X., Sazer, S., & Gould, K. L. (1998). Isolation and characterization of new fission yeast cytokinesis mutants. *Genetics, 149*, 1265-1275.

Breeding, C. S., Hudson, J., Balasubramanian, M. K., Hemmingsen, S. M., Young, P. G., & Gould, K. L. (1998). The cdr2(+) gene encodes a regulator of G2/M progression and cytokinesis in Schizosaccharomyces pombe. *Mol Biol Cell, 9*, 3399-3415.

Burgess, D. R., & Chang, F. (2005). Site selection for the cleavage furrow at cytokinesis. *Trends Cell Biol, 15*, 156-162.

Cadou, A., La Carbona, S., Couturier, A., Le Goff, C., & Le Goff, X. (2009). Role of the protein kinase Kin1 and nuclear centering in actomyosin ring formation in fission yeast. *Cell Cycle, 8*, 2451-2462.

Carnahan, R. H., & Gould, K. L. (2003). The PCH family protein, Cdc15p, recruits two F-actin nucleation pathways to coordinate cytokinetic actin ring formation in Schizosaccharomyces pombe. *J Cell Biol, 162*, 851-862.

Celton-Morizur, S., Bordes, N., Fraisier, V., Tran, P. T., & Paoletti, A. (2004). C-terminal anchoring of mid1p to membranes stabilizes cytokinetic ring position in early mitosis in fission yeast. *Mol Cell Biol, 24*, 10621-10635.

Celton-Morizur, S., Racine, V., Sibarita, J. B., & Paoletti, A. (2006). Pom1 kinase links division plane position to cell polarity by regulating Mid1p cortical distribution. *J Cell Sci, 119*, 4710-4718.

Chang, F. (1999). Movement of a cytokinesis factor cdc12p to the site of cell division. *Curr Biol, 9*, 849-852.

Chang, F., & Nurse, P. (1996). How fission yeast fission in the middle. *Cell, 84*, 191-194.

Chang, F., Woollard, A., & Nurse, P. (1996). Isolation and characterization of fission yeast mutants defective in the assembly and placement of the contractile actin ring. *J Cell Sci, 109 (Pt 1)*, 131-142.

Daga, R. R., & Chang, F. (2005). Dynamic positioning of the fission yeast cell division plane. *Proc Natl Acad Sci U S A, 102*, 8228-8232.

Daga, R. R., Yonetani, A., & Chang, F. (2006). Asymmetric microtubule pushing forces in nuclear centering. *Curr Biol, 16*, 1544-1550.

Fankhauser, C., Reymond, A., Cerutti, L., Utzig, S., Hofmann, K., & Simanis, V. (1995). The S. pombe cdc15 gene is a key element in the reorganization of F-actin at mitosis. *Cell, 82*, 435-444.

Hachet, O., & Simanis, V. (2008). Mid1p/anillin and the septation initiation network orchestrate contractile ring assembly for cytokinesis. *Genes Dev, 22*, 3205-3216.

Huang, Y., Chew, T. G., Ge, W., & Balasubramanian, M. K. (2007). Polarity determinants Tea1p, Tea4p, and Pom1p inhibit division-septum assembly at cell ends in fission yeast. *Dev Cell, 12*, 987-996.

Huang, Y., Yan, H., & Balasubramanian, M. K. (2008). Assembly of normal actomyosin rings in the absence of Mid1p and cortical nodes in fission yeast. *J Cell Biol, 183*, 979-988.

Kamasaki, T., Osumi, M., & Mabuchi, I. (2007). Three-dimensional arrangement of F-actin in the contractile ring of fission yeast. *J Cell Biol, 178*, 765-771.

Kanoh, J., & Russell, P. (1998). The protein kinase Cdr2, related to Nim1/Cdr1 mitotic inducer, regulates the onset of mitosis in fission yeast. *Mol Biol Cell, 9*, 3321-3334.

Krapp, A., Gulli, M. P., & Simanis, V. (2004). SIN and the Art of Splitting the Fission Yeast Cell. *Curr Biol, 14*, R722-730.

La Carbona, S., Allix, C., Philippe, M., & Le Goff, X. (2004). The protein kinase kin1 is required for cellular symmetry in fission yeast. *Biol Cell, 96*, 169-179.

La Carbona, S., Le Goff, C., & Le Goff, X. (2006). Fission yeast cytoskeletons and cell polarity factors: connecting at the cortex. *Biol Cell, 98*, 619-631.

La Carbona, S., & Le Goff, X. (2006). Spatial regulation of cytokinesis by the Kin1 and Pom1 kinases in fission yeast. *Curr Genet, 50*, 377-391.

Le Goff, X., Buvelot, S., Salimova, E., Guerry, F., Schmidt, S., Cueille, N., Cano, E., & Simanis, V. (2001). The protein phosphatase 2A B'-regulatory subunit par1p is implicated in regulation of the S. pombe septation initiation network. *FEBS Lett, 508*, 136-142.

Lord, M., & Pollard, T. D. (2004). UCS protein Rng3p activates actin filament gliding by fission yeast myosin-II. *J Cell Biol, 167*, 315-325.

Lord, M., Sladewski, T. E., & Pollard, T. D. (2008). Yeast UCS proteins promote actomyosin interactions and limit myosin turnover in cells. *Proc Natl Acad Sci U S A, 105*, 8014-8019.

Martin, S. G., & Berthelot-Grosjean, M. (2009). Polar gradients of the DYRK-family kinase Pom1 couple cell length with the cell cycle. *Nature, 459*, 852-856.

Martin, S. G., McDonald, W. H., Yates, J. R., 3rd, & Chang, F. (2005). Tea4p links microtubule plus ends with the formin for3p in the establishment of cell polarity. *Dev Cell, 8*, 479-491.

Mata, J., & Nurse, P. (1997). tea1 and the microtubular cytoskeleton are important for generating global spatial order within the fission yeast cell. *Cell, 89*, 939-949.

Mishra, M., & Oliferenko, S. (2008). Cytokinesis: Catch and Drag. *Curr Biol, 18*, R247-R250.

Morishita, M., & Shimoda, C. (2000). Positioning of medial actin rings affected by eccentrically located nuclei in a fission yeast mutant having large vacuoles. *FEMS Microbiol Lett, 188*, 63-67.

Morrell, J. L., Nichols, C. B., & Gould, K. L. (2004). The GIN4 family kinase, Cdr2p, acts independently of septins in fission yeast. *J Cell Sci, 117,* 5293-5302.

Moseley, J. B., Mayeux, A., Paoletti, A., & Nurse, P. (2009). A spatial gradient coordinates cell size and mitotic entry in fission yeast. *Nature, 459*, 857-860.

Motegi, F., Mishra, M., Balasubramanian, M. K., & Mabuchi, I. (2004). Myosin-II reorganization during mitosis is controlled temporally by its dephosphorylation and spatially by Mid1 in fission yeast. *J Cell Biol, 165*, 685-695.

Nurse, P., Thuriaux, P., & Nasmyth, K. (1976). Genetic control of the cell division cycle in the fission yeast Schizosaccharomyces pombe. *Mol Gen Genet, 146*, 167-178.

Ohkura, H., Hagan, I. M., & Glover, D. M. (1995). The conserved Schizosaccharomyces pombe kinase plo1, required to form a bipolar spindle, the actin ring, and septum, can drive septum formation in G1 and G2 cells. *Genes Dev, 9*, 1059-1073.

Padte, N. N., Martin, S. G., Howard, M., & Chang, F. (2006). The cell-end factor pom1p inhibits mid1p in specification of the cell division plane in fission yeast. *Curr Biol, 16*, 2480-2487.

Paoletti, A., & Chang, F. (2000). Analysis of mid1p, a protein required for placement of the cell division site, reveals a link between the nucleus and the cell surface in fission yeast. *Mol Biol Cell, 11*, 2757-2773.

Roberts-Galbraith, R. H., & Gould, K. L. (2008). Stepping into the ring: the SIN takes on contractile ring assembly. *Genes Dev, 22*, 3082-3088.

Sipiczki, M. (2007). Splitting of the fission yeast septum. *FEMS Yeast Res, 7*, 761-770.

Sipiczki, M., & Bozsik, A. (2000). The use of morphomutants to investigate septum formation and cell separation in Schizosaccharomyces pombe. *Arch Microbiol, 174*, 386-392.

Sohrmann, M., Fankhauser, C., Brodbeck, C., & Simanis, V. (1996). The dmf1/mid1 gene is essential for correct positioning of the division septum in fission yeast. *Genes Dev, 10*, 2707-2719.

Takeda, T., Kawate, T., & Chang, F. (2004). Organization of a sterol-rich membrane domain by cdc15p during cytokinesis in fission yeast. *Nat Cell Biol, 6*, 1142-1144.

Tanaka, K., Petersen, J., MacIver, F., Mulvihill, D. P., Glover, D. M., & Hagan, I. M. (2001). The role of Plo1 kinase in mitotic commitment and septation in Schizosaccharomyces pombe. *Embo J*, *20*, 1259-1270.

Tatebe, H., Nakano, K., Maximo, R., & Shiozaki, K. (2008). Pom1 DYRK regulates localization of the Rga4 GAP to ensure bipolar activation of Cdc42 in fission yeast. *Curr Biol*, *18*, 322-330.

Tatebe, H., Shimada, K., Uzawa, S., Morigasaki, S., & Shiozaki, K. (2005). Wsh3/Tea4 is a novel cell-end factor essential for bipolar distribution of Tea1 and protects cell polarity under environmental stress in S. pombe. *Curr Biol*, *15*, 1006-1015.

Tolic-Norrelykke, I. M., Sacconi, L., Stringari, C., Raabe, I., & Pavone, F. S. (2005). Nuclear and division-plane positioning revealed by optical micromanipulation. *Curr Biol*, *15*, 1212-1216.

Tran, P. T., Marsh, L., Doye, V., Inoue, S., & Chang, F. (2001). A mechanism for nuclear positioning in fission yeast based on microtubule pushing. *J Cell Biol*, *153*, 397-411.

Vavylonis, D., Wu, J.Q., Hao, S., O'Shaughnessy, B., & Pollard, T. D. (2008). Assembly mechanism of the contractile ring for cytokinesis by fission yeast. *Science*, *319*, 97-100.

Wachtler, V., Huang, Y., Karagiannis, J., & Balasubramanian, M. K. (2006). Cell cycle-dependent roles for the FCH-domain protein Cdc15p in formation of the actomyosin ring in Schizosaccharomyces pombe. *Mol Biol Cell*, *17*, 3254-3266.

Wu, J. Q., Kuhn, J. R., Kovar, D. R., & Pollard, T. D. (2003). Spatial and temporal pathway for assembly and constriction of the contractile ring in fission yeast cytokinesis. *Dev Cell*, *5*, 723-734.

Wu, J. Q., & Pollard, T. D. (2005). Counting cytokinesis proteins globally and locally in fission yeast. *Science*, *310*, 310-314.

Wu, J. Q., Sirotkin, V., Kovar, D. R., Lord, M., Beltzner, C. C., Kuhn, J. R., & Pollard, T. D. (2006). Assembly of the cytokinetic contractile ring from a broad band of nodes in fission yeast. *J Cell Biol*, *174*, 391-402.

In: Cell Division: Theory, Variants and Degradation
Editors: Y. N. Golitsin, M. C. Krylov, pp. 107-116
ISBN: 978-1-60876-986-5

Chapter 6

CELL CYCLE CHECKPOINTS AND CANCER

James A. Marcum[1*] and Zachary A. Marcum[2]
[1]Institute of Biomedical Studies, Baylor University, Waco, TX 76798.
[2]Division of Geriatric Medicine, Department of Medicine,
University of Pittsburgh, Pittsburgh, PA 15213.

ABSTRACT

Regulation of eukaryotic cell division is under tight control and includes several checkpoints. The controlling elements consist of cyclin-dependent kinases (CDKs) and their activators (cyclins) and inhibitors (INK4 and CIP/KIP). As the cell progresses through the cell cycle, various cyclins appear and bind to specific CDKs. These heterodimeric protein kinases are responsible for shuttling the cell through different regulatory checkpoints along the cell cycle. The major checkpoints include the G1/S checkpoint, which regulates entrance into the S-phase and the duplication of DNA; the G2/M checkpoint, which regulates entrance into mitosis and the alignment of the chromosomes; and the metaphase checkpoint, which regulates entrance into anaphase resulting in chromosome splitting and eventually in cell division. The connection between the cell cycle checkpoints and carcinogenesis involves checkpoint misregulation. This misregulation can lead to unscheduled cell division and cell proliferation and to genomic and chromosome instability associated with tumorigenesis. It is often the product of CDK mutation, overexpression of cyclins, or inactivation of CDK inhibitors. Finally, the mechanism of checkpoint (mis)regulation provides ample targets for developing drugs to treat cancer and represents a fecund area for future therapeutic developments.

INTRODUCTION

Over a decade ago in commentary on the future of cell division research, Noble Prize Laureate Paul Nurse (1998) encouraged biomedical researchers to investigate cell cycle

[*] Corresponding author: 254-710-3745 (office), 254-710-3838 (fax), E-mail: James_Marcum@baylor.edu.

checkpoint defects in malignant cells in order to understand better carcinogenesis and to develop effective therapies to cancer. Researchers responded to the challenge and identified several mechanisms responsible for regulating checkpoints, in terms of kinases and their activators and inhibitors (Morgan, 2006; Stein & Pardee, 2004). In this paper, recent developments in cell cycle checkpoints and cancer are examined and discussed. To that end, we first discuss briefly the mechanism of cell division and the role of checkpoints in regulating division. We then examine the mechanisms responsible for misregulation of these checkpoints in the generation of tumors and the opportunity these mechanisms afford for therapeutic developments. The paper concludes with comments on future directions for therapeutic developments *vis-à-vis* checkpoint misregulation.

CELL CYCLE CHECKPOINTS

Two major phases compose the eukaryotic cell division cycle: interphase (I) and mitosis (M), including cytokinesis (C), in the following order (Morgan, 2007).

I ⇨ M ⇨ C

During interphase the cell's **genome** doubles, while during mitosis it halves. Cytokinesis represents division of a cell into two cells. The three sequential phases comprising interphase are G1, S, and G2, along with a fourth phase—G0—as depicted diagrammatically.

G0

⇳

G1 ⇨ S ⇨ G2

After cytokenesis, the cell can opt out of the cell cycle by entering the G0 phase. Biologists often call this phase the resting cell phase, although the cells entering it generally differentiate into specific cell types. Cells in G0 can dedifferentiate and reenter the cell cycle, thereby undergoing division. The G1 phase represents the first gap in the cell cycle, after cytokinesis, and involves cell growth, including synthesis of enzymes needed for the duplication of the chromosomes during the next stage of the cell division cycle. The S phase begins with DNA replication and ends when chromosome duplication is complete, although ploidy remains the same. Histone synthesis also increases during this phase, along with duplication of the centrioles—which remain attached until mitosis. The final phase of interphase is G2, the second gap. During this phase, protein synthesis remains high and cell growth continues, especially in terms of microtubule synthesis. This phase, along with interphase, ends when the cell enters mitosis.

The four sequential phases comprising mitosis are prophase, metaphase, anaphase, and telophase, as shown chronologically.

prophase ⇨ metaphase ⇨ anaphase ⇨ telophase

The first phase, prophase, begins with condensation of the loosely coiled chromatin into highly structured chromotid. Since DNA replicated during S phase, each chromosome consists of identical chromotids. In addition, the centrioles split and migrate opposite each other in the cell. Each centriole is the origin for the production of spindle fibers, composed of microtubules. The next phase is metaphase, which begins with dissolution of the nuclear membrane. Each spindle fiber, from opposing centrioles, then binds to a separate pair of chromotids at the centromere to both kinetichore and non-kinetichore microtubules. The chromotids then line up in the center of the cell, with the use of motor proteins, along the metaphase or equatorial plate. At the conclusion of this phase, each pair of chromotids attaches to spindle fibers from each opposing centriole; hence, a dynamic tension exists pulling each chromotid pair in opposite directions. Anaphase begins with the splitting of the chromotid pairs at the centromeres. Each chromotid then migrates along a spindle fiber, by shortening kinetichore microtubules and elongating non-kinetichore microtubules, towards an opposing centriole. Anaphase ends when the chromotids migrate completely to opposite centrioles. The final phase of mitosis is telophase, with the appearance of a nuclear membrane around each set of chromosomes. The chromosomes then unwind to form chromatin again. Finally, cytokinesis, a separate process from mitosis, represents the division of the original cell into two cells. It begins at the same time as telophase. A cleavage furrow develops along the cell's equatorial plate, formed by a ring of contractile proteins, and progresses until the cell splits in two.

Regulation of cell division is under tight control and includes several checkpoints (Morgan, 2007). The controlling elements consist of protein kinases and their activators (cyclins) and inhibitors (INK4/ARF and CIP/KIP). The cyclin-dependent kinases (CDKs) that regulate interphase are CDKs 2, 4, and 6 and the kinase that regulates mitosis is CDK1. They phosphorylate various targets important in cell cycle division events. As the cell progresses through the cell cycle, various cyclins appear and bind to specific CDKs. The D cyclins, in response to external signals such as growth factors, are responsible for activating CDKs 4 and 6 and thereby regulating the G1 phase of the cell cycle by inducing the cyclins important for the S phase. D cyclins represent a class of cyclins, including cyclins D1, D2, and D3. Cyclins A and E activate CDK 2 and are then responsible for regulating the S stage by promoting DNA replication. Cyclins A and E are also classes of cyclins, including cyclins A1 and A2 and cyclins E1 and E2. Finally, the B cyclins activate CDK1 and are thus responsible for regulating events involved in mitosis, such as membrane dissolution. Again, the B cyclins are a class of cyclins, including cyclins B1, B2, and B3. These heterodimeric protein kinase complexes are responsible for shuttling the cell through various regulatory checkpoints along the cell cycle. The inhibitors, INK4/ARF and CIP/KIP, prevent the protein complexes from functioning (Besson, *et al.*, 2008; De Falco, *et al.*, 2002). The INK4/ARF family of inhibitors, such as p15, p16, p18, and p19, binds CDK4 and seizes the cell cycle at the G1 phase. The CIP/KIP family of inhibitors, such as p21, p27, and p 57, binds a broader spectrum of kinase complexes, including CDK2-cyclin E and CDK2-cyclin A, which arrests the cell cycle in the S phase, as well as CDK4-cyclin D.

Regulation of cell division consists of several cell cycle checkpoints (Morgan, 2007). The major checkpoints include the G1/S or the restriction checkpoint, the G2/M checkpoint, and the metaphase or mitotic spindle checkpoint. The G1/S or the restriction checkpoint regulates entrance of the cell from the G1 phase to the S phase and the duplication of DNA. Essentially this checkpoint determines whether the cell is ready to undergo cell division and whether the machinery is in place to replicate its DNA. The inhibitor p16INK4a is mainly responsible for regulating this checkpoint. The inhibitor binds the G1 CDKs and inactivates them. However, increase titer of cyclin D1 competes with the inhibitor and activates the kinases. The activated kinases then phosphorylate the RB tumor suppressor protein, which can no longer inhibit the transcription factor E2F. The transcription factor facilitates the expression of cyclin E, which activates CDK 2 and shuttles the cell into the S phase.

The G2/M checkpoint regulates the cell's entrance into mitosis and the alignment of the chromosomes during metaphase. One of the main functions of the G1/S and G2/M or DNA damage checkpoints is assessment of DNA damage during cell division. Response to this regulation can be either repair of the damaged DNA or, if repair is not possible, then cell death or apoptosis. The chief regulating factor for the G2/M checkpoint is the mitosis or maturation promoting factor (MPF), which consists of CDK1 and cyclin B. MPF functions to promote chromatin condensation, spindle formation, and nuclear membrane dissolution. It also inhibits cytokenesis by phosphorylating myosin.

The metaphase or mitotic spindle assembly checkpoint regulates entrance into anaphase resulting in chromosome splitting and eventually in cell division. The chief function of this checkpoint is to ensure proper alignment of the chromotids along the metaphase plate. Upon proper alignment of the chromotids, CDC25 activates the anaphase-promoting complex (APC), which consists of an E3 ubiquitin ligase. The main function of APC is to promote chromotid splitting through the ubiquinization of securin, an inhibitor of separase. Separase is responsible for degrading cohesin, which binds the chromotid pair at the centromere. APC also degrades MPF by ubiquinating cyclin B, thereby promoting cytokenesis.

Carcinogenesis

The connection between the cell cycle checkpoints and carcinogenesis involves checkpoint misregulation (Dash & El-Deiry, 2004; Hook, *et al.*, 2007; Kastan & Bartek, 2004; Malumbres & Barbacid, 2009). This misregulation can lead to unscheduled cell division and proliferation or to genomic and chromosome instability associated with tumorigenesis (Qi & Yu, 2006). Misregulation is often the product of CDK mutation, cyclin overexpression, or CDK inhibitor inactivation, which can lead to kinase hyperactivity. Such misregulation of cell division may result in cells not stopping at the DNA damage checkpoints, so that cells continue to divide, or at the spindle assembly checkpoint, so that cells' genome and chromosomes become unstable. Both uncontrolled growth and genetic or chromosome instability are main characteristics of cancer cells and tumors.

Misregulation of interphase CDKs is important in oncogenesis in a variety of tissues. Generally, CDK4 misregulation occurs in carcinoma or epithelial cancers while CDK6 misregulation in sarcoma or mesenchymal cancers (Malumbres & Barbacid, 2009). CDK misregulation often results from mutation or overexpression of the kinase. To date, only CDK4 mutation has been observed in human cancers. Generally, CDK mutation results in an inability to modulate CDK activity *via* inhibitors. For example, a miscoding mutation of CDK4 found in certain melanomas results in decrease binding of the INK4 inhibitor to the kinase (Ortega, *et al.*, 2002). Transgenic mice in which the normal CDK4 gene is replaced with a gene, whose kinase is insensitive to INK inhibitors, are prone to spontaneous generation of tumors (Malumbres, *et al.*, 2003). In some cases, CDK misregulation leads to overexpression of the kinase. CDK overexpression is particularly important in such cancers as breast cancer, glioma, leukemia and lymphoma, melanoma, and sarcoma (Malumbres & Barbacid, 2009). For example, overexpression of CDK4 is associated with glioblastoma multiforme, while overexpression of CDK6 occurs in a variety of leukemias and lymphomas (Malumbres & Barbacid, 2009; Sherr & McCormick, 2002).

Although interphase CDKs are important in normal cell division, recent studies demonstrate that the role of these kinases is not essential for cell division (Malumbres & Barbacid, 2009; Santamaria & Ortega, 2006). For example, CDK2 inhibition via p27 failed to prevent the proliferation of cancer cells (Tetsu & McCormick, 2003). There is a tremendous amount of redundancy and promiscuity in the cell cycle, such that CDKs and cyclins are not necessary for driving cell division and development in specific tissues. For example, CDK4, CDK6, and CDK2 are not indispensable for normal embryonic development (Barrière, *et al.*, 2007). In addition, null p53 transgenic mice with ablation of CDK2 developed spontaneous lymphoblastic lymphomas, as well as null p53 cells with loss of CDK4 and CDK6 (Padmakumar, *et al.*, 2009). Although the interphase CDKs are not necessary for regulating cell cycle division, the mitotic CDK1 appears to be essential for normal cell division and organism development (Hoffmann, 2006; Nigg, 2001). For example, CDK1 knockout mice do not develop beyond a 2-cell embryo, while interphase knockout mice embryos do (Malumbres & Barbacid, 2009). Thus, the model for cell cycle division now appears to be comparable to a yeast model in which only one CDK is necessary for driving cell division. This mitotic kinase is thought to be responsible for carcinogenesis and to provide a unique opportunity for treatment.

In addition, misregulation of interphase cyclins is also important in tumorigenesis. Overexpression of cyclin D1 occurs in a number of cancers, including bladder, breast, esophageal, and lung, while overexpression of D2 and D3 occurs in certain leukemias and colorectal cancers. For example, besides cyclin D3 upregulation, which is important in progression through G1/S for lymphocytic leukemia, cyclin D2 upregulation also occurs (Decker, *et al.*, 2002). In addition, overexpression of cyclin A1 in a mouse transgenic model is associated with myeloid leukemia and is found in human leukemias and hematopoietic malignances (Liao, *et al.*, 2001). Besides overexpression of cyclins, ablation of these CDK activators is also important in tumorigenesis. For example, cyclin E ablation in cells bestows resistance to oncogenic transformation since cells are unable to undergo G0/S transition (Geng, *et al.*, 2003). Moreover, in mouse tumor models cyclin D1 ablation, which causes a putative reduction in CDK4 activity, prevents tumor formation in breast tissue driven by ERBB2 and HRAS oncogenes (Landis, *et al.*, 2006; Reddy, *et al.*, 2005; Yu, *et al.*, 2006). However, in similar studies ablation of this cyclin was unable to prevent tumor formation in such tissue driven by MYC and WNT1 oncogenes (Yu, *et al.* 2001).

Finally, misregulation of CDK inhibitors is another important factor in carcinogenesis (Decker, *et al.*, 2002; De Falco, *et al.*, 2002; Diaz-Padilla, *et al.*, 2009; Slingerland & Pagano, 2000). These inhibitors are important in preventing phase transition during cell cycle division and their removal through downregulation or genetic mutation often results in unscheduled cell division and proliferation. The INK4 family of inhibitors plays a critical role in carcinogenesis. For example, p15 is genetically mutated in leukemia, lymphoma, and myeloma, p16 in bladder cancer, leukemia, lymphoma, lung cancer, thyroid cancer, and ovarian cancer, and p18 in meningioma. The CIP/KIP family of CDK inhibitors is also important in oncogenesis for a large variety of tissues. For instance, p21 is downregulated in colon cancer, p27 in breast cancer, colon cancer, leukemia and lymphoma, lung cancer, and prostate cancer, and p57 in bladder and gastric cancer. Finally, p21 and p27 might play a particularly important role in carcinogenesis, since they inhibit the mitotic kinase CDK1 (Malumbres & Barbacid, 2009).

THERAPUETIC DEVLOPMENTS

The mechanism of checkpoint regulation provides multiple targets for developing drugs to treat cancer (Deep & Agarwl, 2008; Malumbres & Barbacid, 2009). Most therapeutic agents include inhibitors of CDKs (Diaz-Padilla, *et al.*, 2009; Shapiro, 2006). The inhibitors can be broad spectrum or specific for a particular CDK. The latter approach appears to be the better approach since experimental studies with CDK regulation demonstrate tissue specificity of CDK-controlled cell cycle checkpoints involvement in carcinogenesis (Malumbres & Barbacid, 2009). First-generation CDK inhibitors were broad spectrum. For example, flavopiridol (HMR 1275) is the best-known panCDK inhibitor and the first used in clinical trials to treat a variety of cancers (Senderowicz, 1999). It inhibits a variety of CDKs, including CDKs 1, 2, 3, 6, 7, and 9. Initially, flavopiridol demonstrated promising potential pre-clinically by blocking G1/S and G2/M transition, inhibiting angiogenesis, and inducing apoptosis or differentiation. However, this inhibitor along with other first generation CDK inhibitors failed to realize their expected clinical potential (Diaz-Padilla, *et al.*, 2009; Malumbres & Barbacid, 2009). Part of the problem are the side effects and toxicities associated with inhibition of CDKs associated with other crucial biological processes. Such side effects and toxicities prevented using the inhibitors at therapeutic dosages.

Another problem with the first-generation CDK inhibitors is that they target CDK2, among other CDKs. However, preclinical trials demonstrate that CDK2 is not essential for mitotic cell division and that other CDKs can compensate for its loss (Ortega, *et al.*, 2003). Currently second-generation CDK inhibitors are being developed that are more specific or selective with respect to the kinase inhibited, especially CDK4 (Diaz-Padilla, *et al.*, 2009; Shapiro, 2006). For example, Pfizer is currently sponsoring clinical trials with an oral CDK inhibitor, PD-033299, which inhibits CDK4 and 6 specifically. Preclinical trials demonstrate that the inhibitor arrests RB-positive cancer cells at the G1 stage (Fry, *et al.*, 2004; Toogood, *et al.*, 2005). Oral administration of the inhibitor in a human colon-cancer mouse model produced a significant regression of the tumor. Currently, a phase I trial (NCT00141297) is being conducted to evaluate the safety and tolerability of the CDK inhibitor. The test subjects are patients with RB-positive advanced solid tumors or diffuse large cell non-Hodgkin lymphomas refractory to established therapy. In addition, a phase I/II trial (NCT00721409) with the inhibitor is being conducted with postmenopausal women exhibiting ER-positive and HER2-negative breast cancer to evaluate its safety and effectiveness, particularly in combination with aromatase inhibitor, letrozole. PD-033299 represents a promising drug for treating cancer because of its unique action of mechanism and oral administration, although much research is still required to determine its efficacy.

Finally, SNS-032 from Sunesis Pharmaceuticals is another unique CDK inhibitor under clinical study (Ali, *et al.*, 2007; Chen, *et al.*, 2009). It specifically inhibits the CDKs 2, 7, and

9, resulting in cell division block through CDKs 2 and 7 inhibition and in impeding transcription through CDKs 7 and 9 inhibition (Conroy, *et al.*, 2009). Preclinical trials demonstrate *in vivo* activity in a variety of cancer animal models, including ovarian and colon cancer. Unfortunately, attempts to determine maximum tolerated and administrated doses, as well as dose limiting toxicity, for phase II trials were unsuccessful (Heath, *et al.*, 2008). The most common side effects during treatment were fatigue and nausea. However, clinical evidence demonstrated the possibility of developing an oral bioavailability of this CDK inhibitor in the near future. Currently, two phase I trials (NCT00446342 and NCT00292864) are under way with SNS-032 to define better the drug's pharmacokinetic profile in patients with B-lymphoid and refractory solid tumors. Other CDK inhibitors are also being developed currently, but the future for this class of drugs remains to be established (Ali, *et al.*, 2009; Kojima, *et al.*, 2009).

FUTURE DIRECTIONS

The future directions for CDK inhibitors include at least two paths. The first is the development of third-generation mitotic CDK inhibitors to address the pharmacodynamic and pharmacokinetic problems associated with the first two generations of CDK inhibitors (De Castro, *et al.*, 2008; Malumbres, *et al.*, 2008). The assumption behind this newer generation of inhibitors is the inhibition of a single CDK in a specific tumor. This approach depends upon the development of technology that will enable researchers to assess the three-dimensional structure of inhibitor-enzyme interaction and to assay large number of potential inhibitors using a more complete battery of mitotic kinases. The second path in the future development of CDK inhibitor therapy is combinatorial drug therapeutics (Deep & Agarwal, 2008; Dickson & Schwartz, 2009). Combinatorial therapeutics takes advantage of the synergy between the actions of several drugs (Marcum, 2009). For example, combination of flavopiridol with cisplatin and carboplatin revealed that cisplatin provides an acceptable combinatorial drug with flavopiridol but not carboplatin (Bible, *et al.*, 2005). In addition, combination of the CDK4/6 inhibitor, PD-0332991, with the proteaosome inhibitor, bortezomib, potentiated the growth inhibition of myeloma cell lines (Menu, *et al.*, 2008). Ideally, safe and effective third-generation CDK inhibitor therapy would possess favorable pharmacodynamic and pharmacokinetic profiles (including good oral bioavailability) in order to maximize therapeutic benefit while minimizing adverse side effects.

In conclusion, cancer is a disease of cell-cycle division misregulation. Although much is currently known about the regulation of the cell cycle checkpoints, much more is certainly needed to provide a comprehensive analysis of misregulation in diseases such as cancer, including information on other components involved in cell cycle regulation, such asCDC25 phosphotase and the mitotic Aurora and Polo-like kinases (De Castro, *et al.*, 2008; Deep & Agarwl, 2008). As biomedical researchers identify the differences between normal and transformed cells, therapeutic regimens can be tailored not only to the specific type of cancer but also to the patient suffering from the disease.

REFERENCES

Ali, M. A., Choy, H., Habib, A. A. & Saha, D. (2007). SNS-032 prevents cell-induced angiogenesis by inhibiting vascular endothelial cell growth factor. *Neoplasia*, *19*, 370-381.

Ali, S., Heathcote, D. A., Kroll, S. H., Jogalekar, A. S., Scheiper, B., Patel, H., Brackow, J., Siwicka, A., Fuchter, M. J., Periyasamy, M., Tolhurst, R. S., Kanneganti, S. K., Snyder, J. P., Liotta, D. C., Aboagye, E. O., Barrett, A. G. & Coombes, R. C. (2009). The development of a selective cyclin-dependent kinase inhibitor that shows antitumor activity. *Cancer Research*, *69*, 6208-6215.

Barrière, C., Santamaria, D., Cerqueira, A., Galán, J., Martin, A., Ortega, S., Malumbres, M., Dubus, P. & Barbacid, M. (2007). Mice thrive without CDK4 and CDK2. *Molecular Oncology*, *1*, 72-83.

Besson, A., Dowdy, S.F. & Roberts, J. M. (2008). CDK inhibitors: cell cycle regulation. *Developmental Cell*, *14*, 159-169.

Bible, K. C., Lensing, J. L., Nelson, S. A., Lee, Y. K., Reid, J. M., Ames, M. M., Isham, C. R., Piens, J., Rubin, S. L., Rubin, J., Kaufmann, S. H., Atherton, P. J., Sloan, J. A., Daiss, M.K., Adjei, A. A. & Erlichman, C. (2005). Phase 1 trial of flavopiridol combined with cisplatin and carboplatin in patients with advanced malignancies with the assessment of pharmacokinetic and pharmacodynamic end points. *Clinical Cancer Research*, *11*, 5935-5941.

Chen, R., Wierda, W. G., Chubb, S., Hawtin, R. E., Fox, J. A., Keating, M. J., Gandhi, V. & Plunkett, W. (2009). Mechanism of action of SNS-032, a novel cyclin dependent kinase inhibitor, in chronic lymphocytic leukemia. *Blood*, *113*, 4637-4645.

Conroy, A., Stockett, D. E., Walker, D., Arkin, M. R., Hoch, U., Fox, J. A. & Hawtin, R. E. (2009). SNS-032 is a potent and selective CDK 2, 7 and 9 inhibitor that drives target modulation in patient samples. *Cancer Chemotherapy and Pharmacology*, *64*, 723-732.

Dash, B. C. & El-Deiry, W. S. (2004). Cell cycle checkpoint control mechanisms that can be disrupted in cancer. *Methods in Molecular Biology*, *280*, 99-161.

De Castro, I. P., de Carcer, G., Montoya, G. & Malumbres, M. (2008). Emerging cancer therapeutic opportunities by inhibiting mitotic kinases. *Current Opinion in Pharmacology*, *8*, 375-383.

Decker, T., Schneller, F., Hipp, S., Miething, C., Jahn, T. & Peschel, C. (2002). Cell cycle progression of chronic lymphocytic leukemia is controlled by cyclin D2, cyclin D3, cyclin-dependent kinase (cdk) 4 and the cdk inhibitor p 27. *Leukemia*, *16*, 327-334.

Deep, G. & Agarwal, R. (2008). New combination therapies with cell cycle agents. *Current Opinion in Investigational Drugs*, *9*, 591-604.

De Falco, G., Soprano, C. & Giordano, A. (2002). Cdk inhibitors: background and introduction. In A. Giordano, & K.J. Soprano (Eds.), *Cell cycle inhibitors in cancer therapy: Current strategies* (pp. 1-10). Totowa, NJ: Humana Press.

Diaz-Padilla, I., Siu, L. L. & Duran, I. (2009). Cyclin-dependent kinase inhibitors as potential targeted anticancer agents. *Investigational New Drugs*, *27*, 586-594.

Dickson, M. A. & Schwartz, G. K. (2009). Development of cell-cycle inhibitors for cancer therapy. *Current Oncology*, *16*, 36-43.

Fry, D. W., Harvey, P. J., Keller, P. R., Elliot, W. L., Meade, M., Trachet, E., Albassam, M., Zheng, X., Leopold, W. R., Pryer, N. K. & Toogood, P. L. (2005). Specific inhibition of cyclin-dependent kinase 4/6 by PD 0332991 and associated antitumor activity in human tumor xenografts. *Molecular Cancer Therapeutics*, *3*, 1427-1438.

Geng, Y., Yu, O., Sicinska, E., Das, M., Schneider, J. E., Bhattacharya, S., Rideout, W. M., Bronson, R. T., Gardner, H. & Sicinski, P. (2003). Cyclin E ablation in the mouse. *Cell*, *114*, 431-443.

Heath, E. I., Bible, K., Martell, R. E., Adelman, D. C. & LoRusso, P. M. (2008). A phase I study of SNS-032 (formerly BMS-387032), a potent inhibitor of cyclin-dependent kinases 2, 7 and 9 administered as a single oral dose and weekly infusion in patients with metastatic refractory solid tumors. *Investigational New Drugs*, *26*, 59-85.

Hoffmann, I. (2006). Protein kinases involved in mitotic spindle checkpoint regulation. *Results and Problems in Cell Differentiation*, *42*, 93-109.

Hook, S. S., Lin, J. J. & Dutta, A. (2007). Mechanisms to control replication and implications for cancer. *Current Opinion in Cell Biology*, *19*, 663-671.

Kastan, M. B. & Bartek, J. (2004). Cell cycle checkpoints and cancer. *Nature*, *432*, 316-323.

Kojima, K., Shimanuki, M., Shikami, M., Andreeff, M., Nakakuma, H. (2009). Cyclin-dependent kinase 1 inhibitor RO-3306 enhances p53-mediated Bax activation and mitochondrial apoptosis in AML. *Cancer Science*, *100*, 1128-1136.

Landis, M. W., Pawlyk, B. S., Li, T., Sincinski, P. & Hinds, P. W. (2006). Cyclin D1-dependent kinase activity in murine development and mammary tumorigenesis. *Cancer Cell*, 9, 13-22.

Liao, C., Wang, X. Y., Wei, H. Q., Li, S. Q., Merghoub, T., Pandolfi, P. P. & Wolgemuth, D. J. (2001). Altered myelopoiesis and the development of acute myeloid leukemia in transgenic mice overexpressing cyclin A1. *Proceedings of the National Academy of Sciences (USA)*, *98*, 6853-6858.

Malumbres, M. & Barbacid, M. (2009). Cell cycle, CDKs and cancer: a changing paradigm. *Nature Reviews Cancer*, *9*, 153-166.

Malumbres, M., Hunt, S. L., Sotillo, R., Martin, J., Odajima, J., Dubus, P., Ortega, S. & Barbacid, M. (2003). Driving the cell cycle to cancer. *Advances in Experimental Medicine and Biology*, 532, 1-11.

Malumbres, M., Pevarello, P., Barbacid, M. & Bischoff, J. R. (2008). CDK inhibitors in cancer therapy; what is next? *Trends in Pharmacological Sciences*, *29*, 16-21.

Marcum, J. A. (2009). Cancer biology: from molecular biology to systems biology. Forthcoming in T. D. Ford (ed.). *New cancer research developments*. Hauppauge, NY: Nova Science Publishers.

Menu, E., Garcia, J., Huang, X., Di Liberto, M., Toogood, P. L., Chen, I., Vanderkerken, K. & Cheng-Kiang, S. (2008). A novel therapeutic combination using PD 0332991 and bortezomib: study in the 5T33MM myeloma model. *Cancer Research*, *68*, 5519-5523.

Morgan, D. O. (2006). *The cell cycle: Principles of control*. New Science Press.

Nigg, E. A. (2001). Mitotic kinases as regulators of cell division and its checkpoints. *Nature Reviews Molecular Cell Biology*, *2*, 21-32.

Nurse, P. (1998). Understanding the cell cycle: past, present and future. *Nature Medicine*, *4*, 1103-1004.

Ortega, S., Malumbres, M. & Barbacid, M. (2002). Cyclin D-dependent kinases, INK4 inhibitors and cancer. *Biochimica et Biophysica Acta*, *1602*, 73-87.

Ortega, S., Prieto, I., Odajima, J., Martin, A., Dubus, P., Sotillo, R., Barbero, J. L., Malumbres, M. & Barbacid, M. (2003). Cyclin-dependent kinase 2 is essential for meiosis but not for mitotic cell division. *Nature Genetics*, *35*, 25-31.

Padmakumar, V. C., Aleem, E., Berthet, C., Hilton, M. B. & Kaldis, P. (2009). Cdk2 and Cdk4 activities are dispensable for tumorigenesis caused by the loss of p53. *Molecular and Cell Biology*, *29*, 2582-2593.

Qi, W. & Yu, H. (2006). The spindle checkpoint and chromosomal stability. *Genome Dynamics*, *1*, 116-130.

Reddy, H. K., Mettus, R. V., Rane, S. G., Grana, X., Litvin, J. & Reddy, E. P. (2005). Cyclin-dependent kinase 4 expression is essential for neu-induced breast tumorigenesis. *Cancer Research*, *65*, 10174-10178.

Santamaria, D. & Ortega, S. (2006). Cyclins and CDKS in development and cancer: lessons from genetically modified mice. *Frontiers in Bioscience*, *11*, 1164-1188.

Senderowicz, A. M. (1999). Flavopiridol: the first cyclin-dependent kinase inhibitor in human clinical trials. *Investigational New Drugs*, *17*, 313-320.

Shapiro, G. I. (2006). Cyclin-dependent kinase pathways as targets for cancer treatment. *Journal of Clinical Oncology*, *24*, 1770-1783.

Sherr, C. J. & McCormick, F. (2002). The RB and p53 pathways in cancer. *Cancer Cell*, *2*, 103-112.

Slingerland, J. & Pagano, M. (2000). Regulation of the Cdk inhibitor p27 and its deregulation in cancer. *Journal of Cellular Physiology*, *183*, 10-17.

Stein G. S. & Pardee, A. B. (eds.) (2004). *Cell cycle and growth control: Biomolecular regulation and cancer* (2nd edition). Hoboken, NJ: John Wiley & Sons.

Tetsu, O. & McCormick, F. (2003). Proliferation of cancer cells despite CDK2 inhibition. *Cancer Cell*, *3*, 233-245.

Toogood, P. L., Harvey, P. J., Repine, J. T., Sheehan, D. J., VanderWel, S. N., Zhou, H., Keller, P. R., McNamara, D. J., Sherry, D., Zhu, T., Brodfuehrer, J., Choi, C., Barvian, M. R. & Fry, D. W. (2005). Discovery of a potent and selective inhibitor of cyclin-dependent kinase 4/6. *Journal of Medicinal Chemistry*, *48*, 2388-2406.

Yu, O., Geng, Y. & Sincinski, P. (2001). Specific protection against breast cancers by cyclin D1 ablation. *Nature*, *411*, 1017-1021.

Yu, O., Sincinski, E., Geng, Y., Ahnström, M., Zagozdzon, A., Kong, Y., Gardner, H., Kiyokawa, H., Harris, L.N., Stål, O. & Sincinski, P. (2006). Requirement for CDK4 kinase function in breast cancer. *Cancer Cell*, *9*, 23-32.

In: Cell Division: Theory, Variants and Degradation
Editors: Y. N. Golitsin, M. C. Krylov, pp. 117-126
ISBN: 978-1-60876-986-5

Chapter 7

Cohesin and Cohesin-Regulator Complexes: From Cell Division to Gene Expression Control

José L. Barbero *

Cell Proliferation and Development Program. Chromosome Dynamics in Meiosis Laboratory. Centro de Investigaciones Biológicas (CSIC), Ramiro de Maeztu 9, E-28040 Madrid, Spain.

Abstract

About a decade ago, a four-protein complex denominated the cohesin complex emerged as a key player on the control of sister chromatid cohesion during cell division. In addition, during the last 2-3 years, new findings have implicated the cohesin complex in the control of gene expression, development and other essential cell functions in mammals.

The function of cohesin complex in chromosome segregation is mediated by the formation of a ring-like structure, which entrapped replicated DNA. The dynamic of the cohesin ring is regulated by a more and more large number of cohesin-interacting proteins. Cohesin-regulators were essentially identified and studied in relation with the cohesion function of cohesin complexes. However, recent results on the phenotype of mouse KO models and the discovery that mutations in some cohesin-regulator genes are the molecular causes of Cornelia de Lange and Roberts syndrome/Phocomelia human disorders suggested that these proteins are also involved in other important biological tasks of cohesins.

Keywords: Chromosome segregation, cohesin, cohesin–regulators, cohesinopathies, CTCF, gene expression control, insulators, neuron development, sister chromatid cohesion, viral transcription control.

* Corresponding author: E-mail: jlbarbero@cib.csic.es, Tel.: +34 918373112 ext 4311, Fax: +34 915360432

INTRODUCTION

Rigorous control of sister chromatid cohesion during cell division ensures proper distribution of genetic material to daughter cells. Sister chromatid cohesion is mediated by a multiprotein cohesin complex, which was firstly characterized in *Saccharomyces* and *Xenopus* [1-3]. Based on biochemical and immunocytological results, it was proposed that the canonical cohesin complex was composed of four evolutionarily conserved core subunits; two that belong to the structural maintenance of chromosomes family of proteins (SMC1 and SMC3), one kleisin α (from the Greek word for closure) subunit SCC1/RAD21, and stromalin SCC3/SA/STAG. According to structural characteristic of SMC proteins and electronic microscopy results, it was suggested that these complexes form a ring-like structure and mediate cohesion by embracing chromatin fibers from the two sister chromatids [4,5]. Sister chromatid cohesion is maintained until metaphase/anaphase transition when the activation of a specific protease, separase, cleaves the Scc1 subunit allowing chromatid segregation [6].

In parallel with the studies on cohesin role, different genetic approaches carried out in yeast showed the requirement of the function of an ever-increasing number of proteins for correct control of sister chromatid cohesion. Cohesin-regulators include Ctf4, a protein associated with DNA polymerase and the clamp-loader RFC complex proteins Ctf8 and Ctf18; kinases such polo-like kinase 1, Aurora B and Haspin/Gsg2, phospatase PP2A, proteases as separase, etc. [for a review see 7]. Adherin complex, a two-subunits, Scc2/Scc4, is required for the cohesin loading into chromosomes [8,9]. Eco1/Ctf7p acetyltransferase [10-13] is essential for the establishment, but dispensable for the maintenance of cohesion. Shugoshins Sgo1 and Sgo2 [14] protect the centromeric cohesion. Another three cohesion-regulator proteins PDS5 [15-17], WAPL [18,19] and sororin [20] are involved in the control of the association/dissociation of cohesin complexes to chromatin.

In addition to their canonical role as "chromosome glue" during cell division, cohesins are involved in additional cellular mechanisms including centromeric heterochromatin formation, post-replicative double-strand break repair and gene expression in interphase. A number of recent studies report cohesin expression and function in post-mitotic cells, as well as the involvement of cohesin and cohesin-interacting protein gene mutations in human pathologies.

Recently, new reported results are improving our knowledge about the molecular mechanisms by which cohesin-regulator complexes modulate the cohesin ring dynamic during cell cycle. These findings are changing our concept of the cohesin complexes, indicating that the name "cohesin" is probably a partial reflection of the many functions of these proteins in the cell.

COHESIN COMPLEX LOADING, COHESION ESTABLISHMENT AND COHESINOPATHIES

In *Saccharomyces cerevisiae* mitosis, the cohesin complexes are loaded near G1 to S phase, but cohesins bind to chromatin in telophase in most organisms studied [21]. The loading of cohesin complex to chromosomes depends on the Scc2/Scc4 adherin complex

[8,9]. The loading of cohesin to chromatin is not sufficient for the cohesion function in chromosome segregation and the Eco1/Ctf7p acetyltransferase is required for the establishment of cohesion [10,11]. A substrate of Eco1 acetylase is SMC3 and this cohesin subunit is acetylated in an Eco1-dependent manner during replication to promote sister chromatid cohesion [22,23]. This mechanism is conserved from yeast to man [23]. Human SMC3 is acetylated at K105 and K106 by the human Eco1 homolog ESCO1; these acetylation sites are located in the middle of the N-terminal head domain, which contains the "Walker A" nucleotide-binding domain and it could be important in the interactions of SMC1/SMC3 heterodimer with SCC1 for closing the ring.

Recently, new findings by independent groups addressed the mechanism by which cohesin-regulator complexes modulate the cohesin ring dynamic during cell cycle. In yeast *S. cerevisiae* mitosis, studies with different cohesin and cohesin-regulator mutants suggest the presence of a tripartite cohesin complex, formed by Smc1/Smc3 heterodimer and Scc1/Rad21 (Figure 1A) and a controlling complex composed by Scc3/STAG, Rad61/WAPL and PDS5 (it is designated as *security* complex in figure 1A), that regulates the opening/closing of cohesin ring [24]. Acetylation of SMC3 cohesin complex subunit modulates the on/off stage of security complex allowing the cohesion establishment (Figure 1B) similar to the working mechanism of a mountain climbing locking carabiner (Figure 1C). More recently, Heidinger-Pauli et al. 2009 [25] showed that Eco1 acetylates a different target, the cohesin subunit Sccl/Mcd1p, to generate cohesion after double strand break (DBS) in G2/M. Tacking into account that other two related proteins Scc3 and Pds5 have been reported as Eco1 substrates *in vitro*, perhaps the acetylation of a specific target by Eco1 controls the generation of cohesion in distinct DNA dynamic processes.

The loading of cohesin complex and the generation of cohesion are key processes in cell life. Mutations in genes encoding adherin SCC2, cohesin subunits SMC1 and SMC3 [reviewed in 26] and cohesin regulator PDS5B [27] are involved in the different phenotypes of human Cornelia de Lange Syndrome (OMIM: 122470, 300590, 610759). Mutations in the gene encoding for human ESCO1, the homolog to yeast Eco1 acetyltransferase, were found as responsible for the human Roberts syndrome/phocomelia (OMIM: 268300) [28]. These two syndromes have been recently described as cohesinophaties.

Cohesin Complex, Insulator CTCF Factor and Control of Gene Expression

Several groups have recently studied cohesin localization in mammalian chromosomes and found that numerous cohesin-binding sites overlap the CCCTC-binding factor (CTCF), an insulator protein that participates in blocking enhancer-promoter interactions [29-31]. In addition, they demonstrate that cohesins are required for the CTCF insulation function and for control of *H19/IGF2* locus imprinting in G2 and G1 phases in mice. Because there is no sister chromatid cohesion in G1 phase, the function of cohesins in the control of *H19/IGF2* transcription is independent of their role in sister chromatid cohesion.

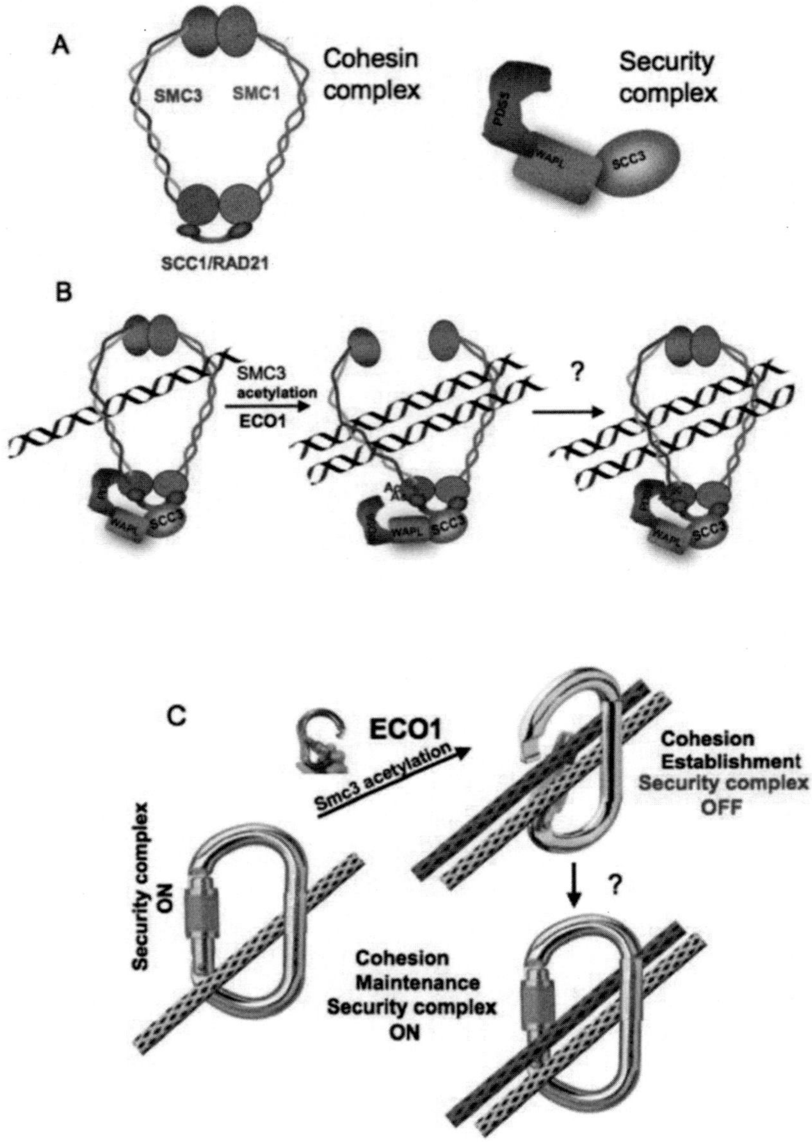

Figure 1. Cohesin and cohesin-regulator complexes. A. Ring-like cohesin complex formed by SMC subunits and closed by SCC1/RAD21 and heterotrimer "security" complex formed by SCC3/STAG, WAPL and PDS5 proteins. B. ECO1-dependent acetylation of SMC3 subunit modulates the opening of cohesin complex, allowing to de novo synthesized chromatid to enter through the cohesin ring. The security complex-dependent mechanism by which cohesin ring is again closed is unknown. C. Example of mechanism showed in B using locking carabiners and ropes employed in mountain climbing.

Two groups have shown evidence that cohesin complex subunits are needed for morphogenesis of non-dividing neurons in *Drosophila.* In a genetic screening using a modified *piggyBac* vector for insertional mutagenesis, Schuldiner et al. [32] identified two cohesin subunits SMC1 and SA/STAG as essential for axon pruning. Similar conclusions were reached in a study by Pauli et al. [33], who generated flies expressing a modified version of cohesin subunit RAD21, RAD21^{TEV}, a substrate of tobacco etch virus (TEV) protease.

Seeking the putative role of cohesins in these neuron effects, Schuldiner et al. [32] analyzed the expression of the steroid hormone receptor *EcR*, which encodes EcR-B1 protein, an essential regulator of axon pruning in the mushroom body. They observed that EcR-B1 expression is reduced in SMC1-depleted γ-neurons and that the pruning defect is reversed by EcR-B1 overexpression, suggesting that in this case cohesins facilitate *EcR* transcription. This is the opposite of the effect previously described for cohesin function in insulators, but is not the only evidence of positive regulation of gene transcription by cohesins. In human cells, SA2/STAG2 co-activates a multimeric NF-κB reporter construct and enhances activity of the p65/RelA transactivation domain [34]. Zebrafish embryos lacking cohesin subunit RAD21 or SMC3 do not express *runx3* and lose *runx1* expression in early embryonic development [35]. These findings suggest that the role of cohesin in transcription regulation might be gene-dependent.

CTCF/cohesin-mediated insulators maintain the chromatin loop formation and the localization of transcriptional apparatus at the promoters at the human apolipoprotein gene cluster [36]. Using chromatin immunoprecipitation, Degner et al. 2009 [37] showed a lineage and stage –specific RAD21 recruitment to CTCF sites in all Ig loci during B lymphocyte development, in form that the binding of cohesin to CTCF sites may promote multiple loop formation and thus effective V(D)J recombination.

In order to analyze the cohesin-mediated enhancer-blocking mechanisms in depth Hadjur et al. 2009 [38] studied the contribution of cohesin to long-range chromosomal interactions at the mouse *Ifng* locus, which encodes the cytokine interferon-γ (IFN-γ). This locus contains several putative cis-regulatory elements located at considerable distances from the coding region and that can function as enhancer or insulators. In this study the authors found that the binding of cohesin defines the spatial conformation of specific regions that are the basis for cell-type-specific long-range chromosomal interactions *in cis* at the developmentally controlled *IFNG* locus. Recently Liu et al. 2009 [39] in a study of 16 mutant cell lines from severely affected CdLS probands identified specific gene expression profiles for CdLS. Cohesin preferentially binds to promoter regions of the actively expressed genes, suggesting a role as a general transcription factors. These binding sites are significantly reduced in *SCC2/NIPBL* mutants CdLS samples. However out of the dysregulated genes in CdLS samples about 60% were upregulated and 40% are downregulated suggesting that SCC2/NIPBL and cohesin can result in both negative and positive effects on expression. This architectural function of cohesin would modulate the interaction of positive or negative regulatory elements (Figure 2) in gene transcription during development, providing the first link between genotype and phenotype of above-mentioned cohesinopathies.

In protozoa, a recent study showed that cohesin complex regulates variant surface glycoprotein (*VSG*) monoallelic expression in trypanosomes [40]. The authors demonstrated that the active *VSG* ES (expression site) locus is associated with the single ESB (RNA polymerase I-dependent transcription site ES body) during S, G2 and early mitosis and that this site exhibits a delay in the separation of sister chromatid which is dependent of cohesin complex providing a new function of cohesin complex in the epigenetic modulation of mono-allelic expression of *Trypanosma brucei VSG* ES [40].

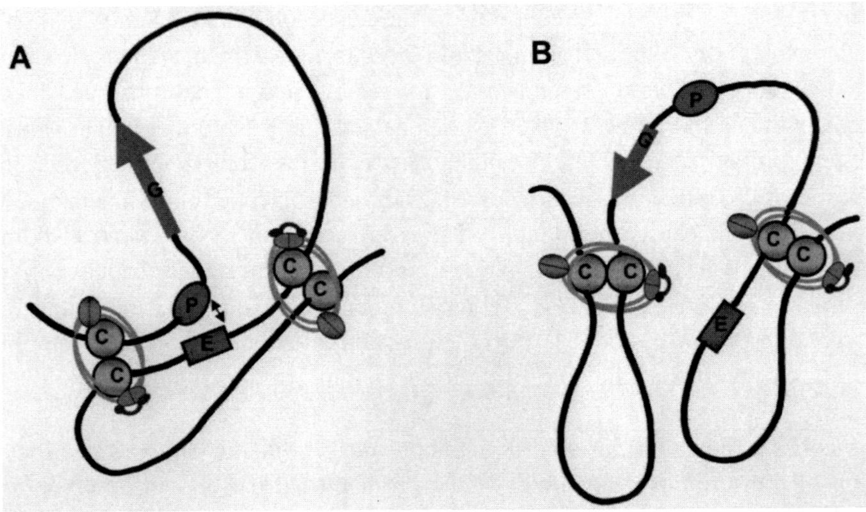

Figure 2. Putative mechanism of CTCF and cohesin cooperation in the control of gene expression. The interactions of cohesin complexes with chromatin-bound CTCF could act as local chromatin architect in two ways: A. bringing regulatory elements (E, P) nearer and promoting transcription of gene G or B. maintaining a chromatin structure in which the enhancer E could not interact with the promoter P and behaving as an insulator, repressing G gene expression.

Cohesins and Viral Transcription Control

CTCF is also a boundary factor for the latent cycle gene expression programs of Epstein-Barr virus and herpes simplex virus-1, emerging as a good system for understanding chromatin structure and regulatory elements. During latency, most of viral genes are repressed, but a few viral genes essential for genome maintenance and host-cell survival must be expressed. Using an array of the Kaposi´s sarcoma-associated herpesvirus (KSHV) genome and chromatin immunoprecipitation (ChIP), Stedman *et al.*, 2008 [29], found several CTCF enriched sites within the KSHV genome and, interestingly, a colocalization of CTCF and cohesins (SMC1, SMC3 and RAD21) at the KSV major latency control regions, which regulate the transcription of a cluster of latency gene products. In addition, depletion of RAD21 from KSVH-infected cells caused an increase in ORF74 expression, similar to depletion of CTCF binding sites from KSVH genomes, suggesting that cohesins are essential to control viral transcription program.

In a posterior study, this laboratory found that the KSHV genes regulated by CTCF-cohesin are under cell cycle control. CTCF subcellular localization altered significantly at different stages of cell cycle; cohesin interact with CTCF in mid-S phase and repress CTCF-regulated genes in a cell cycle-dependent manner [41]. The authors propose that CTCF would repress transcription when bound cohesin in S phase, but would allow active transcription when cohesin dissociated in G_2/M.

CONCLUDING REMARKS

Cohesins emerged a decade ago as central protagonists in chromosome segregation during cell division regulating sister chromatid cohesion. During this period, a lot of effort has been developed on the study of cohesin complex structure and on the characterization of the cohesin-interacting proteins that modulate cohesin complex function. In addition, in the last four years, two different approaches based on the generation of mouse deficient in cohesin function on one hand and, the identification and characterization of mutations of cohesin and cohesin-regulator genes in human syndromes, on the other hand, have revealed new and important roles for cohesins in gene expression control and development. Thus, recently, cohesins are coming up as key molecules in the maintenance of specific chromatin structures in specific chromosome locations. These cohesin-dependent chromatin conformations are required for the activation or repression of subsequent cellular machineries that control several aspects of DNA dynamics such as DNA-repair, enhancing or silencing the expression of determined cellular genes according to cellular and development stage and even controlling the transcriptional program of some viral cellular hosts.

These new cohesin complex functions open novel questions about the molecular mechanisms that drive cohesins in these multiple cellular processes. The future research on molecular signals and molecular partners of cohesins that modulate the function of cohesin complex is an exciting and essential task in our aspiration to know the molecular bases of cell growth, differentiation and development.

REFERENCES

[1] Michaelis, C., Ciosk, R. & Nasmyth, K. (1997). Cohesins: chromosomal proteins that prevent premature separation of sister chromatids. *Cell, 91*, 35-45.

[2] Losada, A., Hirano, M. & Hirano, T (1998). Identification of *Xenopus* SMC protein complexes required for sister chromatid cohesion. *Genes Dev., 12*, 1986-1997.

[3] Guacci, V., Koshland, D. & Strunnikov, A. (1997). A direct link between sister chromatid cohesion and chromosome condensation revealed through the analysis of MCD1 in *S. cerevisiae*. Cell 91, 47-57.

[4] Gruber, S., Haering, C. H. & Nasmyth, K. (2003). Chromosomal cohesin forms a ring. Cell 112, 765-777.

[5] Ivanov, D. & Nasmyth, K. (2005). A topological interaction between cohesin rings and a circular minichromosome. *Cell, 122*, 849-860.

[6] Uhlmann, F., Lottspeich, F. & Nasmyth, K. (1999). Sister-chromatid separation at anaphase onset is promoted by cleavage of the cohesin subunit Scc1. *Nature, 400*, 37-42.

[7] Barbero, J. L. (2009). Cohesins: Chromatin architects in chromosome segregation, control of gene expression and much more. *Cell. Mol. Life Sci., 66*, 2025-2035.

[8] Ciosk, R., Shirayama, M., Shevchenko, A., Tanaka, T., Toth, A., Shevchenko, A. & Nasmyth, K. (2000). Cohesin's binding to chromosomes depends on a separate complex consisting of Scc2 and Scc4 proteins. *Mol. Cell, 5*, 243-254.

[9] Watrin, E., Schleiffer, A., Tanaka, K., Eisenhaber, F., Nasmyth, K. & Peters, J. M. (2006). Human Scc4 is required for cohesin binding to chromatin, sister-chromatid cohesion, and mitotic progression. *Curr. Biol.*, *16*, 863-874.

[10] Skibbens, R. V., Corson, L. B., Koshland, D. & Hieter, P. (1999). Ctf7p is essential for sister chromatid cohesion and links mitotic chromosome structure to the DNA replication machinery. *Genes Dev.*, *13*, 307-319.

[11] Toth A., Ciosk R., Uhlmann F., Galova M., Schleiffer A. & Nasmyth K. (1999). Yeast cohesin complex requires a conserved protein, Eco1p(Cft7), to establish cohesion between sister chromatids during DNA replication. *Genes Dev.*, *13*, 320-323.

[12] Tanaka, K., Yonekawa, T., Kawasaki, Y., Kai, M., Furuya, K., Iwasaki, M., Murakami, H., Yanagida, M. & Okayama, H. (2000). Fission yeast Eso1p is required for establishing sister chromatid cohesion during S phase. *Mol. Cell. Biol.*, *20*, 3459-3469.

[13] Ivanov, D., Schleiffer, A., Eisenhaber, F., Mechtler, K., Haering, C. H. & Nasmyth, K. (2002). Eco1 is a novel acetyltransferase that can acetylate proteins involved in cohesion. *Curr. Biol.*, *12*, 323-328.

[14] Kitajima, T. S., Kawashima, S. A. & Watanabe, Y. (2004). The conserved kinetochore protein shugoshin protects centromeric cohesion during meiosis. *Nature*, *427*, 510-517.

[15] Sumara I., Vorlaufer E., Gieffers C., Peters B. H. & Peters J.M. (2000). Characterization of vertebrate cohesin complexes and their regulation in prophase. *J. Cell Biol., 151*, 749-762

[16] Wang, F., Yoder, J., Antoshechkin, I. & Han, M. (2003). *Caenorhabditis elegans* EVL-14/PDS-5 and SCC-3 are essential for sister chromatid cohesion in meiosis and mitosis. *Mol. Cell. Biol., 23*, 7698-7707.

[17] Zhang, Z., Ren, Q., Yang, H., Conrad, M. N., Guacci V., Kateneva A.,and Dresser M. E. (2005). Budding yeast PDS5 plays an important role in meiosis and is required for sister chromatid cohesion. *Mol. Microbiol.*, 56, 670-680.

[18] Gandhi, R., Gillespie, P. J. & Hirano, T. (2006). Human Wapl is a cohesin-binding protein that promotes sister-chromatid resolution in mitotic prophase. *Curr. Biol.*, *16*, 2406-2417.

[19] Kueng, S., Hegemann, B., Peters, B. H., Lipp, J .J., Schleiffer, A., Mechtler, K. & Peters, J. M. (2006). Wapl controls the dynamic association of cohesin with chromatin. *Cell*, 127, 955-967.

[20] Rankin, S., Ayad, N. G. & Kirschner, M. W. (2005). Sororin, a substrate of the anaphase-promoting complex, is required for sister chromatid cohesion in vertebrates. *Mol Cell.*, *18*, 185-200.

[21] Nasmyth, K. (2001). Disseminating the genome: joining, resolving, and separating sister chromatids during mitosis and meiosis. *Annu. Rev. Genet.*, *35*, 673-745.

[22] Ben-Shahar, T. R., Heeger, S., Lehane, C., East, P., Flynn, H., Skehel, M. & Uhlmann, F. (2008). Eco1-dependent cohesin acetylation during establishment of sister chromatid cohesion. *Science*, *321*, 563-566.

[23] Zhang, J., Shi, X., Li, Y., Kim, B.J., Jia, J., Huang. Z., Yang, T., Fu, X., Jung, S. Y., Wang, Y., Zhang, P., Kim, S. T., Pan, X. & Qin, J. (2008). Acetylation of Smc3 by Eco1 is required for S phase sister chromatid cohesion in both human and yeast. *Mol. Cell*, *31*, 143-151.

[24] Rowland, B. D., Roig, M. B., Nishino, T., Kurze, A., Uluocak, P., Mishra, A., Beckouët, F., Underwood, P., Metson, J., Imre, R., Mechtler, K., Katis, V. L. and Nasmyth, K.

(2009). Building sister chromatid cohesion: smc3 acetylation counteracts an antiestablishment activity *Mol. Cell*, *33*, 763-774.

[25] Heidinger-Pauli, J. M., Unal, E. and Koshland, D. (2009). Distinct targets of the Eco1 acetyltransferase modulate cohesion in S phase and in response to DNA damage. *Mol. Cell.*, *34*, 311-321.

[26] Liu, J. and Krantz, I. D. (2008). Cohesin and human disease. *Annu. Rev. Genomics Hum. Genet.*, *9*, 303-20

[27] Zhang, B., Chang, J., Fu, M., Huang, J., Kashyap, R., Salavaggione, E., Jain, S., Shashikant, K., Deardorff, M. A., Uzielli, M. L., Dorsett, D., Beebe, D. C., Jay, P. Y., Heuckeroth. R. O., Krantz, I. and Milbrandt, J. (2009). Dosage effects of cohesin regulatory factor PDS5 on mammalian development: implications for cohesinopathies. *PLos ONE*, 4, e5232.

[28] Vega, H., Waisfisz, Q., Gordillo, M., Sakai, N., Yanagihara, I., Yamada, M., van Gosliga, D., Kayserili, H., Xu, C., Ozono, K., Jabs, E. W., Inui, K. and Joenje. H. (2005). Roberts syndrome is caused by mutations in ESCO2, a human homolog of yeast ECO1 that is essential for the establishment of sister chromatid cohesion. *Nat. Genet.*, *37*, 468-470.

[29] Stedman, W., Kang, H., Lin, S., Kissil, J. L., Bartolomei, M. S. and Lieberman, P. M. (2008). Cohesins localize with CTCF at the KSHV latency control region and at cellular c-myc and *H19/Igf2* insulators. *EMBO J.*, *27*, 654-666.

[30] Wendt, K. S., Yoshida, K., Itoh, T., Bando, M., Koch, B., Schirghuber, E., Tsutsumi, S., Nagae, G., Ishihara, K., Mishiro T., Yahata, K., Imamoto, F., Aburatani, H., Nakao, M., Imamoto, N., Maeshima, K., Shirahige, K. and Peters, J. M. (2008). Cohesin mediates transcriptional insulation by CCCTC-binding factor. *Nature*, *451*, 796-801.

[31] Parelho, V., Hadjur, S., Spivakov, M., Leleu, M., Sauer, S., Gregson, H. C., Jarmuz, A., Canzonetta, C., Webster, Z., Nesterova, T., Cobb, B. S., Yokomori, K., Dillon, N., Aragon, L., Fisher, A. G. and Merkenschlager, M. (2008). Cohesins functionally associate with CTCF on mammalian chromosome arms. *Cell*, *132*, 422-433.

[32] Schuldiner, O., Berdnik, D., Levy, J. M., Wu, J. S., Luginbuhl, D., Gontang, A. C. and Luo, L. (2008). *piggyBac*-based mosaic screen identifies a postmitotic function for cohesin in regulating developmental axon pruning: Dev. *Cell*, *14*, 227-238.

[33] Pauli, A., Althoff, F., Oliveira, R. A., Heidmann, S., Schuldiner, O., Lehner, C. F., Dickson, B. J. and Nasmyth, K. (2008). Cell-type-specific TEV protease cleavage reveals cohesin functions in *Drosophila* neurons. Dev. *Cell*, *14*, 239-251.

[34] Lara-Pezzi, E., Pezzi, N., Prieto, I., Barthelemy, I., Carreiro, C., Martínez, A., Maldonado-Rodríguez, A., López-Cabrera, M. and Barbero, J.L. (2004). Evidence of a transcriptional co-activator function of cohesin STAG/SA/Scc3. *J. Biol. Chem.*, *279*, 6553-6559.

[35] Horsfield, J. A., Anagnostou, S. H., Hu, J. K., Cho, K. H. Y., Geister, R., Lieschke, G., Crosier, K. E. and Crosier, P. S. (2007). Cohesin dependent regulation of *Runx* genes. *Development*, *134*, 2639-2649.

[36] Mishiro, T., Ishihara, K., Hino, S., Tsutsumi, S., Aburatani, H., Shirahige, K., Kinoshita, Y. and Nakao, M. (2009). Architectural roles of multiple chromatin insulators at the human apolipoprotein gene cluster. *EMBO J.*, *28*, 1234-1245.

[37] Degner, S. C., Wong, T. P., Jankevicius, G. and Feeney, A. J. (2009). Cutting edge: developmental stage-specific recruitment of cohesin to CTCF sites throughout immunoglobulin loci during B lymphocyte development. *J. Immunol.*, *182*, 44-48.

[38] Hadjur, S., Williams, L. M., Ryan, N. K., Cobb, B. S., Sexton, T., Fraser, P., Fisher, A. G. and Merkenschlager, M. (2009). Cohesins form chromosomal cis-interactions at the developmentally regulated IFNG locus. *Nature*, *460*, 410-413.

[39] Liu, J., Zhang, Z., Bando, M., Itoh, T., Deardorff, M. A., Clark, D. Kaur, M., Tandy, S., Kondoh, T., Rappaport, E., Spinner, N. B., Vega, H., Jackson, L. G., Shirahige, K. and Krantz, I. D. (2009). Transcriptional dysregulation in NIPBL and cohesin mutant human cells. *PLos Biol.*, *7*, e1000119.

[40] Landeira, D, Bart, J. M., Van Tyne D & Navarro, M. (2009). Cohesin regulates *VSG* monoallelic expression in trypanosomes. *J. Cell Biol.*, *186*, 243-254.

[41] Kang, H. and Lieberman, P. M. (2009). Cell cycle control of Kaposi's sarcoma-associated herpesvirus latency transcription by CTCF-cohesin interactions. *J. Virol.*, *83*, 6199-6210.

In: Cell Division: Theory, Variants and Degradation ISBN: 978-1-60876-986-5
Editors: Y. N. Golitsin, M. C. Krylov, pp. 127-132

Chapter 8

THE ROLE OF DM NXF1 IN CONTROLLING EARLY EMBRYONIC MITOSES IN DROSOPHILA MELANOGASTER

E. V. Golubkova and L. A. Mamon
Department of Genetics, St. Petersburg State University.

ABSTRACT

The known function of the evolutionary conservative NXF1 (Nuclear eXport Factor) is the nuclear-cytoplasmic transport of the most mRNAs. On our data Dm NXF1 is involved in control of cell division. By immunostaining of early embryos with antibodies to C-terminal part of Dm NXF1 we have shown that the intensity of the staining depends on the cell cycle stage. The cytoplasmic Dm NXF1 is abundant on prometaphase and it almost disappears on anaphase. It is possible that Dm NXF1 can be involved in RNP-complexes including mRNAs which translation is regulated during cell cycle. Such complexes dissociate to resolve the translation of according mRNAs.

INTRODUCTION

The *small bristles* (*sbr*) gene of *Drosophila melanogaster* belongs to the evolutionary conserved family of nuclear export factor (NXF) genes. Since the *sbr* gene is orthologous to the main gene of the *NXF* family, it has another name, *Dm NXF1*. *NXF1* genes are involved in controlling the active transport of most, if not all, mRNAs from the nucleus to the cytoplasm [13]. This is the universal function of *NXF1* genes, and one of the reasons for pleiotropic effects of *sbr* gene mutations. Among such effects are the disruption of the synthesis of HSP (heat shock proteins) as a response to a heat shock in species homozygous with the thermosensitive *l(1)ts403* allele or sbr^{10} [7], the high frequency of aneuploid progenies in sbr^{10} females exposed to a heat shock [17], disruptions of the first meiotic spindle in sbr^{10} and *sbr*^{5} females [10] and disruptions of embryonic mitoses in their progenies [9], male sterility, and disruptions in the sexual behavior of *sbr*^{12} males.

The disruption of the synthesis of HSP in *sbr*^{10} mutants is a recessive manifestation [23]. It may be the result of the defect of the nuclear export of *Hsps* mRNA in mutant cells [26; 28]. The other effects are dominant. The dominant allele-specific effects of some *sbr* alleles suggest that the *sbr* gene has specialized functions in addition to universal function. One such function of the *sbr* (*Dm NXF1*) gene may be to control chromosome segregation during cell division.

Results

It is known that NXF1 protein is localized in the nucleus or in the nuclear envelope, according to the universal function of this factor [3]. Specific functions may be evident in a specific distribution of Dm NXF1 in a cell during cell division. Using the antibodies to C-terminal domains of Dm NXF1 (Ivankova et al, unpublished), we have localized this factor in embryos of the Oregon-R wild stock at different stages of cell cycle.

For the analysis, we used early embryos (no older than 2 hours after oviposition). We were able to detect Dm NXF1 protein not only in the nucleus, but also in the cytoplasm (Figure1). Moreover, the intensity of the coloration of immunostaining varies throughout the cell cycle (Figure1). The highest concentration of SBR protein is during the prometaphase. The granules of the protein distribute evenly, occupying the cytoplasm around the nucleus. During early embryonic mitoses, *D. melanogaster* has no cell membranes; cell boundaries are formed by vacuole-like structures containing no SBR protein. Such structures are usually referred to as youlk bodies [15]. During transition from the metaphase to the anaphase, the staining intensity decreases (Figure 1).

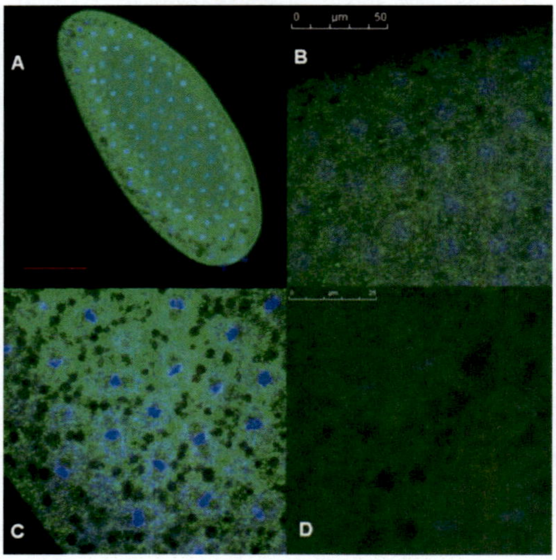

Figure 1. Immunostaining of the SBR (Dm NXF1) protein in the different stages of cell cycle during *D.melanogaster* embryogenesis. Wild-type embryos were stained with both anti-SBR antibody (green) and DAPI (DNA, blue). The synchronous dividing nuclei: A, C – pro-metaphase; B – interphase; D – anaphase.

Discussion

The early embryogenesis of *D. melanogaster* is characterized by the fact that mitoses are managed by products that the maternal organism had reserved during oogenesis [30]. Zygotic genes begin to work 1.5–2 hours after fertilization [6]. During early stages of embryogenesis of *D. melanogaster*, the cell cycle is restricted to M and S phases: the DNA replication period is followed by the sister chromatid segregation [16]. The transition to the division of the nucleus requires the activation or synthesis of factors for the building of the spindle and for the processes of chromosome segregation. The products during one stage of the cell cycle must be deactivated or destroyed during another stage, and activated or synthesized again during the transition to the next stage of the cell cycle. The regulation of gene expression at the level of translation of maternal mRNA, synthesized during oogenesis, plays an important role in such transitions [25; 2]. This allows for the synthesis of the factors that have degraded during the transition to the respective stage of the cell cycle. The cell cycle progression is regulated at the level of translation of *Cyclin B* mRNA during early embryogenesis [11; 12]. The control of translation of *Cyclin B* mRNA is regulated by cytoplasmic polyadenylation [20]. mRNA *sbr* (*Dm NXF1*) has been found among the stored maternal mRNAs in ovaries and in early embryos [14]. The broad band of mRNA *sbr* has been found in both early embryos (0–2 h) and in ovaries. There are *cis*-**acting sequences in the 3′ untranslated region** (UTR) of mRNA *sbr* (Figure 2), the cytoplasmic polyadenilation element (CPE,) and the hexanucleotide AAUAAA, which are important for the cytoplasmic polyadenylation [19; 8]. The presence of cytoplasmic polyadenylation elements in 3′UTR of *sbr* mRNA further indicates that the *sbr* gene expression can be regulated at the translation level via adenylation/deadenylation. From this we derive that the maternally provided *sbr* transcripts are translationally regulated during early embryogenesis, contributing to the control of synchronous nuclear divisions at this stage of development [14]. **In addition, 3′UTR of** mRNA *sbr* includes AU-rich elements (AREs) (Figure 2), which are characteristic of mRNA cell-cycle regulatory proteins [22; 27].

This leads us to the conclusion that the cyclic nature of the intensity of coloration, observed when using immunostaining with anti-SBR proteins, may be connected with the regulation of expression of the *sbr* gene at the translational level.

5′ - AUCGCAUAGGAGUUUCCGUAGGACAGAGCCGCGUGCCAC
AUCCACAUAAUCGAAUGCUGUUUUUUUUUUUUUUGGUUUUGUAA
UUAAAUUUUAAAAUUAUUAGAGAAACCUCUAUAUAAUAAUAAU
AAUUAAUAUUAUUAAGCUGCGAAGUUGUGUGCACAUUCGGGCA
GUAGCAAUUAUUAUCCCAGCACUGCGGGCAAUGUGCAUCAACG
AUCACAGUUCUUCGAUAGAUUAGUUUAGCUCUCUUUAAGUUCC
GUCCGCAGAUCCGCUGGUCUACAUUGAGGCCAGGACGAGUCUG
CGAACGGUAGUCCCUUUAGAGUUAAAGUUGUUUUAGAUUCCUA
AGCCAAACACCUUCAAACACACACAACACGACAACACUAUUAA
ACGUAAUGCAACAAUGUUGUCGAAUCGAAAGAAACCCAA**UUUU**
UAUUUUAAUAUAUACGACGAUACCGAAACCAAGGCGAUGGUCG
AAAAGCAUGGAUCGCGCCAAUAAUUCUAUAUUCCCCGCUUUCC
CAGAUCCUCGACUCGCCUUACAUUUUGUAUACAAAUACCAUAG
AAUAAAAAGAAACAUUUUGACCACUGUAAAAAUUUUGUAACGC
UCGGAAACCAAAAUUACCUUUAUUUCUUAAUAGAAAAAAAAUUA
UUCG**AUUUA**CAAUACACGCUUAGCCGUAAAUUCAAUUGA**AUUU**
AAGUGUAAGAUAUAUAAAAAUUAUAUACAUUAAGACAAAAGUG
UAGAUUCAUA**AAUAAA**UUUUUCAGAAUAGAAU - 3′

Figure 2. 3′UTR of the gene *Dm nxf1*. **Marked**: CPE – cytoplasmic polyadenylation element – UUUUUAU, two hexanucleotides AAUAAA and two AREs (AU-rich elements) - AUUUA.

```
mpkrgggssq rynnnvgngg grynapedfd dfdvedrqrr
kdrnkrrvsf kpsqclhnkk diklrpedlr rwdedddmsd
mttavkdrpt srrrgspipr gkfgklmpns fgwyqvtlqn
aqiyeketll sallaamsph vfipqywrve rncvifftdd
yeaaeriqhl gknghlpdgy rlmprvrsgi plvaiddafk
ekmkvtmakr yniqtkaldl srfhadpdlk qvfcplfrqn
vmgaaidimc dnipdlealn lndnsissme afkgvekrlp
nlkilylgdn kipslahlvv lrnlsilelv lknnpcrsry
kdsqqfisev rrkfpklvkl dgetlepqit fdlseqgrll
etkasylcdv agaevvrqfl dqyfrifdsg nrqalldayh
ekamlsismp sasqagrlns fwkfnrnlrr llngeenrtr
nlkygrlacv stldewpktq hdrrtftvdl tiyntsmmvf
tvtglfkeln detnnpasme lydvrhfart yvvvpqnngf
cirnetifit natheqvref krsqhqpapg ampstssavt
spqagaaagl qgrlnalgva tgpvailsgd plaatapvns
gsaaisttav apgaqdestk mqmieamsaq sqmnviwsrk
cleetnwdfn haafvfeklf kenkippeaf mk
```

Figure 3. SBR protein sequence. Domains: RBD (RNA-binding) – grey; 4xLRR (leucine-rich repeats) – yellow; NTF2-like (nuclear transport factor 2 – like) – green; UBA-like (ubiquitin associated like) – cyan. Marked RXXL – D-box; KEN-box

Such cyclic changes in coloration allow us to assume the degradation of the SBR protein during the transition to the anaphase. The presence of D-box and KEN-box sequences in the amino-acid sequence of SBR protein (Figure 3) suggests that SBR protein can potentially degrade, mediated by the anaphase-promoting complex/cyclosome (APC/C) during the metaphase-anaphase transition [24; 5]. These sequences are localized in the C-terminal domain of SBR protein, which, we believe, are important for controlling cell division [10].

The cytoplasmic localization of the RNA-binding SBR protein (Figure 1) indicates that this protein interacts with some mRNAs, not only during their transition from the nucleus to the cytoplasm, but also after the mRNAs leave the nucleus. RNA-binding proteins allow for nuclear export, and dictate the functional program of cytoplasmic mRNAs [21]. The SBR may be a part of cytoplasmic mRNP granules (P-granules), which contain mRNAs programmed for delayed translation [4; 1]. This is particularly important during transcriptional silencing in early embryogenesis. It is possible that SBR protein interacts with mRNAs whose translation is regulated in the cell cycle, including mRNA *sbr*. The dissociation of mRNP complexes is a necessary stage in activating the translation of mRNAs that are part of these complexes. A characteristic feature of actively dividing cells is the absence of cytoplasmic P-granules [29]. Cytoplasmic granules containing SBR protein were usually absent in the regions of actively dividing cells, if organs were stained in their entirety.

Conclusion

The SBR protein can be identified as cytoplasmic granules in early embryos of *D. melanogaster*. The concentration of this protein depends on the stage of the cell-cycle stage. This is easy to observe due to the synchronous nature of cell division during early embryogenesis in *D. melanogaster*. The transcript of the *sbr* gene has sequences that allow for the regulation of gene expression at the translational level. The SBR protein has sequences that allow for the regulation of the amount of this protein in APC/C-mediated cell cycle.

The cytoplasmic localization of the RNA-binding SBR protein suggests that the cytoplasmic functions of this protein and its possible interaction with mRNAs are involved in the regulation of cell-cycle progression. The lowering of staining intensity during the transition from the metaphase to the anaphase suggests that SBR protein is destroyed during translation, when mRNPs granules disassemble. It is possible that the oscillation of SBR protein concentration during the cell cycle reflects the cyclic behavior of mRNP granules. The regulated synthesis of SBR protein is perhaps necessary to form RNP granules during the next cell cycle as a means of preventing the translation of mRNAs at the stage of degradation of their respective protein products.

The study has been supported by grant CRDF-Ministry of education ST-012, awarded by the leading schools; by grants RFBR-09-04-00697 and SciSch-197.2008.4.

REFERENCES

[1] Anderson, P; Kedersha, N. RNA granules. *J.Cell Biol.*, 2006, 172, 803-808.

[2] Bashirullah, A; Cooperstock, RL; Lipshitz, HD. RNA localization in development. *Annu. Rev.Biochem.,* 1998, 67, 335-394.

[3] Braun, IC; Herold, A; Rode, M; Izaurralde, E. Nuclear Export of mRNA by TAP/NXF1 Requires Two Nucleoporin-Binding Sites but Not p15. *Mol Cell Biol.,* 2002, 22, 5405-5418.

[4] Brengues, M; Teixeira, D; Parker, R. Movement of eukaryotic mRNAs between polysomes and cytoplasmic processing bodies. *Science.,* 2005, 310, 486-489.

[5] Crane, R; Gadea, B; Littlepage, L; Wu, H; Ruderman, JV. Aurora A, meiosis and mitosis. *Biol. Cell.,* 2003, 96, 215-229.

[6] Edgar, BA; Schubiger, G. Parameters controlling transcriptional activation during early *Drosophila* development. *Cell.,* 1986, 44, 871-877.

[7] Evgen'ev, MB; Denisenko, ON. The effect of a higher temperature on expression of the heat shock-inducible genes in Drosophila melanogaster: III. Synthesis of HSP70-related protein. *Russian J of Genetics.* 1990, 26, 266-271.

[8] Fox, CA; Sheets, MD; Wickens, MP. Poly(A) addition during maturation of frog oocytes: distinct nuclear and cytoplasmic activities and regulation by the sequence UUUUUAU. *Genes Develop.*, 1989, 3, 2151-2162.

[9] Golubkova, EV; Nokkala, S; Mamon, LA. The nuclear export factor gene *small bristles* is involved in the control of early embryonic mitoses in *Drosophila melanogaster. Drosophila Inform. Serv.*, 2006, 89, 31-39.

[10] Golubkova, EV; Markova, EG; Markov, AV; Avanesyan, EO; Nokkala, S; Mamon, LA. *Dm nxf1/sbr* Gene Affects the Formation of Meiotic Spindle in female *Drosophila melanogaster. Chromosome Research.* 2009 (in press).

[11] Groisman, I; Huang, YS; Mendez, R; Cao, Q; Theurkauf, W; Richter, JD. CPEB, maskin, and cyclin B1 mRNA at the mitotic apparatus: implications for local translational control of cell division. *Cell*, 2000, 103, 435-447.

[12] Groisman, I; Jung, MY; Sarkissian, M; Cao, Q; Richter, J. Translational control of the embryonic cell cycle. *Cell*, 2002, 109, 1-20.

[13] Herold, A; Teixeira, L; Izaurralde, E. Genome-wide analysis of nuclear mRNA export pathways in *Drosophila. EMBO J.,* 2003, 22, 2472-2483.

[14] Ivankova, NA; Tretyakova, IV; Lyozin, GT; Avanesyan, EO; Evgen'ev, MB; Mamon, LA. Ubiquitous and specific transcripts of evolutionary conservative gene *Dm nxf1* (*sbr – small bristles*) *Drosophila melanogaster. Vest. SPU.*, 2009 (in press).

[15] Ji, JY; Squirrell, JM; Schubiger, G. Both Cyclin B levels and DNA-replication checkpoint control the early embryonic mitoses in Drosophila. *Development*, 2004, 131, 401-411.

[16] Murray, AW. Remembrance of things past. *Nature.*, 1991, 349, P.367-368.

[17] Mamon, LA; Mazur, EL; Churkina, IV; Barabanova, LV. Influence of high temperature on frequency nondisjanctions and losses of sexual chromosomes at females of *Drosophila melanogaster* lines *l(1)ts403* with defect in system of heat shock protein. *Russian J. Genetics*, 1990, 26, 554-556.

[18] Mamon, LA; Bondarenko, LV; Tretyakova, IV; Komarova, AV; Nikitina, EA; Pugatchova, OM; Golubkova, EV. Consequences of cell stress in conditions of disturbed synthesis of heat shock proteins in *Drosophila melanogaster. Vest. SPU.*, 1999, 4, 100-114.

[19] McGrew, LL; Dworkin-Rasti, E; Dworkin, MB; Richter, JD; Poly(A) elongation during *Xenopus* oocyte maturation is required for translation recruitment and is mediated by a short sequence element. *Genes Develop.*, 1989, 3, 803-815.

[20] Mendez, R; Richter, JD. Translational control by CPEB: a means to the end. *Nat. Rev. Mol. Cell. Biol.* 2001 2, P.521-529.

[21] Moore, MJ. From birth to death: the complex lives of eukaryotic mRNAs. *Science.*, 2005, 309, 1514-1518.

[22] Nemer, M; Stuebing EW. WEE1-like CDK tyrosine kinase mRNA level is regulated temporally and spatially in sea urchin embryos. *Mech. Dev.*, 1996, 58, 75-88.

[23] Nikitina, E.A; Komarova, AV; Golubkova, EV; Tretyakova, IV; Mamon, LA. Dominant effects of *l(1)ts403* (*sbr10*) mutation at the disjunction of sex chromosomes in meiosis of *Drosophila melanogaster* females after heat shock. *Russian J. Genet.*, 2003, 39, 341-348.

[24] Pfleger, CM; Krischner, MW. The KEN box: an APC recognition signal distinct from the D box targeted by Cdh1. *Genes Dev.*, 2000, 14, 655-665.

[25] Raff, JW; Whitfield, WGF; Glover, DM. Two distinct mechanisms localise cyclin B transcripts in syncytial *Drosophila* embryos. // *Development*, 1990, 110, 1249-1261.

[26] Tretyakova, IV; Lyozin, GT; Markova, EG; Evgen'ev, MB; Mamon, LA. The *sbr* gene product in *Drosophila melanogaster* and its orthologs in yeast (Mex67p) and human (TAP*). Russian J. Genet.,* 2001, 37, 593-560.

[27] Wang, W; Caldwell MC; Lin S; Furneaux H; Gorospe M. HuR regulates cyclin A and cyclin B1 mRNA stability during cell proliferation. *EMBO J.*, 2000, 19, 2340-2350.

[28] Wilkie, GS; Zimyanin, V; Kirby, R; Korey, C; Francis-Lang, H; Van Vactor, D; Davis, I. *small bristles*, the *Drosophila* ortholog of *NXF-1,* is essential for mRNA export throughout development. RNA 7, 1781-1792.

[29] Yang, Z; Jakymiw, A; Wood, MR; Eystathioy, T; Rubin, RL; Marvin, JF; Chan, EKL. GW182 is critical for the stability of GW bodies expressed during the cell cycle and cell proliferation. *J.Cell Sci.*, 2004, 117, 5567-5578.

[30] Zalokar, M. Autoradiographic studies of protein and RNA during early development of *Drosophila* eggs. *Dev. Biol.*, 1976, 49, 425-437.

In: Cell Division: Theory, Variants and Degradation
Editors: Y. N. Golitsin, M. C. Krylov, pp. 133-171
ISBN: 978-1-60876-986-5

Chapter 9

CYANOBACTERIAL CELL DIVISION: GENETICS, COMPARATIVE GENOMICS AND PROTEOMICS*

Olga A. Koksharova
A.N. Belozersky Institute of Physico-Chemical Biology,
M.V. Lomonosov Moscow State University, Moscow 119992, Russian Federation.

ABSTRACT

Division in cyanobacteria, ancient phototrophic relatives of chloroplasts, may serve as a model for study of plant chloroplast division. Cyanobacterial mutants impaired in cell division were identified after chemical mutagenesis, by random cassette mutagenesis and by transposon mutagenesis. Analysis of such mutants appears to be an effective strategy for investigating cyanobacterial cell division. In addition, the availability of the complete genomic sequences of many cyanobacteria, bacteria, some plants and algae facilitates comparative genomic analysis. Some of the cyanobacterial cell division genes have homologues among cyanobacteria, green algae and higher plants, some genes are specific only for cyanobacteria. Finding of cyanobacterial *ftn2* gene, for example, helped to study the function of its plant homologoes that encoding Arc6 protein, a nuclear-encoded protein of chloroplast inner envelope membranes that is required for organelle division. Cell division is a highly co-ordinated and fine-tuned process, and the precise regulation and positioning of the cell division apparatus requires a number of both structural and regulatory components, of which many are still unidentified. Mutagenic disruption of proper regulation in the cell division machinery often leads to the formation of elongated and/or mini cells and may impose a strong internal stress, altering cell physiology. Metabolic pathways that are regulated by the cell cycle may also be affected. The first proteomic comparative study of two cyanobacterial cell division mutants has been initiated. Quantitative differences in the protein maps were detected and proteins with significant quantitative changes were identified. The upregulated proteins include

---

* A version of this chapter was also published in Handbook of Cell Proliferation, edited by Andre P. Briggs and Jacob A. Coburn, Nova Science Publishers. It was submitted for appropriate modifications in an effort to encourage wider dissemination of research.

proteins involved in cell division/cell morphogenesis, protein synthesis and processing, oxidative stress response, amino acid metabolism, nucleotide biosynthesis, and glycolysis, as well as unknown proteins. Among the downregulated proteins are those involved in chromosome segregation, protein processing, photosynthesis, redox regulation, carbon dioxide fixation, nucleotide biosynthesis, the biosynthetic pathway to fatty acids, and energy production. Identification of such differentially expressed proteins provides new targets for future studies that will allow assessment of their physiological roles and significance in cyanobacterial cell division.

INTRODUCTION

Most known bacteria divide symmetrically during normal growth. Although superficially simple, bacterial cell division is a complex regulatory process about which much is being learned. Discovery of bacterial *fts* and other genes [Bouche & Pichoff, 1998; Bramhill, 1997; Levin & Losick, 2000; Margolin, 2000; Shapiro & Losick, 2000; Howard & Kruse, 2005; Dajkovic & Lutkenhaus, 2006] has helped enhance understanding of cell division: how the bacterial cell forms the membrane-associated FtsZ ring that mediates septation, how a cell determines the site of division, how division is coordinated with chromosome replication, and how regulation of proteolysis assists cell division.

Despite their small size (typically 1-3 μm) and normal lack of the specialized organelles and cytoskeletal elements that are found in eukaryotic cells, bacterial cells are highly organized. In recent ten-fifteen years, it has become clear that many proteins and specific parts of the chromosome are localized to specific subcellular regions [Shapiro & Losick, 2000; Dajkovic & Lutkenhaus, 2006.]. Hirota *et al.* [Hirota *et al.*, 1968] identified conditionally lethal mutants of *E. coli* affected in cell division by screening for the formation of long, non-septate filaments at a restrictive temperature. This approach relied on the ability of the bacteria to continue elongation of the cylindrical portion of the cell in the absence of division. Later, additional such mutations and genes were described [Bramhill, 1997; Margolin, 2000]. Bacteria possess a number of cytoskeletal elements [Mayer, 2003], including FtsZ, a bacterial tubulin homologue [Carballido-López & Errington, 2003; Michie & Löwe, 2006; Klint *et al.*, 2007], MreB coiled structures similar to F-actin, the physiological polymer of eukaryotic actin [van den Ent *et al.*, 2001], MinCDE coiled arrays [Shih *et al.*, 2003] and intracellular protofilaments containing bacterial elongation factor Tu (EF-Tu) [Löwe *et al.*, 2004]. All of them may form cytoskeletal webs, which are important for the organization of intracellular structures and cell function [Mayer, 2003]. Dividing bacteria use a cytoskeletal structure at the division site for the mechanical constriction of the cell. The major component of this structure in most species is FtsZ [Bi & Lutkenhaus, 1991], a tubulin-like GTPase [Löwe & Amos, 1998] that shares many properties with eukaryotic cytoskeletal molecules. FtsZ assembles at the site of division and orchestrates cell division [Lutkenhaus & Addinall, 1997]. In the presence of GTP, purified FtsZ molecules self-assemble into long filamentous structures that are depolymerized rapidly when all of the GTP has been hydrolysed [Mukherjee & Lutkenhaus, 1998]. After a ring of molecules of FtsZ is formed, a dozen other cell-division proteins are recruited sequentially to the site of future division, forming additional ring structures [Rothfield, *et al.*, 1999; Dajkovic & Lutkenhaus, 2006]. In most bacterial species, the septum is formed at the midpoint of the cell. The mechanism of midsite selection is still not completely investigated, but in *E. coli*, the minicell genes *minC, minD* and *minE* are implicated in this process [de Boer, *et al.*, 1989; Jacobs & Shapiro, 1999; Raskin & de Boer. 1999a,b; Sullivan & Maddock, 2000; Jensen & Shapiro, 2000; Kruse *et al.*, 2007; Loose *et al.*, 2008]. Donachie and Begg [Donachie & Begg, 1996] confirmed that the number of septa formed per generation per *E. coli* cell length is fixed and that "division potential" is directly proportional to cell length. In a *minC* mutant, septa form with equal probability at the poles, centers, and 1/4- and 3/4-cell positions. These same authors showed that the time to next division is inversely related to cell length and that division is asynchronous in long cells, suggesting that a single cell can form only one septum at a time.

Since the discovery of the Z ring, immunofluorescence microscopy and fusion to green fluorescent protein (GFP) have been used for visualization of FtsZ and other cell division proteins. Most associate with the Z ring to form a complete septal apparatus (divisome or septal ring) capable of carrying out cell division [Lutkenhaus & Addinall, 1997; Errington *et al.*, 2003; Dajkovic & Lutkenhaus, 2006].

Cell-cycle processes, such as DNA replication, chromosome segregation and cell division must be strictly coordinated to ensure efficient proliferation. To understand how all of these processes are coordinately regulated in the bacterial cell, the complete set of related regulatory genes must be identified and their roles understood.

Cyanobacterial cell division mutants can aid in the search for such genes. Cyanobacteria, ancient relatives of chloroplasts and structurally similar to Gram-negative prokaryotes, perform plant-type photosynthesis; some of them are able to fix nitrogen and to cell differentiation. All methods of molecular biology are available for study of cyanobacteria [Koksharova & Wolk, 2002a]. Genomic DNA sequences are available for more than 40 different strains and spiecies of cyanobacteria for the moment of this review writing (http://www.ncbi.nlm.nih.gov/sutils/genom_table.cgi). However, the genetical control of cell division has been studied much less in cyanobacteria than it has in heterotrophic bacteria, such as *Escherichia coli*, *Bacillus subtilis* or *Caulobacter crescentus*. Morphologically aberrant mutants of cyanobacteria presumably impaired in cell division, recovered with high frequency after chemical mutagenesis [Ingram & Thurston, 1970; Ingram & Van Baalen. 1970; Ingram, *et al.*, 1972; Ingram & Fisher, 1973a,b; Zhevner *et al.*, 1973; Ingram *et al.*,1975], were described many years ago. This is surprising, but so far only limited information has been obtained about cyanobacterial genes that are involved in the regulation of cell division. Study of cyanobacterial cell division can help to investigate molecular mechanisms of plastid division and plastid evolution. To study the cyanobacterial cell division methods of genetics, genomics and proteomics could be applied.

Genetical Approach to Study Cyanobacterial Cell Division

Which genes are important for cyanobacterial cell division? One tool that should be able to provide an answer to this question is forward genetics, which aims to identify and clone mutant genes responsible for a phenotype of an interest. By using forward genetics approaches first we conduct mutant screens of a new quality and quantity and then proceed to new gene identification. Reverse genetic analysis for cyanobacterial genes encoding cell division proteins could be also applied after comparative genomic and proteomic analysis. Identification of cyanobacterial mutants and genes that are involved in cell division and cell differentiation can enhance understanding of the regulation of morphogenesis of bacteria and plant chloroplasts.

The first cyanobacterial mutants impaired in cell division were described in the seventies [Ingram & Thurston, 1970; Ingram & Van Baalen. 1970; Ingram, *et al.*, 1972; Ingram & Fisher, 1973a,b; Zhevner *et al.*, 1973; Ingram *et al.*,1975]. Filamentous mutants showed two distinct phenotypes [Ingram & Fisher, 1973a]: septate filaments containing cross-walls apparently impaired in the terminal stages of cell separation; and serpentine forms that divide sporadically to produce multinucleoidal long cells. The gene mutated in a septate mutant of *Synechococcus* sp. strain PCC 7942 as a consequence of insertional inactivation [Dolganov & Grossman, 1993] was identified and characterized. Dolganov and Grossman by using "random cassette mutagenesis", i.e. the random insertion of an antibiotic resistance gene into the genome upon homologous recombination of genomic restriction fragments fused to that gene [Broedel & Wolf, 1990; Labarre, *et al.*, 1989], identified seven filamentous mutants of *Synechococcus* PCC 7942 as a result of insertional inactivation [Dolganov & Grossman, 1993]. In one of the mutants, the lesion may have been in an *flm3* region in *orf3* (Synpcc7942_*2006*), which encoded hypothetical protein. We applied transposon mutagenesis to the study of cell division. By use of transposon Tn*5*-692, which provides large numbers of transposon mutants in *Synechococcus* sp. PCC 7942, could have identified the mutants of the second, serpentine type [Koksharova & Wolk, 2002b; Miyagishima *et al.*, 2005].

Transposon mutagenesis and analysis of ftn genes, of Synechococcus sp. strain PCC 7942. Mutagenesis by transposition was first reported in *Synechococcus* sp. PCC 7942 (PCC 7942) when Tandeau de Marsac *et al.* [Tandeau de Marsac *et al.*, 1982] used transposition of Tn*901* from a plasmid to the chromosome to mutagenize a chromosomal locus. Transposon mutagenesis with Tn*901* from plasmid pUH24 of PCC 7942 [van den Hondel *et al.*, 1980] has been used to identify a cluster of genes involved in nitrate assimilation [Madueño, *et al.*, 1988; Luque, *et al.*, 1992]. Limiting the utility of Tn*901* is its low frequency of transposition [Golden, 1988]. Tn*5* was later used in *Anabaena* sp. strain PCC 7120 [Borthakur & Haselkorn, 1989], but became much more effective with the introduction of variants, e.g., Tn*5*-1058 and its progeny, that had (i) a much stronger promoter driving the antibiotic-resistance operon, (ii) enhanced transposition, and (iii) an *Escherichia coli* origin of replication within the transposon that facilitates recovery of the mutated gene. This vector allows the cloning of sequences contiguous with the transposon, by cutting genomic DNA with a restriction endonuclease that does not cut within the transposon, recircularizing *in vitro* and transforming *E. coli* with the resulting ligation mixture [e.g., Wolk *et al.*, 1991; Cohen *et al.*, 1998]. We introduce the use of transposon Tn*5*-692, whose ca. 100-fold increase in the rate of transposition provides large numbers of transposon mutants of *Anabaena variabilis* strain ATCC 29413 (PCC 7937) (C.P. Wolk & O.A. Koksharova, unpublished data) and of *Synechococcus* sp. PCC 7942. Two new transposition-derived cell division mutants of PCC 7942 have been characterized and two new cell division genes have been sequenced (GenBank accession AF421196 and AF421197) [Koksharova & Wolk, 2002b].

When *Synechococcus* sp. strain PCC 7942 was mutagenized with transposon Tn*5*-692, ca. 3000 Em^rSp^r, dense, round mutant colonies with regular margins were accompanied by 39 spreading colonies with irregular borders (Figure 1) that were comprised of very elongated cells. In classical studies of *f*ilamentous *t*emperature-*s*ensitive mutants of *E. coli* affected in cell division [Bramhill, 1997], the corresponding genes were designated *fts*; by analogy, we designated the mutants that we isolated, FTN-mutants (Filamentous, TransposoN-derived) and the corresponding genes, *ftn*. Two such mutants, FTN2 and FTN6, whose irregular colonies are composed of cells that are longer than wild-type cells (Figure 2). Cells of mutants FTN2 and FTN6 of *Synechococcus* sp. strain PCC 7942 have the appearance of long filaments that divide occasionally, at variable positions along the cell (Figure 3). The cells of both mutants usually divided asymmetrically, sometimes produce branches. It appears that inactivation of *ftn2* or *ftn6* blocks cell division at an early stage or, alternatively, that the coordination of cell elongation and cell division is disrupted. Mutants FTN2 and FTN6 of *Synechococcus* sp. PCC 7942 are completely segregated (Figure 4A,B). In FTN2 and FTN6, the transposon was inserted in single-copy (Figure 4C,D) open reading frames that we denote *ftn2* and *ftn6*. *ftn2* predicts a 631-amino acid protein that shows greatest similarity to the predicted products of other cyanobacterial and plants (Table 1).

Table 1. Ftn2-like proteins and their accession numbers.

Organism	Accession Number/Open Reading Frame Name
Synechococcus sp PCC 7942	AF421196/Synpcc7942_*1943*
Thermosynechococcus elongatus BP-1	NP_681547/ *tlr0758*
Synechococcus sp. WH 7803	YP_001225456/SynWH7803_*1733*
Synechocystis sp PCC 6803	NP_441990/*Sll0169*
Anabaena/Nostoc sp PCC 7120	NP_486747/*all2707*
Nostoc punctiforme PCC 73102	YP_001868827/Npun_*R5579*
Anabaena variabilis ATCC 29413	YP_324769/Ava_*4275*
Trichodesmium erythraeum IMS101	YP_724444/Tery_*5067*
Protochlorococcus marinus MIT 9211	YP_001551219/P9211_*13341*
Protochlorococcus marinus MT9313	NP_894181/PMT*0348*
Chlamydomonas reinhardtii	XP_001690917/CHLREDRAFT_*169875*
Paulinella chromatophora	YP_002048788/PCC_*0126*
Arabidopsis thaliana	AAQ18646/*ARC6*
Oryza sativa	DAA01472/*Arc6*
Zea mays	ACF86369.1/BT041364.1:53…2338

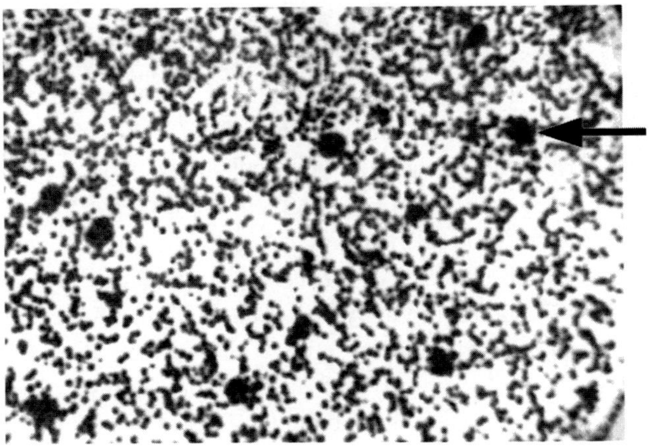

Figure 1. When the unicellular cyanobacterium, *Synechococcus* sp. strain PCC 7942, was mutagenized with transposon Tn*5*-692, dense, round mutant colonies with regular margins were accompanied by spreading colonies with irregular borders (one of them is indicated by an arrow).

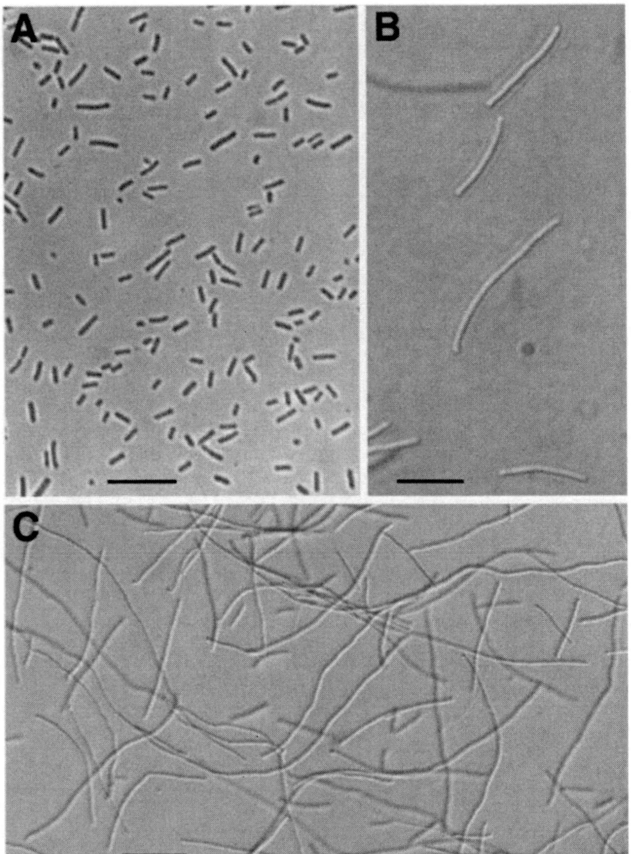

Figure 2. Morphology of wild-type *Synechococcus* sp. PCC 7942 (A) and of mutants FTN2 (B) and FTN6 (C) grown in liquid, and visualized by light microscopy. Scale bars represent 12.5 μm (A,B) or 25.6 μm (C) [Koksharova & Wolk, 2002b].

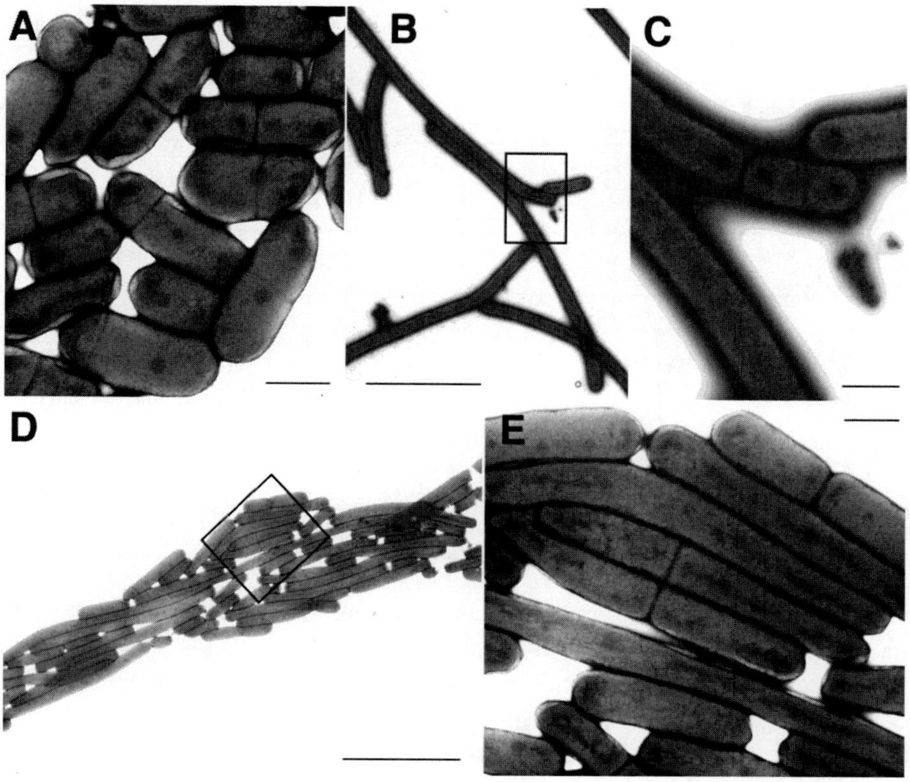

Figure 3. Structure of wild-type PCC 7942 (A), and of mutants FTN2 (C, see box in panel B) and FTN6 (E, see box in panel D), negatively stained with uranyl acetate, and examined by electron microscopy. The cells of both mutants usually divided asymmetrically. Scale bars represent 1 μm (A,C,E) or 10 μm (B,D) [Koksharova & Wolk, 2002b].

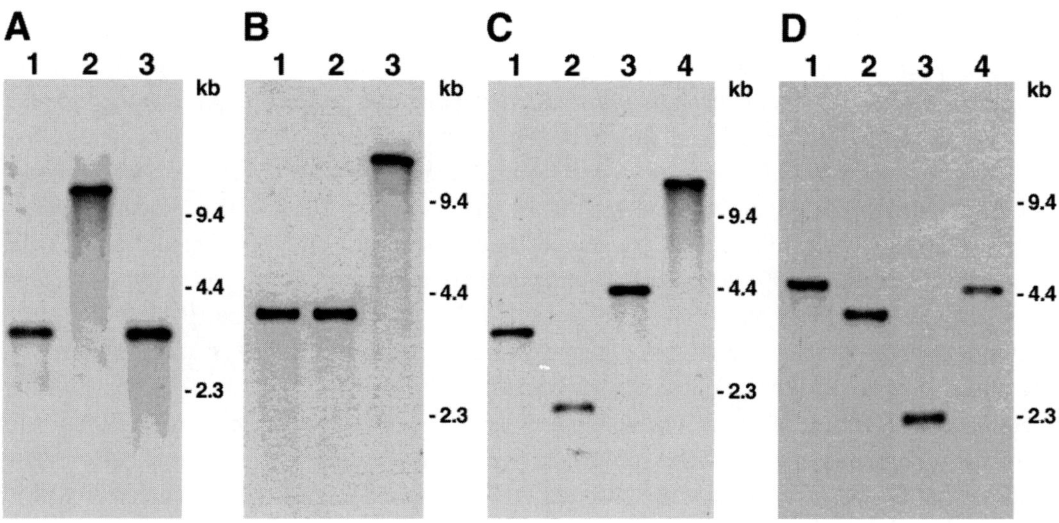

Figure 4.Southern blots, hybridized with an *ftn2* probe (A, C) or an *ftn6* probe (B, D). (A,B) Genomic DNA of wild-type Synechococcus sp. PCC 7942 (lanes 1) or mutants FTN2 (lanes 2) or FTN6 (lanes 3), digested with *Sal*I and blotted. (C, D) Genomic DNA of wild-type PCC 7942 digested with *Sal*I (C, lane 1; D, lane 2), *Eco*RI (C, lane 2; D, lane 3), *Hind*III (C, lane 3; D, lane 4), or *Xho*I (C, lane 4; D, lane 1), and blotted.

Table 2.Characteristics of Ftn2 protein of *Synechococcus* sp. PCC 7942 and its homologs

Protein and organism	Number of aa	MW (kDa)	pI	Domains or pattern
Ftn2 *Synechococcus* sp. PCC 7942 AF421196/Synpcc7942_*1943*	648	72.4	5	1. DnaJ N-terminal domain (aa 6-70) 2. TPR repeat (aa 136-169) 3. Leucine zipper (aa 234-255)
Anabaena sp. PCC 7120 NP_486747/*all2707*	798	90.1	6.3	1. DnaJ N-terminal domain (aa 16-80)
Nostoc Punctiforme YP_001868827/Npun_*R5579*	768	87.4	6.8	1. DnaJ N-terminal domain (aa 16-80) 2. ATP/GTP binding site motif A (P-loop) (aa 566-573)
Synechocystis PCC 6803 NP_441990/*Sll0169*	714	79.4	4.7	1. DnaJ N-terminal domain (aa 6-70)
Arabidopsis thaliana AAQ18646/*ARC6*	801	88.3	4.6	1. DnaJ domain profile (aa 89-153) 2. Myb DNA-binding domain (aa 677-690)

The InterProScan program (http://www.ebi.ac.uk/interpro/scan.html) shows the presence in Ftn2 of a DnaJ N-terminal domain (aa 6-70) and a single TPR repeat (aa 136-169). The Prosite-Protein against PROSITE program (http://ca.expasy.org/tools/scnpsite.html/) shows the presence in Ftn2 of a leucine zipper pattern (aa 234-255; Table 2). Ftn2 and its cyanobacterial and plant orthologs show the presence of a DnaJ N-terminal domain, but are otherwise, as are Ftn6 and its orthogs, dissimilar from the products of known division-related genes [Bramhill, 1997]. *ftn6* predicts a 152-amino acid protein and specific to cyanobacteria (Table3).

The presence of a DnaJ domain, a (single) tetratricopeptide repeat (TPR) and a leucine zipper motif suggest that Ftn2 may function as part of a complex with one or more other proteins and may be regulatory. DnaJ domains are characteristic of a family of chaperonins. Proteins in this family, from bacterial to human, have three distinct domains: (i) a highly conserved J domain of approximately 70 amino acids, often found near the N-terminus, which mediates interaction of DnaJ (a.k.a., Hsp40) with Hsp70 (DnaK) and regulates the ATPase activity of the latter; (ii) a glycine and phenylalanine (G/F)-rich region of unknown function that may act as a flexible linker; and (iii) a cysteine-rich region (C domain) that contains four CXXCXGXG motifs, and resembles a zinc-finger domain [Ohtsuka & Hata, 2000]. Although not originally identified as an *fts* gene, *dnaJ* shares with *fts* genes the property that its inactivation leads to a filamentous phenotype [Paciorek *et al.*, 1997]. Cheetham and Caplan [Cheetham & Caplan, 1998] classified DnaJ/Hsp40 homologs into three groups: type I have all three of these domains; type II have only the J and G/F domains; and type III, like Ftn2, have only a J domain. DnaK proteins are highly versatile chaperones that assist a large variety of processes [Bukau, 1999; Bukau & Horwich, 1998; Bukau & Walker, 1989; Fink, 1999; Gething, 1997; Hartl, 1996], from folding of newly synthesized proteins to facilitation of proteolytic degradation of unstable proteins [Laufen *et al.*, 1999]. This functional diversity requires that DnaK proteins associate promiscuously with misfolded proteins or selectively with folded substrates, including with regulatory proteins of low abundance.

Table 3. Genes involved in cell division by the example of *Synechococcus* sp. PCC 7942

Gene	Protein	Function	Reference	Bacterial homolog	Plant homolog (in *Arabidopsis* genome)
Synpcc7942_*2378*	FtsZ	GTP-binding cell division protein; septum ring formation	Bi & Lutkenhaus. 1991	FtsZ	FtsZ1-1 AT5G55280 FtsZ2-1 AT2G36250
Synpcc7942_*2377*	FtsQ	cell division protein that is part of the divisome complex	van den Ent *et al.*, 2008	FtsQ	absent
Synpcc7942_*0580* Synpcc7942_*0482*	FtsI	peptidoglycan glycosyltransferase	Pogliano *et al.*, 1997	FtsI	absent
Synpcc7942_*0564* Synpcc7942_*1414*	FtsE	cell division protein	Corbin etal., 2007	FtsE	absent
Synpcc7942_*2580* Synpcc7942_*2468* Synpcc7942_*2073*	dnaK molecular chaperone	Heat shock protein 70; assists in folding of nascent polypeptide chains; refolding of misfolded proteins.	Bukau & Walker, 1989; Nimura *et al.*,2001	dnaK	CPHSC70-1 (chloroplast heat shock protein 70-1 NP_194159.1
Synpcc7942_*1943*	Ftn2	may function in a chaperone system	Koksharova & Wolk, 2002b; Vitha *et al.*, 2003	absent	Arc6 AAQ18646/ARC6
Synpcc7942_*1707*	Ftn6	hypothetical protein	Koksharova & Wolk, 2002b	absent	absent
Synpcc7942_*0897*	MinE	cell division topological specificity factor	Lutkenhaus, 2007; Loose *et al.*, 2008	MinE	AtMinE1 AT1G69390 BAB79236
Synpcc7942_*0896*	MinD	septum site-determining protein	Lutkenhaus, 2007; Kerr *et al.*, 2006; Loose *et al.*, 2008	MinD	MIND AT5G24020
Synpcc7942_*1104* Synpcc7942_*0324*	FtsW	cell division protein	Mercer & Weiss, 2001	FtsW	absent

Table 3. (*Continued*)

Gene	Protein	Function	Reference	Bacterial homolog	Plant homolog
Synpcc7942_*2001*	MinC	septum formation inhibitor	Lutkenhaus, 2007; Zhou & Lutkenhaus, 2005; Loose *et al.*, 2008	MinC	absent
Synpcc7942_*0653* *cdv1*	Peptidyl-prolyl cis-trans isomerase (rotamase) - cyclophilin family-like	unknown	Miyagishima *et al.*, 2005		CYP38 (Cyclophilin 38); peptidyl-prolyl cis-trans isomerase AT3G01480
Synpcc7942_*0644*	CikA GAF sensor hybrid histidine kinase	a regulator of the *Synechococcus elongatus* PCC 7942 circadian clock	Schmitz *et al.*, 2000 Miyagishima *et al.*, 2005	Several histidine kinases (Score 98-160 bits)	AHK3 NP_564276
Synpcc7942_*2059* *cdv2*	hypothetical protein; cell division protein SepF	Cell division protein that is part of the divisome complex and is recruited early to the Z-ring. Probably stimulates Z-ring formation, perhaps through the cross-linking of FtsZ protofilaments. Its function overlaps with FtsA.	Miyagishima *et al.*, 2005	BSU15390 *B subtilis*	absent
Synpcc7942_*2006* *cdv3*	hypothetical protein	unknown	Dolganov & Grossman, 1993; Miyagishima *et al.*, 2005	absent	absent

Table 3. (*Continued*)

Gene	Protein	Function	Reference	Bacterial homolog	Plant homolog
S 6803 *slr1471* Synpcc7942_*1617*	Putative inner membrane protein translocase component YidC NP441564.1	member of the Alb3/Oxa1/YidC protein family	Fulgosi *et al.*, PNAS, 2002,99:11501-11506	absent	ARTEMIS locus of *Arabidopsis* (NP_173858) envelope membrane integrase
Slr1223 S6803 Synpcc7942_*2477*	SulA cell division inhibitor	Predicted nucleoside-diphosphate sugar epimerase	Raynaud *et al*, 2004	SulA	(GC1) (Giant chloroplast1); NP_565505
murC Synpcc7942_*1741* murE Synpcc7942_*1484* murD Synpcc7942_*1667* murI Synpcc7942_*2361*	UDP-N-acetylmuramate--L-alanine ligase UDP-N-acetylmuramoylalanyl-D-glutamate-2,6-diaminopimelate ligase UDP-N-acetylmuramoyl-L-alanyl-D-glutamate synthetase glutamate racemase	involved in cell wall formation; peptidoglycan synthesis; involved in cell wall formation; peptidoglycan synthesis; catalyzes the addition of meso-diaminopimelic acid to the nucleotide precursor UDP-N-aceylmuramoyl-l-alanyl-d-glutamate involved in peptidoglycan biosynthesis; catalyzes the addition of glutamate to the nucleotide precursor UDP-N-acetylmuramoyl-L-alanine during cell wall formation converts L-glutamate to D-glutamate, a component of peptidoglycan	Smith, 2006; Deva *et al.*, 2006; El Zoeiby *et al.*, 2003; Meroueh *et al.*, 2006	*E. coli* ZP_03071496 NP_414627.1 NP_414630 NP_418402	absent absent absent absent

The tetratricopeptide repeat (TPR) of, typically, 34 amino acids was first described in the yeast cell division cycle regulator Cdc23p [Sikorski *et al.*, 1990] and was later found in many other proteins [Das *et al.*, 1998, Goebl & Yanagida, 1991; Lamb *et al.*, 1995]. TPRs are frequently present in tandem arrays of 3-16 copies, although single (as in Ftn2) or paired TPRs are also common [Lamb *et al.*, 1995]. Processes involving TPR proteins include cell-cycle control, repression of transcription, response to stress, protein kinase inhibition, mitochondrial and peroxisomal protein transport, and neurogenesis [Goebl & Yanagida, 1991]. There appears to be no common biochemical function connecting TRP-containing proteins, although the TRP forms scaffolds that mediate protein-protein interactions and, often, the assembly of multiprotein complexes.

A web-based program (http://HypothesisCreator.net/iPSORT/) predicts that an *Arabidopsis* ortholog of *ftn2* has a chloroplast transit peptide (MEALS HVGIG LSPFQ LCRLP PATTK LRRSH); according to ProfileScan (http://www.isrec.isb-sib.ch/software/PFSCAN_form.html), this protein possesses a DnaJ domain profile; and according to InterProScan (http://www.ebi.ac.uk/interpro/scan.html), the protein possesses a Myb DNA-binding domain. A role of this ortholog in chloroplast cell division has been shown [Vitha *et al.*, 2003].

Reverse genetic analysis for homologous cyanobacterial genes encoding cell division proteins Ftn2 [Koksharova & Wolk, 2002b; Mazouni *et al.*, 2004] and Ftn6 [Koksharova & Wolk, 2002b] in *Anabaena* sp. PCC 7120 (Figure 5) and in *Synechocystis* sp. PCC 6803 has been applied. Mutants show significant cell division defects. However, in contrast to *Synechococcus* sp. PCC 7942 FTN2 mutant, corresponding mutants of *Anabaena* and *Synechocystis* failed to segregate completely [Koksharova & Wolk, 2002b; Mazouni *et al.*, 2004]. The presence of the greatly enlarged cells, which by their shape and frequent contiguity to heterocysts somewhat resemble akinetes (Figure 5), suggests that *Anabaena* sp. PCC 7120 Ftn2 and Ftn6 homologues may be involved not only in the regulation of cell growth, but also in cellular differentiation.

In order to identify other genes involved in cyanobacterial cell division, *Synechococcus* sp. PCC 7942 has been mutagenized [Miyagishima *et al.*, 2005] by the introduction of pRL692, which carries a derivative of transposon Tn5 (Tn5-692; [Koksharova & Wolk, 2002b]). Seven loci have been selected for study. These included *ftn2* (Synpcc7942_*1943*) and *minE* (Synpcc7942_*0897*), whose roles in cyanobacterial cell division have been lately investigated [Koksharova & Wolk, 2002b; Mazouni *et al.*, 2004]; *flm3* region *orf3* (Synpcc7942_*2006*) and *ftn6* (Synpcc7942_*1707*), previously identified as possible cell division loci [Dolganov & Grossman, 1993; Koksharova & Wolk, 2002b]; and three genes, Synpcc7942_*0653*, Synpcc7942_*0644* and Synpcc7942_*2059*, not previously associated with cell division in cyanobacteria [Miyagishima *et al.*, 2005]. Synpcc7942_*0644* encodes CikA, a regulator of the *Synechococcus elongatus* PCC 7942 circadian clock [Schmitz *et al.*, 2000; Mutsuda *et al.*, 2003]. Synpcc7942_*0653* (named as *cdv1*, [Miyagishima *et al.*, 2005]) encodes *p*eptidyl-prolyl cis-trans isomerase and Synpcc7942_*2059* (named as *cdv2*, [Miyagishima *et al.*, 2005] encodes cell division protein SepF.

Now all these genes are placed on the list of the known genes that control of cyanobacteria cell prolifiration (Table3). By using Tn mutagenesis as a molecular genetical experimental tool we can add more new cell division genes to this list in the nearest future.

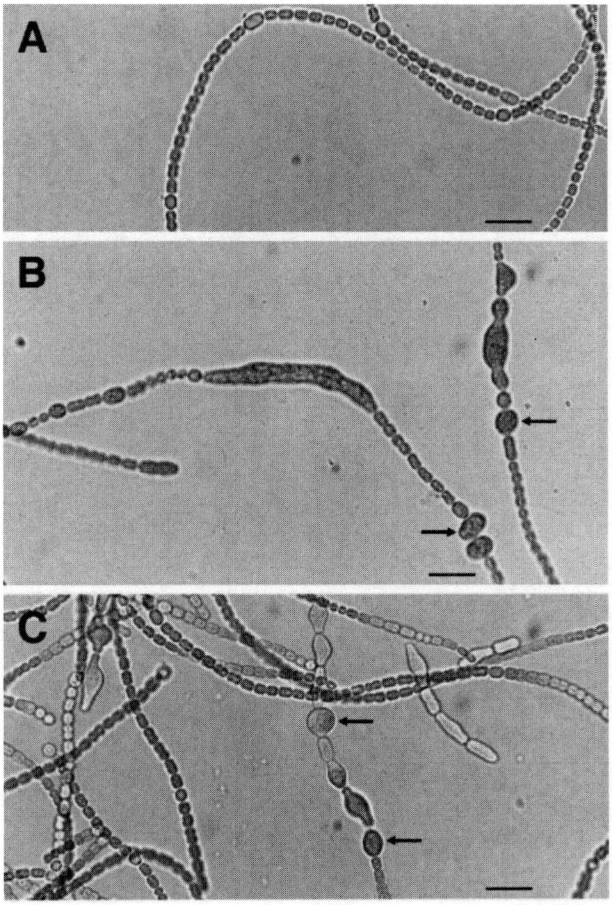

Figure 5. Morphology of *Anabaena* sp. PCC 7120 wild type (A) and mutants $FTN2_A$ (B) and $FTN6_A$ (C) grown in liquid medium free of combined nitrogen (AA/8). Scale bars represent 12.5 μm. Division defective akinete-like cells are indicated by arrows (adapted from [Koksharova & Wolk, 2002b]).

Genomic Studies of Cyanobacterial Cell Division Genes

By mutational and comparative analysis, the list of genes known or predicted to influence cell division in *Synechococcus* sp. PCC 7942 has been extended. The availability of whole bacterial genome sequences has revealed that cyanobacteria encode homologues of cell division genes originally identified in *E. coli*: *ftsE*, *ftsI*, *ftsK*, *ftsQ*, *ftsW*, *ftsZ*, *minC*, *minD* and *minE* [Doherty & Adams, 1995; Mazouni *et al.*, 2004; Miyagishima *et al.*, 2005]. Studies in *Synechococcus* and in *Synechocystis* have confirmed a role for six further cell division genes, *ftn2*, *ftn6*, *cdv1*, *cdv2* and *cdv3*, *sulA*, [Koksharova *et al.*, 2002; Raynaud *et al.*, 2004; Miyagishima *et al.*, 2005] (Table 3). A cyanobacterial gene that encodes an ortholog of cell division protein FtsZ has been cloned and sequenced so far from *Anabaena* PCC 7120 [Doherty & Adams, 1995; Zhang, *et al.*, 1995]. This protein, present in vegetative cells [Kuhn, *et al.*, 2000], forming a ring structure [Sakr *et al.*, 2006; Klint *et al.*, 2007], as well as some amount of FtsZ present in non-dividing, differentiated cells called heterocysts. This protein may have a cytoskeletal function [Klint *et al.*, 2007]. FtsZ gene was insertion-inactivated in *Synechococcus* sp. PCC 7942 and in *Synechocystis* sp. PCC 6803 [Sarcina & Mullineaux, 2000]. Mutation was lethal, only heteroplasmic (that is, they retained both wild-type and transformed chromosomes) cells can survive. One more example of the successful application of reverse genetics in the characterization of chloroplast functions is the targeted mutagenesis of plant homologues of the bacterial cell division protein FtsZ [Osteryoung *et al.*, 1998; Strepp *et al.*, 1998; Stokes *et al.*, 2000]. This protein was shown to have a functional chloroplast targeting transit peptide, and subsequent studies demonstrated that, by contrast with most bacteria encoding a single FtsZ protein, *Arabidopsis* and other plant species harbour two families of plastid-targeted FtsZs. FtsZ proteins from both of these families were found to co-localize into a Z ring at the division site in *Arabidopsis*, pea, and tobacco [Fujiwara & Yoshida, 2001; McAndrew *et al.*, 2001; Vitha *et al.*, 2001].

Comparative genomic approach permitted to discover some new common cyanobacterial and plastid division genes. Cell division in cyanobacteria serves as a model for the study of chloroplast division. The morphological similarities between dividing cyanobacteria and dividing chloroplasts are striking and knowledge of cyanobacterial division will undoubtedly benefit plastid division research. Plastids are descended from a cyanobacterial symbiosis which occurred over 1.2 billion years ago. The first hypothesis that plastids are derived from endosymbiotic cyanobacteria had been made by Mereschkowsky C. [Mereschkowsky, 1905; Martin & Kowallik, 1999]. During the course of endosymbiosis, most genes were lost from the cyanobacterium's **genome** and many were relocated to the host nucleus through endosymbiotic gene transfer (EGT) [Raven & Allen, 2003]. According recent estimations, 16-18% of plant nucleus genes are transferred from cyanobacteria [Martin *et al.*, 2002; Deusch *et al.*, 2008]. Among them some chloroplast division genes/proteins have been found: Arc6; ARTEMIS and GC1 (also called AtSulA) (Table 3) [Koksharova & Wolk, 2002b; Vitha *et al.*, 2003; Fulgosi *et al.*, 2002; Raynaud *et al.*, 2004; Maple *et al.*, 2004], ptCpn60α and ptCpn60β [Suzuki *et al.*, 2009].

Plant nuclear gene *arc6* is a descendant of the cyanobacterial cell division gene *ftn2* [Koksharova & Wolk, 2002; Vitha *et al.*, 2003], and ARC6 and its orthologs are only found in cyanobacteria, eukaryotic algae and higher plants. ARC6 was originally identified through cloning of the arc6 mutant (Pyke *et al.*, 1994; Vitha *et al.*, 2003). ARC6 is an inner envelope membrane protein that acts as a positive regulator of Z-ring formation [Vitha *et al.*, 2003]. ARC6-GFP localizes to a ring-like structure at the mid-plastid [Vitha *et al.*, 2003]. ARC6 and Ftn2 proteins possess a conserved region at their N-termini with sequence similarity to J-domains, implicating them as possible Hsp70-associated co-chaperones. arc6 mutants have short FtsZ filaments within a single large chloroplast. In plants overexpressing ARC6, FtsZ filaments are more numerous and form spiral patterns around the enlarged chloroplast. These phenotypes suggest that ARC6 could play a role in bundling of short FtsZ filaments into a ring at the chloroplast division site. The N-terminus of ARC6 resides in the stroma [Vitha *et al.*, 2003] and a conserved N-terminal segment of ARC6 interacts with FtsZ2-1 but not FtsZ1-1 [Maple *et al.*, 2005]. ARC6 has been shown to interact with the CORE domain of AtFtsZ2-1 [Maple *et al.*, 2005]. In *E. coli*, the CORE domain of FtsZ mediates the interaction with both FtsA and ZipA proteins. FtsA and ZipA could be involved in controlling the FtsZ polymerization. No homologues of these bacterial proteins have been identified in the genomes of cyanobacteria or higher plants and ARC6 may play a role analogous to that of FtsA and ZipA, stabilizing or anchoring the Z-ring [Maple & Møller, 2007.]. Actually Z-ring formation by either FtsZ protein is dependent on functional ARC6 since in the *arc6* background both AtFtsZ1-1 and AtFtsZ2-1 form short filaments [Vitha *et al.*, 2003]. This is especially interesting in connection with the discovery that ARC6 interacts specifically with

AtFtsZ2-1, and it is possible that inner membrane-bound AtFtsZ2-1 is stabilized though its interactions with ARC6 and that, subsequently, AtFtsZ1-1 polymerizes and interacts with AtFtsZ2-1, allowing further protein recruitment to the site of division. Quantitative yeast two-hybrid assays using truncated forms of the ARC6 stromal domain revealed that the conserved domain was sufficient for the interaction between ARC6 and AtFtsZ2-1 and that this interaction was not dependent on the presence of the J-domain [Maple *et al.*, 2005]. In contrast, Ftn2 is reported to require the J-domain for interaction with cyanobacterial FtsZ [Mazouni *et al.*, 2004] but the significance of this difference is not yet understood.

ARTEMIS (*Arabidopsis thaliana* envelope membrane integrase) was identified in a search for proteins involved in chloroplast biogenesis [Fulgosi *et al.*, 2002]. The role of ARTEMIS in chloroplast division was discovered from studies using transposon insertion *Arabidopsis* plants with greatly reduced levels of the ARTEMIS protein [Fulgosi *et al.*, 2002]. These plants have similar growth characteristics to wild-type plants, but ultrastructural analysis revealed extended, duplicated, or triplicated, undividing chloroplasts. Whereas the envelope membranes fail to complete constriction, the thylakoid membranes are visibly constricted at the centre of the chloroplasts and are apparently portioned between the two halves of the organelle. ARTEMIS protein has a unique molecular structure combining a C-terminal domain similar to the Alb3 and Oxa1 proteins with conserved YidC translocase elements and an N-terminal region similar to receptor protein kinases. Using the YidC/Alb3-like translocase domain, a homologue of ARTEMIS has been identified in *Synechocystis* PCC6803 (*slr147*). Deletion mutant for this gene has altered cell morphology, with the formation of tetrameric or hexameric clusters of cells indicative of late cell division arrest [Fulgosi *et al.*, 2002]. Cells also seem to initiate their fission events unevenly, leading to cells of irregular shape. The evolutionary conservation of ARTEMIS has been demonstrated by the rescue of wild-type division characteristics in the *slr1471* cyanobacterial mutant with the YidC/Alb3-like domain of ARTEMIS [Fulgosi *et al.*, 2002].

GIANT CHLOROPLAST 1 (GC1) (also called AtSulA) was originally identified based on its similarity to putative cell division inhibitor SulA proteins in *Anabaena* sp. PCC 7120 (*all2390*) and *Synechocystis* sp. PCC 6803 (*slr1223*), although no function had been reported for the cyanobacterial proteins [Maple *et al.*, 2004; Raynaud *et al.*, 2004]. GC1 is located on chromosome II and encodes a protein of 347 amino acids which has an N-terminal plastid-targeting transit peptide absent in the cyanobacterial protein. Phylogenetic analysis of GC1 homologues indicates a clear cyanobacterial origin of GC1. The analysis of a *Synechocystis slr1223* deletion mutant, showing that *slr1223* is essential for cell survival as complete segregaton of this mutant could not be achieved [Raynaud *et al*, 2004]. Microscopic analysis of heteroploid clones revealed that up to 40% initiated but failed to complete cell division, resulting in cloverleaf-like structures, demonstrating that *slr1223* is required for correct cell division in *Synechocystis*. GC1 was shown to be associated with the inner envelope and is likely to be a key regulator of the division process, although its exact function is still unknown. In a subset of bacterial systems, induction of SulA is one of many responses to DNA damage; SulA inhibits cell division by binding directly to FtsZ and occluding the protofilament interface, preventing FtsZ polymerization [Mizusawa & Gottesman, 1983; Cordell *et al.*, 2003]. However, unlike SulA, GC1 does not appear to possess an FtsZ-binding domain identical to that in *Pseudomonas aeruginosa* SulA [Cordell *et al.*, 2003] nor does it bind FtsZ1 or FtsZ2 directly [Maple *et al.*, 2004]. Although SulA inhibits cell division in bacteria, the published effects of GC1 on chloroplast division are contradictory: work from one group suggests that GC1 acts as a positive regulator of chloroplast division [Maple *et al.*, 2004]; while work from another indicates that it acts as a negative regulator [Raynaud *et al.*, 2004]. Further work on GC1 is needed to clarify its role in the division process.

CHAPERONIN PROTEINS ptCpn60α and ptCpn60β are required for proper plastid division in *A. thaliana.* These new plastid division proteins have been identified recently by characterizing plastid division mutants obtained by using forward genetics approach [Suzuki *et al.*, 2009]. Phylogenetic analysis showed that both ptCpn60 proteins are derived from ancestral cyanobacterial proteins and have a similarity with chaperonin GroEL. Early it has been shown that the filamentous phenotypes were observed in GroEL-depleted *Escherichia coli* [Fujiwara & Taguchi, 2007], *Caulobacter crescentus* and *Streptococcus* mutans, suggesting [Susin *et al.*, 2006; Lemos *et al.*, 2007] that GroEL plays a universal role in cell division in bacteria. Notably, a level of Gro EL protein has been upshifted in the proteomes of the FTN2 and FTH6 cell division mutants of *Synechococcus* sp. PCC 7942 [Koksharova *et al.*, 2007] (see also below). No more cell division function had been reported for the cyanobacterial GroEL proteins so far.

Despite its significance to our understanding of plastid division, till now only a few studies have identified components of the cyanobacterial cell division apparatus [Koksharova & Wolk, 2002; Fulgosi *et al.*, 2002; Raynaud *et al.*, 2004; Miyagishima at al., 2005]. It is important that the identification and analysis of division components may be more efficient in cyanobacteria rather than *Arabidopsis* or other model systems because of the easy cultivation, the short cyanobacterial generation time, the ability to obtain a near-synchronous culture, availability of many genetic tools [Koksharova & Wolk, 2002a]. One more of the experimental tools for functional study cyanobacterial cell division could be comparative proteomic analysis.

FUNCTIONAL PROTEOMICS FOR STUDY OF CYANOBACTERIAL CELL DIVISION

Cell division is a highly co-ordinated and fine-tuned process, and the precise regulation and positioning of the cell division apparatus require a number of both structural and regulatory components, of which many are still unidentified. Mutagenic disruption of proper regulation in the cell division machinery often leads to the formation of elongated and/or mini cells and may impose a strong internal stress altering the cellular physiology. In addition, metabolic pathways, which are regulated by the cell cycle, will be affected. Also, compensatory mechanisms to overcome the impaired cell division are expected. Although the cell division is impaired, for example, in the FTN2 and FTN6 cell division mutants, they have comparable growth rates [Koksharova & Wolk, 2002; Miyagishima *et al.,* 2005].

Fueled by ever-growing DNA sequence information, proteomics – the large scale analysis of proteins – has become one of the most important disciplines for characterizing gene function, for building functional linkages between protein molecules, and for providing insight into the mechanisms of biological processes in a high-throughput mode. In particular, proteomic analysis is vital, as the observed phenotype is a direct result of the action of the proteins rather than the genome sequence. Two-dimensional polyacrylamide gel electrophoresis (2-D gels) (Figure 6) is the pre-eminent tool for monitoring proteomic changes for example during bacterial stress responses [for review Neidhardt & VanBogelen, 2000]. However, proteomic studies of stress responses in cyanobacteria, including the potentially stressful condition that a blocked cell division may impose, are so far limited. Proteome analysis has been successfully used for identifying periplasmic proteins of salt-stressed *Synechocystis* sp. strain PCC 6803 cells, and resulted in the identification of proteins responding strongly to salt stress [Fulda *et al.*, 2000; Fulda *et al*, 2006; Huang *et al.*, 2006]. Proteomic analysis of the heat shock response of wild-type and a mutant of the histidine kinase 34 gene has been performed in the cyanobacterium *Synechocystis* sp. strain PCC 6803 [Slabas *et al.*, 2006]. Moreover, 2-D gel electrophoresis with *in vivo* [^{35}S] methionine labelling has been applied for investigating long-term chlorotic cells of *Synechococcus* [Sauer *et al.*, 2001].

The unicellular *Synechococcus* sp. strain PCC 7942 belongs to the ancient cyanobacterial group of photoautotrophic prokaryotes [Rippka *et al.,* 1979], and has been used as a model organism for studying the genetic control of cyanobacterial cell division [Dolganov & Grossman, 1993; Koksharova & Wolk, 2002; Miyagishima *et al.,* 2005] as well as plastid division in higher plants [Vitha *et al.*, 2003]. In *Synechococcus* sp. strain PCC 7942, the first proteomic overview has been initiated recently [Koksharova *et al.*, 2006]. The proteome was analyzed by two-dimensional gel electrophoresis with subsequent MALDI-TOF mass spectroscopy and database analysis. Of the 140 analyzed protein spots, 110 were successfully identified as 62 different proteins, many of which occurred as multiple spots on the gel (Figure 7). The identified proteins participate in the major metabolic and cellular processes in cyanobacterial cells during the exponential growth phase. In addition, 14 proteins which were previously either unknown or considered to be hypothetical were shown to be true gene products in *Synechococcus* sp. strain PCC 7942 [Koksharova *et al.*, 2006]. These results may be helpful for the annotation of the recently sequenced genome of this cyanobacterium, as well as for biochemical and physiological studies of *Synechococcus*.

In the next proteomic study of this cyanobacteria [Koksharova *et al.*, 2007] proteomes of the two cell division mutants FTN2 and FTN6 mutants were compared to the wild-type in order to widen our knowledge about the cell division machinery using a new approach. Quantitative differences in the protein maps were detected and proteins with significant quantitative changes were identified.

Comparative Proteomics of Cyanobacterial Cell Division Mutants FTN2 and FTN6 of *Synechococcus* sp. PCC 7942

Two new cell division genes, *ftn2* and *ftn6*, were discovered in *Synechococcus* sp. strain PCC 7942 by transposon Tn*5*-692 mutagenesis, followed by mutant DNA cloning and sequencing [Koksharova & Wolk, 2002]. The Ftn2 protein contains a DnaJ domain, a single tetratricopeptide repeat (TPR) and a leucine zipper pattern suggesting that Ftn2 may associate as a component in a protein complex and have a regulatory function. The Ftn6 protein was found to be specific for cyanobacteria and, as no detectable conserved domains have been found within the protein, knowledge about its precise function is still lacking [Koksharova & Wolk, 2002; Miyagishima *et al.,* 2005]. Occasionally FTN2 and FTN6 mutant cells divide and septum formation takes place irregularly [Koksharova & Wolk, 2002] but only a slight and

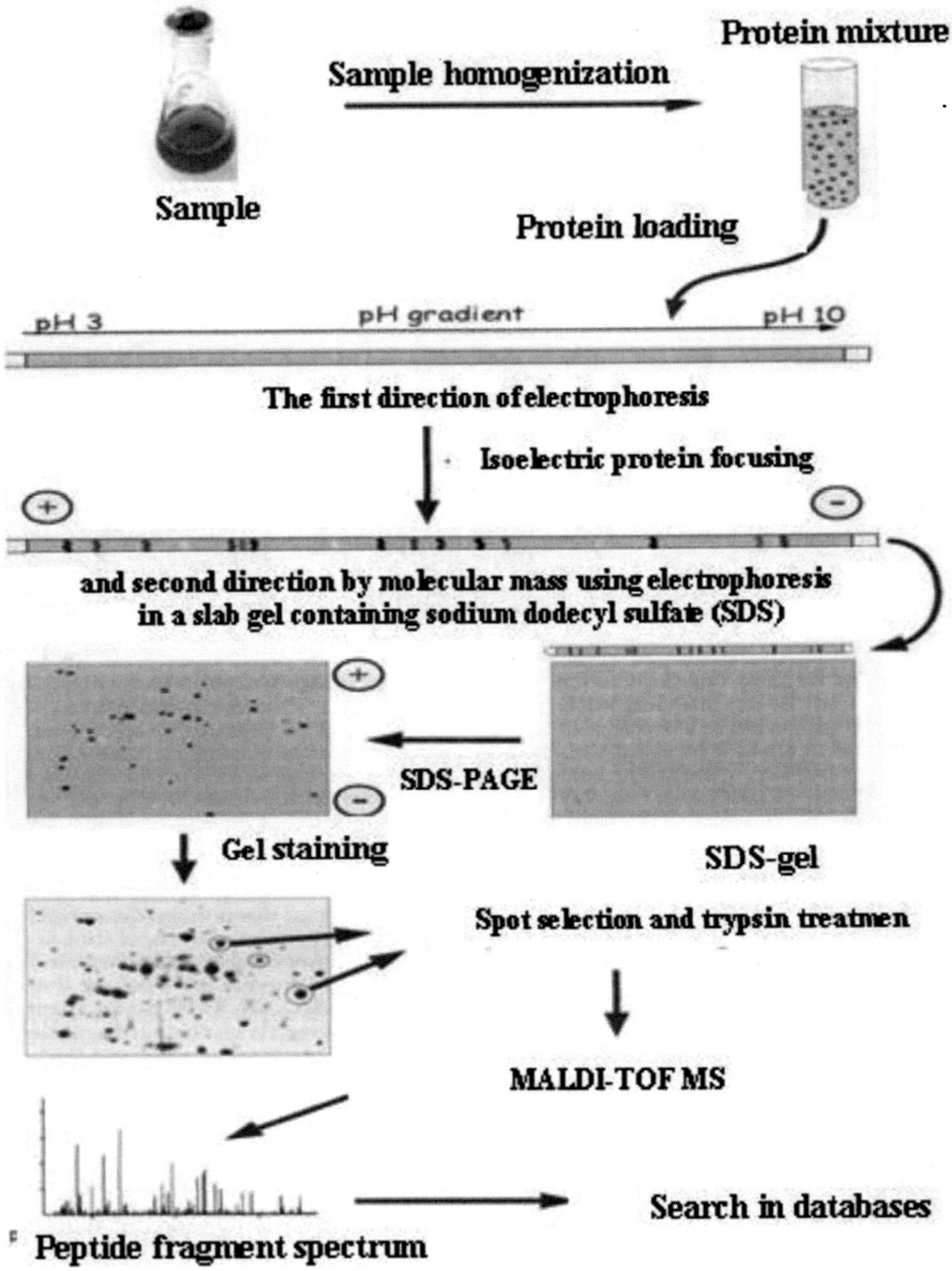

Figure 6. Scheme of a proteomic analysis is based on Two-dimensional polyacrylamide gel electrophoresis and MALDI-TOF mass spectroscopy.

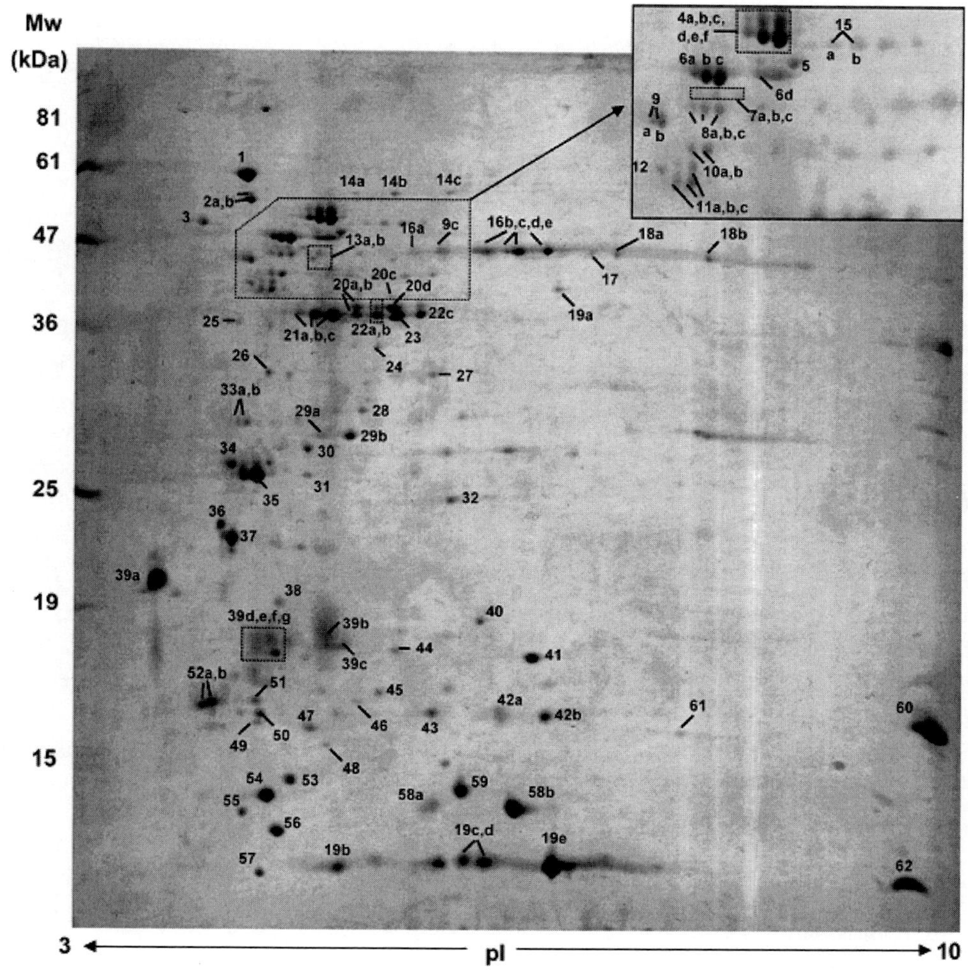

Figure 7. Two-dimensional electrophoresis protein profile (Coomassie-stained gel) of total protein of *Synechococcus* sp. strain PCC 7942. The protein molecular weight standard (Mw) (y axis) and isoelectric points (pI) (x axis) are shown [Koksharova *et a*l., 2006].

diffuses localization of the key cell division protein FtsZ, homologous of tubulin [Bi & Lutkenhaus, 1991], has been detected at these rare cell division constriction sites. However, only a small difference in FtsZ protein levels could be detected between the mutants and the wild-type strain using immunoblot analysis of total soluble protein extracts [Koksharova, Klint, Rasmussen, 2003, unpublished results; Miyagishima *et al.,* 2005]. Therefore it has been suggested that these mutants are defective in recruitment of FtsZ to the division site or in subsequent assembly of the Z ring. Investigations of the Ftn2 protein orthologs in *Arabidopsis thaliana* (ARC6) and in the cyanobacterium *Synechocystis* sp. strain PCC 6803 (ZipN) have shown that a direct interaction between Ftn2 and FtsZ is most likely [Vitha *et al.*, 2003; Mazouni *et al.*, 2004]. Ftn2 may function in a chaperone system, probably to stabilize FtsZ filaments. Whether the Ftn6 protein in cyanobacteria interacts directly or indirectly with FtsZ is not known, but a loss of the *ftn6* gene results in aberrant cell division, similar to the FTN2 mutant [Koksharova & Wolk, 2002; Mazouni *et al.*, 2004; Miyagishima *et al.,* 2005].

For the first proteomic study of cyanobacterial cell division total soluble proteins extracted from the wild-type *Synechococcus* sp. strain PCC 7942 and the two cell division mutants FTN2 and FTN6 were analyzed by separation on 2-D gels in the pH range 3-10 and 4-7, followed by staining with SYPRO Ruby (representative gels from the eighteen gel series are presented on Figure 8). Fluorescent chromophore-staining (SYPRO Ruby) dye is very sensitive [Berggren *et al.*, 2000] and permits to obtain digital image of the gel that can be analyzed by using PDQuest software. More than 800 protein spots on each gel were visualized, among which 76 protein spots in total were changed in quantity between the wild-type and the mutants as resolved by using the PDQuest software. These protein spots were subjected to MALDI-TOF mass spectroscopy resulting in the identification of 53 protein spots representing 44 unique proteins, which were grouped into seven main functional categories. Fifteen proteins were up-shifted or induced in both cell division mutants, and 13 proteins were down-shifted or repressed. The changed proteins included a general increased level of proteins involved in cell cycle and regeneration as well as protein synthesis, posttranslational processing and modification. Besides of eliciting common responses, the inactivation of *ftn2* and *ftn6* in the mutants may result in different responses in protein levels between the mutants [Koksharova *et al.*, 2007]. Among identified differentially affected proteins, 80% (8/10) of the spots affected in the FTN2 mutant were up-shifted, whereas in the FTN6 mutant 70% (7/10) of the affected protein spots were down-shifted (Table 5). These results indicate that the Ftn2 protein may have a negative effect and the Ftn6 protein may have a positive effect on the level of some proteins in *Synechococcus* sp. PCC 7942, either directly or indirectly.

Mutations in genes *ftn2* and *ftn6* influence on level of 44 idetified proteins that are represent different physiological processes:

1. Cell cycle and morphogenesis
2. Synthesis and modification of proteins
3. Photosynthesis
4. Oxidative stress defense
5. CO_2 fixation and carbon concentrating mechanism
6. Energy production and different biosynthetic processes
7. Processes that involve unknown and hypothetical proteins

Possible functions of some of these proteins are discussed below to assess the impact of impaired cell division on cell physiology at the protein level.

Cell Cycle and Morphogenesis

Several proteins involved in cell cycle control were affected in the cell division mutants FTN2 and FTN6. The beta subunit (DnaN) of the multi-chain enzyme, DNA polymerase III, a key enzyme in the replicative synthesis of bacteria, was two fold up-shifted in the FTN2 mutant (Table 4, 5) DnaN is required for the initiation of DNA replication and regulates the chromosomal replication cycle [Katayama *et al.*, 1998]. The rhythmical expression of *dnaN* gene in *Synechococcus* sp. strain PCC 7942 suggests that DNA replication could be under circadian control in this organism [Liu & Tsinoremas, 1996]. Chromosome replication and cell division are highly co-ordinated processes, and the early stages of DNA replication play a key role in the precise positioning of the Z ring at mid-cell and between replicating daughter chromosomes [Harry *et al.*, 1999]. In *Escherichia coli*, the function of DnaA is negatively regulated by DnaN [Katayama *et al.*, 1998], and an interaction between the replication initiator DnaA and DnaN is required to regulate the chromosomal replication cycle [Katayama *et al.*, 1998; Kawakami *et al.*, 2001]. It is likely that the increased amount of DnaN in cells of the FTN2 mutants may affect DNA replication and consequently disturbs cell division.

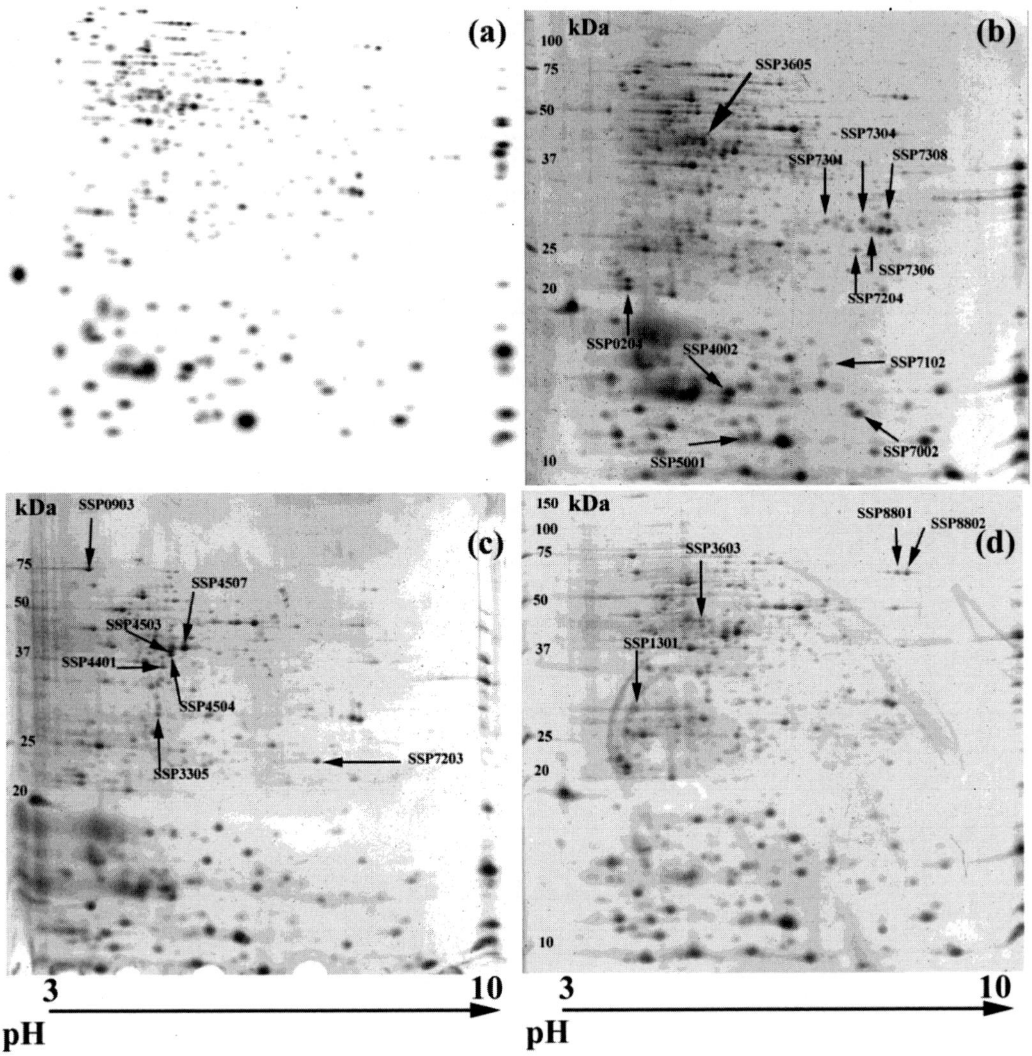

Figure 8. Protein patterns of *Synechococcus* sp. strain PCC 7942 revealed by 2D gel electrophoresis (pH range 3–10). (a) Synthetic gel created by using PDQuest software, (b) wild-type cells, (c) FTN2 mutant, (d) FTN6 mutant. Protein molecular mass standards (y -axis) and pHs (x-axis) are shown. Arrows show the protein spots that were cut out from the gels and processed for identification. The gels were stained with SYPRO Ruby. [Koksharova et al., 2007]

Table 4. Identified proteins that are differently expressed in the wild-type and cell division mutants of *Synechococcus* sp. strain PCC 7942

NCBI Acces. no.	Gene no.	Encoded protein	Protein level (arbitrary units)*		
			WT	FTN2	FTN6
Group 1. Cell cycle/cell morphogenesis					
974615	0001	DNA polymerase III β subunit	1474	3005	1911
46129703	1139	Chromosome segregation ATPase	557	621	274
81299111	0300	Actin-like ATPase involved in cell morphogenesis (MreB)	1857	3094	3291
46130530	2468	Molecular chaperone (Hsp70)	4781	6240	5158
46129574	0928	Outer-membrane protein	138	482	281
Group 2. Protein synthesis and processing					
46129550	0884	GTPase translation elongation factor	3687	7040	6077
46130513	2440	Polyribonucleotide nucleotidyltransferase	0	1123	541
22002498	1591	Ribosomal protein S1	1313	1974	2121
45512376	0790	RNA-binding protein (RRM domain)	1673	5300	293
53762838	0685	Chaperonin GroEL	0	372	127
45513516	2072	Molecular chaperone GrpE	2726	5463	3667
53762820	0712	Periplasmic protease	1257	2627	1328
53762940	0531	TPR domain	1133	1352	2154
46129730	1190	Leucyl aminopeptidase	1201	0	0
53762913	0565	FHA domain	715	444	0
Group 3. Photosynthesis					
226392	1002	PsaD protein, PSI	3808	231	111
45512096	0240	Hypothetical protein Selo03002341	1336	304	0
46129650	1050	Hypothetical protein Selo03000334	787	169	142
45512619	1053	Hypothetical protein Selo03000332	9154	697	457
142156	0294	Mn-stabilizing protein precursor	1692	3254	7312
Group 4. Oxidative stress response and redox control					
45513728	2309	Peroxiredoxin	6063	12477	10824
46130096	1793	Thioredoxin	917	779	44
53763070	0304	Ubiquinone biosynthesis protein Coq4	886	7673	461
Group 5. Carbon dioxide concentrating mechanism and fixation					
45513432	1980	Transcriptional regulator	514	716	195
576253	1426	Chain A, RuBisCO, oxygenase	1406	0	0
46129874	1427	RuBisCO small subunit	7609	1606	2921
46129871	1423	Carbonic anhydrase/ acetyltransferase	883	536	1227
Group 6. Energy production and different biosynthetic processes					
53763249	0003	FGAM synthase (PurL)	735	354	220
53763017	0396	AICAR transformylase (PurH)	354	1241	433

Table 4. (*Continued*)

NCBI Acces. no.	Gene no.	Encoded protein	Protein level (arbitrary units)*		
			WT	FTN2	FTN6
45512432	0851	Phosphoribosylaminoimidazole synthase (PurM)	1600	1473	2125
46130119	1831	IMP dehydrogenase/GMP reductase	1229	2474	899
46130337	2156	Glutamine synthetase	1330	470	0
46130191	1927	Diaminopimelate epimerase	1315	2910	3943
46130169	1896	N-Acetylglutamate synthase	437	1002	566
53763244	0009	Argininosuccinate synthase	1391	1473	522
46129889	1443	Fructose/tagatose bisphosphate aldolase	2904	6058	3932
46129736	1198	Pyruvate/2-oxoglutarate dehydrogenase complex, dihydrolipoamide dehydrogenase (E3) component	286	0	0
53763057	0335	F_0F_1-type ATP synthase, δ subunit	987	417	385
45513409	1956	Acetyl-CoA carboxylase β subunit	1961	771	525
53762839	0684	Dehydrogenase with different specificities	2258	1081	1877
Group 7. Unknown and hypothetical proteins					
53763101	0259	Hypothetical protein Selo03002321	3310	5999	6071
46129994	1613	Hypothetical protein Selo03000898	4052	8130	6301
25019695	2483	Unknown	0	338	276
24414820	0443	Hypothetical protein	163	732	167

* These values were calculated by PDQuest software as an average from three independent experiments [Koksharova *et al.*, 2007]

Table 5. Proteins up- or downregulated differently between the FTN2 and FTN6 mutants.

Protein	Protein expression changes*	
	FTN2 mutant	FTN6 mutant
Carbonic anhydrase/acetyltransferase	0.5	NS
Dehydrogenase with different specificities	0.5	NS
DNA polymerase III β subunit	2	NS
Molecular chaperone (Hsp70)	1.3	NS
Periplasmic protease	2	NS
AICAR transformylase (PurH)	3.5	NS
Hypothetical protein	4.5	NS
RNA-binding protein (RRM domain)	3	0.2
Ubiquinone biosynthesis protein Coq4	9	0.5
IMP dehydrogenase/GMP reductase	2	0.7
Chromosome segregation ATPase	NS	0.5
Thioredoxin	NS	0.05
Transcriptional regulator	NS	0.4
Argininosuccinate synthase	NS	0.4
TPR domain	NS	1.9
Phosphoribosyl-aminoimidazole synthase (PurM)	NS	1.3

*A minimum of 1.3-fold change was considered for the upregulated proteins and 0.7-fold for downregulated proteins compared to wild- type. NS, Not significantly changed compared to wild-type [Koksharova et al., 2007].

A protein identified as chromosome segregation ATPases was two fold down-shifted in the FTN6 mutant (Table 4, 5). However, how the chromosome segregation ATPase contributes to the process of cyanobacterial chromosome segregation and how it can be connected functionally with Ftn6 protein are presently unknown. Since MreB was also affected in the mutants (see below), the processes of chromosome segregation and cell septation may be co-regulated at some level in cyanobacteria *Synechococcus* sp. PCC 7942.

Chromosome segregation has been well studied in the heterotrophic bacteria *E. coli, Bacillus subtilis,* and *Caulobacter crescentus* [Kruse *et al.*, 2003; Sherratt, 2003] where proteins such as the Min system [Åkerlund *et al.*, 2002], Par A and Par B [Easter & Gober, 2002], DivIVA [Thomaides *et al.*, 2001], SMC proteins [Graumann, 2001], and SpoIIIE [Bath *et al.*, 2000] have been proposed to be involved. Cell division normally follows the completion of each round of chromosome replication in *Escherichia coli.* Transcription of the essential cell division genes clustered at the *mra* region (*ftsL, ftsI, ftsW, ftsQ, ftsA*) is shown to depend on continuing chromosomal DNA replication [Liu *et al.*, 2001]. W.D.Donachie and his colleagues suggested the existence of SOS-independent co-ordination of cell division and chromosome replication. In *Caurobacter crescentus* response regulator of the cell cycle, CtrA, coordinates the cell cycle-dependent expression of genes including *ftsZ* [Wortinger *et al.*, 2000]. Little is known about cyanobacterial cell cycle and about a coordination of DNA replication and cell division. In some cyanobacteria these processes are reported to be under the control of a circadian clock [Sweeney & Borgese.1989; Mori *et al.*, 1996; Kondo *et al.*, 1997]. Study of expression of cell cycle-related genes (*ftsZ* and *dnaA*) in synchronized cultures of *Prochlorococcus* sp. strain PCC 9511 has shown that both genes exhibited clear expression patterns with mRNA maxim a during the replication (S) phase. Western blot experiments indicated that the peak of FtsZ concentration occurred at night, i.e., at the time of cell division. Thus, the transcript accumulation of genes involved in replication and division is coordinated in *Prochlorococcus* sp. strain PCC 9511 [Holtzendorff *et al.*, 2001]. Other study was performed for the bloom forming cyanobacteria *Microcystis aeruginosa* [Yoshida T. *et al.*, 2005]. In this research authors have shown that when either nalidixic acid (an inhibitor of DNA gyrase) or hydroxyurea (an inhibitor of ribonucleotide reductase) was added to a synchronized culture of *Microcystis aeruginosa* to block DNA replication, cell division did not occur and FtsZ transcription was repressed. However, the increased amount of DNA, in DAPI-DNA-stained tubulin inhibitor, such as thiabendazole (TBZ), treated *Synechococcus* 7942 cells, indicates that DNA replication still occurs in the presence of TBZ, which block cell division [Sarcina & Mullineaux, 2000].

MreB, an actin homologue, is involved in shape determination in rod-shaped prokaryotic cells [Wachi *et al.*, 1987; Jones *et al.*, 2001; Figge *et al.*, 2004; Gitai *et al.*, 2004] and may or may not be involved in DNA replication in some bacterial species [Kruse *et al.*, 2003, 2006; Gitai *et al.*, 2005; Hu *et al.*, 2007]. Very little is known about MreB function in cyanobacterial cells. Recently it has been suggested [Hu *et al.*, 2007] that in *Anabaena* sp. PCC 7120 this protein involved in shape determination, but not in DNA segregation. A previous study revealed that cell division in *E. coli* is under negative control of the *mreB* gene [Wachi & Matsuhashi, 1989]. While overexpression of wild-type MreB has been shown to inhibit cell division but not perturb chromosome segregation, overexpression of mutant forms of MreB causes, in addition to the inhibition of cell division, abnormal MreB filament morphology and induces severe localization defects of the nucleoid in *E. coli* [Kruse *et al.*, 2003]. This fact, together with enhanced expression of the cell division gene *ftsI* in *mreB* mutant *E. coli* cells [Wachi & Matsuhashi, 1989], may indicate a function of the *mreB* gene as a regulator for determining progression to cell division or elongation in *E. coli*. At the same time, in *Synechococcus* sp. strain PCC 7942, the upshift of the MreB protein in the two cell division mutants could reflect a direct or indirect negative regulation of MreB by the *ftn2* and *ftn6* genes and explain the filamentous phenotype of the mutant cells [Koksharova *et al.*, 2007].

Bacteria possess a number of cytoskeletal elements [Mayer, 2003], including FtsZ, a bacterial tubulin homologue [Carballido-López & Errington, 2003; Michie & Löwe, 2006; Klint *et al.*, 2007], MreB coiled structures similar to F-actin, the physiological polymer of eukaryotic actin [van den Ent *et al.*, 2001], MinCDE coiled arrays [Shih *et al.*, 2003] and intracellular protofilaments containing bacterial elongation factor Tu (EF-Tu) [Löwe *et al.*, 2004]. All of them may form cytoskeletal webs, which are important for the organization of intracellular structures and cell function [Mayer, 2003]. Two of these proteins, MreB and EF-Tu were notably upshifted in the cell division mutants FTN2 and FTN6 (Table 4). It is likely that filamentous cells of the mutants may require an extended cytoskeletal web.

A molecular chaperone, heat shock protein Hsp70 was up-regulated in the FTN2 mutant (Table 4, 5). This 634 amino acid protein has an N-terminal MreB (amino acid 1-371) region, and the protein show 94% sequence identity with the chaperone protein K2 (heat shock protein 70-2) of *Synechococcus* sp. strain PCC 7942 (gi|1706478|sp|P50021|DNK2_SYNP7). Overproduction of DnaK2 has resulted in defects in cell septation and formation of cell filaments [Nimura *et al.*, 2001], suggesting an interaction with key cell septation protein(s).

An outer membrane protein containing one transmembrane helix in the N-terminus was up-regulated in both cell division mutants (Table 4). This protein show homology with the chloroplast import-associated channel IAP75 protein of *Synechocystis* sp. PCC 6803 (Gene ID: 954135 IAP75) and with *Arabidopsis thaliana* outer envelope protein of 80 kDa (Gene ID: 832082 OEP80), wich involved in protein import as one of the translocation channel protein at the chloroplast outer envelope membrane [Baldwin *et al.*, 2005]. The location of this protein in the outer membrane may suggest its involvement in cyanobacteria cell envelope biogenesis and/or secretion. Presumably, elongated mutant cells require an increased synthesis of cell membrane as well as an intensive intracellular traffic.

Protein Synthesis and Processing

Three proteins (GTPase translation elongation factor, Polyribonucleotide nucleotidyltransferase, Ribosomal protein S1) involved in protein synthesis were up-shifted in both mutants. The GTPase–translation elongation factor has been mentioned above in the context of cytoskeletal webs, but this protein also has a role in protein translation [Rodnina *et al.*, 2000]. Polyribonucleotide nucleotidyltransferase was identified exclusively in the mutant cells (Table 4). In addition, the protein abundance was two fold higher in FTN2 mutant compared to FTN6 mutant (Table 4). Polyribonucleotide nucleotidyltransferase possesses four 3' exoribonuclease family domains and three RNA binding domains. The polynucleotide phosphorylase is a 3'-5' key exonuclease for mRNA decay and part of a multicomponent mRNA-protein complex (the "degradosome") [Coburn & Mackie, 1999] that orchestrates mRNA decay in bacteria. Under stress conditions, polyribonucleotide nucleotidyltransferase has been shown to be up-regulated in bacteria [Len *et al.*, 2004], which may also be the situation in the FTN2 and FTN6 mutant cells.

The ribosomal protein S1 involved in ribosome binding to mRNA during translation was up-regulated in the mutants (Table 4). Moreover, the RNA-binding protein (RRM domain-RNA Recognition Motif) was three fold up-shifted in FTN2 cells and almost six fold down-shifted in FTN6 mutant (Table 4, 5). There is no information available so far about the regulation of RNA-binding proteins during the impaired cell division condition; however, it is known that *Rbps* (*R*NA-*b*inding *p*roteins) of cyanobacteria are under stress-responsive regulation, reacting to e.g. the temperature and nitrogen status [Maruyama *et al.*, 1999; Mori *et al.*, 2003].

In the cell division mutants, three proteins involved in posttranslational protein processing and modifications (chaperonin GroEL, molecular chaperone GrpE, and periplasmic protease) were up-shifted (Table 4). GroEL and GrpE are chaperones, which may additionally reflect that the mutants are under a stressed condition; notably chaperonin GroEL was exclusively found in the mutant cells (Table 4). The GroEL/GroES system is a major chaperone system in all bacteria and its involvement in cyanobacterial stress responses have been extensively studied [Hihara *et al.*, 2001; Kovacs *et al.*, 2001; Mary *et al.*, 2004]. Some new data appeared suggesting involvement of GroEL in bacterial cell division [Kerner *et al.*, 2005; Susin *et al.*, 2006; Fujiwara & Taguchi, 2007; Lemos *et al.*, 2007]. In addition, new plastid division proteins, ptCpn60α and ptCpn60β, have been identified recently [Suzuki *et al.*, 2009]. These two proteins have a similarity with cyanobacterial chaperonin GroEL. It is possible that cyanobacterial chaperonin GroEL also may be involved in cell division and therefore in the mutants FTN2 and FTN6 its level noticeably increased due to impaired cell division.

The two fold up-shift of periplasmic protease was only obvious for the FTN2 mutant (Table 4, 5).

One protein, identified as TPR repeat-containing protein was distinctly up-shifted in the FTN6 (Table 4, 5). The tetratricopeptide repeat (TPR) is a degenerate 34-amino-acid sequence, present in tandem arrays of 1–16 motifs mediating protein–protein interactions, was found for the first time by Sikorski and co-authors in the cell division control protein Cdc23 [Sikorski *et al.*, 1990]. TPR motifs are important for the function of chaperones, cell-cycle, transcription, and protein-transport complexes [Blatch & Lässle, 1999]. Interestingly, the TPR repeat is present also in the cell division protein Ftn2 in *Synechococcus* sp. strain PCC 7942 [Koksharova & Wolk, 2002b].

Two proteins, possibly involved in protein-protein interactions and protein processing/degradation, were, in contrast to the other proteins in this group, down-shifted in both mutants. One, the leucyl aminopeptidase (Table 4), was only detected in the wild-type. A second protein, containing the FHA domain, was absent in FTN6 mutant and down-shifted in cells of FTN2 mutant (Table 4). FHA domains are implicated in many bacterial processes, including the regulation of cell shape, type III secretion, sporulation, pathogenic and symbiotic host-bacterium interactions, carbohydrate storage and transport, signal transduction [Pallen *et al.*, 2002].

Cell Metabolism Changes in the Cell Division Mutants

Four photosynthetic proteins were down-regulated in one or both mutants. Protein PsaD, a small extrinsic polypeptide located on the stromal side of the photosystem I reaction center complex, was strongly down-shifted in both cell division mutants. Three hypothetical proteins (Selo03002341, Selo03000334 and Selo03000332) homologous to light-harvesting pigment-proteins were also down-shifted in the mutant cells. In contrast to the photosynthetic pigmented proteins, Mn-stabilizing protein precursor associated with the oxygen evolving photosystem II was strongly up-shifted in both mutants (Table 4).

The up-shift in the oxygen evolving Mn-stabilizing protein precursor may result in the production of reactive oxygen species and free radicals. Consequently, a protein involved in oxidative stress response, peroxiredoxin [Wood *et al.*, 2003] was identified as up-regulated in both mutants (Table 4). Additionally, an uncharacterized protein involved in ubiquitine biosynthesis was up-shifted in the FTN2 mutant (Table 4, 5). This protein possesses a region named Coenzyme Q (ubiquinone) biosynthesis protein Coq4. Ubiquinones are essential redox components of the photosynthetic electron-transport chain in photoautotrophic organisms. They play vital roles in the management of oxidative stress and gene regulation [Soballe & Poole, 1999].

Thiol-disulfide isomerase (thioredoxin) was down-shifted in both mutants, most pronounced (more than 20 fold) in the FTN6 mutant (Table 4). Earlier by using a proteomic approach, Kumar and co-authors [Kumar *et al.*, 2004] identified in total 80 bacterial proteins associated with thioredoxin, implicating the involvement of thioredoxin in at least 26 distinct cellular processes including transcriptional regulation, cell division, energy transduction, and several biosynthetic pathways. Our data show that the protein level of thioredoxin may also have a direct or indirect connection with cell division in cyanobacteria.

A transcriptional regulator belonging to the lysR family [Henikoff *et al.*, 1988] was slightly up-shifted in FTN2 and more then 2.5 fold down-shifted in FTN6 cells (Table 4, 5). The closest homologous proteins were found in *Nostoc* sp. strain PCC 7120 (gi|17133087|dbj|BAB75652.1| ORF_ID:all3953~transcriptional regulator, RbcR homolog, 83% sequence identity). Hence, this protein is possibly involved in regulation of RuBisCO expression.

The protein identified as chain A of RuBisCO was not detected in protein extracts from the mutants and the small subunit of RuBisCO was down-shifted in both mutants (Table 4). The activity, synthesis and degradation of this enzyme are regulated by several mechanisms; one of them being by the redox potential [Marcus *et al.*, 2003]. Stress conditions, provoked by nitrate deprivation, also decrease the RuBisCO contents [Marcus *et al.*, 2003]. The interpretations for the low abundance of RuBisCO proteins in the cell division mutants FTN2 and FTN6 are speculative. Potentially, some changes in general cell redox status of the division mutants as well as possible deficiency of nitrogen can induce degradation of this protein.

A carbonic anhydrases/acetyltransferase [Badger & Price, 2003] was down-shifted in FTN2 and slightly up-shifted in FTN6 mutant (Table 4 and 5).

Four proteins involved in purine biosynthesis were affected in the mutants, among them are FGAM synthase (PurL), AICAR transformylase (PurH), Phosphoribosylaminoimidazole synthase (PurM), and IMP dehydrogenase/GMP reductase (Table 4). Phosphoribosylformylglycinamidine (FGAM) synthase (PurL) is the fourth enzyme in the purine nucleotide biosynthesis pathway. The *purL* gene in *Synechococcus* sp. strain PCC 7942 is expressed under circadian cycle control in the same gene cluster as *dnaN* (see above) [Liu *et al.*, 1996]. The PurL protein was down-regulated in the FTN2 and FTN6 cell division mutants. On the contrary, two other purine biosynthesis enzymes were up-regulated in both mutants (Table 4). The protein AICAR transformylase/IMP cyclohydrolase PurH catalyzes the last two steps in *de novo* purine biosynthesis [Kappock *et al.*, 2000], whereas IMP dehydrogenase/GMP reductase (*guaB*) catalyzes the rate-limiting reaction of *de novo* GTP biosynthesis. The latter enzyme is another example of different regulation of Ftn2 and Ftn6 in *Synechococcus.* This enzyme was up-regulated in FTN2 mutant cells and down-regulated in FTN6 mutant cells (Table 5). Guanine nucleotides are important substrates for macromolecular synthesis, cell signalling and have an evolutionary conserved role during differentiation, proliferation, and apoptosis [Yalowitz & Jayaram, 2000]. An important observation is that these four nucleotide synthesis proteins and a component of DNA polymerase III (DnaN) involved in replicative synthesis (see above) were affected in FTN2 and FTN6 mutants. This could be an indication of that the cell cycle in the FTN2 and FTN6 mutants is affected in some stages prior to cell division and/or the cell cycle is arrested due to the mutations, and thus expression of cell cycle dependent genes is modified. In addition, a chromosome segregation ATPase and MreB were affected (see above), also pointing in this direction.

A key enzyme of nitrogen metabolism, glutamine synthase (GS), was strongly down-shifted in both mutants (Table 4). Inhibition of GS in *Synechococcus* sp. strain PCC 7942 leads to a rapid decrease of allophycocyanin mRNA and increase of *nblA* (the gene essential for degradation of the phycobilisome) levels, which is characteristic for nitrogen deprivation [Sauer *et al.*, 1999]. The low level of GS, phycobiliproteins (Group 3) and RuBisCO proteins (Group 5) are indications for nitrogen starvation and/or deficiency in amino acids in the mutants.

Three additional proteins involved in amino acid metabolism (Diaminopimelate epimerase, N-Acetylglutamate synthase, Argininosuccinate synthase; Table 4) were significantly changed in the cell division mutants, although different behavior between the proteins was seen. Diaminopimelate epimerase is involved in peptidoglycan synthesis by catalyzing the isomeriazation of L,L- to D,L-meso-diaminopimelate in the biosynthetic pathway leading from aspartate to lysine, [Mirelman, 1979]. N-acetylglutamate synthase (N-acetylornithine aminotransferase) is a member of the ArgJ family involved in arginine biosynthesis [Caldovic & Tuchman, 2003]. These two enzymes are up-regulated in both cell division mutants (Table 4). A second enzyme involved in arginine biosynthesis, argininosuccinate synthase is down-shifted in FTN 6 cells (Table 4, 5).

Two proteins (Pyruvate/2-oxoglutarate, dihydrolipoamide dehydrogenase (E3) component and F_0F_1-type ATP synthase, δ subunit) involved in energy production and conversion were down-shifted in both cell division mutants (Table 4).

The first enzyme of the biosynthetic pathway to fatty acids, beta subunit of acetyl-CoA carboxylase, was also identified as down-shifted in both cell division mutants (Table 4). As fatty acids are primarily precursors of phospholipids, acetyl coenzyme A (CoA) carboxylase activity can be correlated to cell growth and division, as well as to cell development [Gornicki *et al.*, 1993].

The glycolytic enzyme fructose/tagatose bisphosphate aldolase (Table 4) was up-shifted in both cell division mutants. Such up-shift in a glycolytic enzyme(s) could possibly be a way to somehow compensate for deficit of energy in the mutant cells, caused by the down-regulation of many proteins involved in general cell metabolism.

Unknown and Hypothetical Proteins

A hypothetical protein possessing three S-layer homology (SLH) domains was up-shifted 4.5 fold in the FTN2 mutant. Three proteins (Selo03002321; Selo03000898, and Unknown) were up-shifted in both cell division mutants (Table 4), but do not show any significant homology to proteins with known function. The unknown protein was found only in the mutants (Table 4). Targeted inactivation of the genes encoding unknown and hypothetical proteins identified in this proteomic study may elucidate roles of these proteins in relation to cyanobacterial cell division.

Identification of such differentially expressed proteins provides new targets for future genetical studies that will allow assessment of their physiological roles and significance in cyanobacterial cell division. Moreover, as evident from the presented proteomic data, cell division mutants FTN2 and FTN6 may be useful for study of diferent sides of cyanobacterial cellular metabolism and physiology as well.

Conclusion

Cyanobacteria, prokaryotic photoautotrophes and ancient relatives of chloroplasts, can assist analysis of cell division and its regulation more easily than can studies with higher plants. Identification and study of cyanobacterial genes could help to discover their plant homologues and to investigate functions of these genes. A fruitful genetical approach to understanding of the division process in both cyanobacteria and chloroplasts is created. High efficient transposon mutagenesis helps to identified new cell division genes. The availability of the complete genomic sequences of many cyanobacteria, bacteria, some plants and algae facilitates comparative genomic and proteomic analysis. The results show that mutations only in two cell division genes *ftn2* and *ftn6* affect the cellular quantity of many different proteins. Identification of these proteins provides the new targets for coming studies that will allow assessments of their functions and importance in cell division of cyanobacteria. For a fruitful study of molecular biology of cyanobacterial cell division, integration of genetic, genomic, proteomic and future transcriptomic data are required.

Acknowledgements

I would like to thank kindly Professor S.V.Shestakov and Dr. Mikheeva L.E. at M.V. Lomonosov Moscow State University, who were my first teachers in cyanobacterial genetics. I express my sincere gratitude to Professor C. Peter Wolk at Michigan State University, which supported me in our cyanobacteria cell division research. I would like to thank my wonderful colleagues Ulla Rasmussen and Johan Klint at Botanical Department of Stockholm University for the joy of our work in the cell division proteomic project. I thank very much my colleagues Baulina O.I. and Gorelova O.A. at the M.V. Lomonosov Moscow State University for their help and support during study cyanobacterial cell division mutants. My love and gratitude is to my parents and brother, to my lovely children and dear husband. This work was supported by The Royal Swedish Academy of Sciences and by grants from the Russian Foundation for Basic Research (number 03-04-49332 and 08-04-00878).

REFERENCES

Åkerlund, T., Gullbrand, B. & Nordström, K. (2002). Effects of the Min system on nucleoid segregation in *Escherichia coli*. *Microbiology, 148*, 3213-3222.

Badger, M. R. & Price, G. D. (2003). CO_2 concentrating mechanisms in cyanobacteria: molecular components, their diversity and evolution. *J Exp Bot, 54,* 609-622.

Baldwin, A., Wardle, A., Patel, R., Dudley, P., S. Ki Park, Twell, D., Inoue, K., & Jarvis, P. (2005). A molecular-genetic study of the *Arabidopsis* Toc75 gene family. *Plant Physiology, 138*, 715-733.

Bath, J., Wu, L. J., Errington, J. & Wang, J. C. (2000). Role of *Bacillus subtilis* SpoIIIE in DNA transport across the mother cell-prespore division septum. *Science, 290*, 995-997.

Berggren, K., Chernokalskaya, E., Steinberg, T. H., Kemper, C., Lopez, M. F., Diwu, Z., Haugland, R. P. & Patton, W. F. (2000). Background-free, high sensitivity staining of proteins in one- and two-dimensional sodium dodecyl sulfate-polyacrylamide gels using a luminescent ruthenium complex. *Electrophoresis, 21*, 2509-2521.

Bi, E., & Lutkenhaus, J. (1991). FtsZ ring structure associated with division in *Escherichia coli*. *Nature*, *354*, 161-164.

Blatch, G. L. & Lässle, M. (1999). The tetratricopeptide repeat: a structural motif mediating protein-protein interactions. *Bioessays, 21*, 932-939.

Borthakur, D. & Haselkorn, R. (1989). Tn*5* mutagenesis of *Anabaena* sp. strain PCC 7120: isolation of a new mutant unable to grow without combined nitrogen. *J. Bacteriol*, *171*, 5759- 5761.

Bouche, J. P. & Pichoff, S. (1998). On the birth and fate of bacterial division sites. *Mol. Microbiol. 29*, 19-26.

Bramhill, D. (1997). Bacterial cell division. *Annu. Rev. Cell. Dev. Biol*, *13*, 395-424.

Broedel, S. E., & Wolf, R. E. (1990). Genetic tagging, cloning, and DNA sequence of the *Synechococcus* sp. strain PCC 7942 gene (*gnd*) encoding 6-phosphogluconate dehydrogenase. *J. Bacteriol.*, *172*, 4023-4031.

Bukau B. Molecular Chaperones and Folding Catalysts-Regulation, Cellular Function and Mechanisms. Amsterdam. Hardwood. 1999.

Bukau, B., & Horwich, A. L. (1998). The Hsp70 and Hsp60 chaperone machines. *Cell*, *92*, 351-366.

Bukau, B., & Walker, G. C. (1989). Cellular defects caused by deletion of the *Escherichia coli dnaK* gene indicate roles for heat shock protein in normal metabolism. *J. Bacteriol.*, *171*, 2337- 2346.

Caldovic, L. & Tuchman, M. (2003). N-Acetylglutamate and its changing role through evolution. *Biochem J.*, *372*, 279-290.

Carballido-López, R. & Errington, J. (2003). A dynamic bacterial cytoskeleton. *Trends Cell Biol*, *13*, 577-583.

Cheetham, M. E., & Caplan, A. J. (1998). Structure, function and evolution of DnaJ: conservation and adaptation of chaperone function. *Cell Stress Chaperones*, *3*, 28-36.

Coburn, G. A. & Mackie, G. A. (1999). Degradation of mRNA in *Escherichia coli*: an old problem with some new twists. *Prog Nucleic Acid Res Mol Biol*, *62*, 55-108.

Cohen, M. F., Meeks, J. C., Cai, Y. A., & Wolk, C. P. (1998). Transposon mutagenesis of heterocyst-forming filamentous cyanobacteria. *Methods Enzymol.*, *297*, 3-17.

Corbin, B. D., Wang, Y., Beuria, T. K., & Margolin, W. (2007). Interaction between cell division proteins FtsE and FtsZ. *J. Bacteriol.*, *189*, 3026-3035.

Cordell, S. C., Robinson, E. J., Lowe, J. (2003).Crystal structure of the SOS cell division inhibitor SulA and in complex with FtsZ. *Proc Natl Acad Sci U S A*; *100*, 7889-7894.

Dajkovic, A. & Lutkenhaus, J. 2006. Z ring as executor of bacterial cell division. *J. Mol. Microbiol. Biotechnol.*, *11*, 140-151.

Das, A. K., Cohen, P. W., & Barford, D. (1998). The structure of the tetratricopeptide repeats of protein phosphatase 5: implications for TPR-mediated protein-protein interactions. *EMBO J.*, *17*, 1192-1199.

de Boer, P. A., Crossley, R. E., & Rothfield, L. I. (1989). A division inhibitor and a topological specificity factor coded for by the minicell locus determine proper placement of the division septum in *E. coli*. *Cell*, *56*, 641-649.

Deusch, O., Landan, G., Roettger, M., Gruenheit, N., Kowallik, K. V., Allen, J. F., Martin, W., & Dagan, T. (2008). Genes of cyanobacterial origin in plant nuclear genomes point to a heterocyst-forming plastid ancestor. *Mol. Biol. Evol.*, *25*, 748-761.

Deva, T., Baker, E. N., Squire, C. J. & Smith, C. A. (2006). Structure of *Escherichia coli* UDP-N-acetylmuramoyl: L-alanine ligase (MurC). *Acta Crystallogr D Biol Crystallogr*, *62*, 1466-1474.

Doherty, H. M., & Adams, D. G. (1995). Cloning and sequence of *ftsZ* and flanking regions from the cyanobacterium *Anabaena* PCC 7120. *Gene*, *163*, 93-99.

Dolganov, N., & Grossman, A. R. (1993). Insertional inactivation of genes to isolate mutants of *Synechococcus* sp. strain PCC 7942: isolation of filamentous strains. *J. Bacteriol.*, *175*, 7644-7651.

Donachie, W. D., & Begg, K. J. (1996). "Division potential" in *Escherichia coli*. *J. Bacteriol.*, *178*, 5971-5976.

Easter, J., & Gober, J. W. (2002). ParB-stimulated nucleotideexchange regulates a switch in functionally distinct ParA activities. *Mol Cell*, *10*, 427-434.

El Zoeiby, A., Sanschagrin, F. & Levesque, R. C. (2003). Structure and function of the Mur enzymes: development of novel inhibitors. *Mol Microbiol*, *47*, 1-12.

Errington, J., Daniel, R. A. & Scheffers, D. J. (2003). Cytokinesis in bacteria. *Microbiol Mol Biol Rev*, *67*, 52-65.

Figge, R. M., Divakaruni, A. V. & Gober, J. W. (2004). MreB, the cell shape-determining bacterial actin homologue, co-ordinates cell wall morphogenesis in *Caulobacter crescentus*. *Mol Microbiol*, *51*, 1321-1332.

Fink, A. (1999). Chaperone-mediated protein folding. *Physiological Rev*. 79, 425-449.

Fujiwara, K., & Taguchi, H. (2007). Filamentous morphology in GroE-depleted *Escherichia coli* induced by impaired folding of FtsE. *J.Bacteriol.*, *189*, 5860-5866.

Fujiwara, M. & Yoshida, S. (2001). Chloroplast targeting of chloroplast division FtsZ2 proteins in *Arabidopsis*. *Biochemical and Biophysical Research Communications*, *287*, 462-467.

Fulda, S., Huang, F., Nilsson, F., Hagemann, M. & Norling, B. (2000). Proteomics of *Synechocystis* sp. strain PCC 6803. Identification of periplasmic proteins in cells grown at low and high salt concentrations. *Eur J Biochem*, *267*, 5900-5907.

Fulda, S., Mikkat, S., Huang, F., Huckauf, J., Marin, K., Norling, B. & Hagemann, M. (2006). Proteome analysis of salt stress response in the cyanobacterium *Synechocystis* sp. strain PCC 6803. *Proteomics*, *6*, 2733-2745.

Fulgosi, H., Gerdes, L., Westphal, S., Glockmann, C. & Soll, J. (2002). Cell and chloroplast division requires ARTEMIS. *Proceedings of the National Academy of Sciences USA*, *99*, 11501-11506.

Gething, M. J. (1997). Protein folding. The difference with prokaryotes. *Nature*, *388*, 329-331.

Gitai, Z., Dye, N. A. & Shapiro, L. (2004). An actin-like gene can determine cell polarity in bacteria. *Proc Natl Acad Sci U S A*, *101*, 8643-8648.

Gitai, Z., Dye, N. A., Reisenauer, A., Wachi, M. & Shapiro, L. (2005). MreB actin-mediated segregation of a specific region of a bacterial chromosome. *Cell*, *120*, 329-341.

Goebl, M., & Yanagida, M. (1991). The TPR snap helix: a novel protein repeat motif from mitosis to transcription. *Trends Biochem. Sci.*, *16*, 3-177.

Golden, S. S. (1988). Mutagenesis of cyanobacteria by classical and gene-transfer based methods. *Methods Enzymol.*, *167*, 714-727.

Gornicki, P., Scappino, L. A. & Haselkorn, R. (1993). Genes for two subunits of acetyl coenzyme A carboxylase of *Anabaena* sp. strain PCC 7120: biotin carboxylase and biotin carboxyl carrier protein. *J. Bacteriol.*, *175*, 5268-5272.

Graumann, P. L. (2001). SMC proteins in bacteria: condensation motors for chromosome segregation? *Biochimie*, *83*, 53-59.

Harry, E. J., Rodwell, J. & Wake, R. G. (1999). Co-ordinating DNA replication with cell division in bacteria: a link between the early stages of a round of replication and mid-cell Z ring assembly. *Mol Microbiol*, *33*, 33-40.

Hartl, F. U. (1996). Molecular chaperones in cellular protein folding. *Nature*, *381*, 571-579.

Henikoff, S., Haughn, G. W., Calvo, J. M. & Wallace, J. C. (1988). A large family of bacterial activator proteins. *Proc Natl Acad Sci U S A*, *85*, 6602-6606.

Hihara, Y., Kamei, A., Kanehisa, M., Kaplan, A. & Ikeuchi, M. (2001). DNA microarray analysis of cyanobacterial gene expression during acclimation to high light. *Plant Cell*, *13*, 793-806.

Hirota, Y., Ryter, A., & Jacob, F. (1968). Thermosensitive mutants of *E. coli* affected in the processes of DNA synthesis and cellular division. *Cold Spring Harb. Symp. Quant. Biol.*, 33, 677-693.

Holtzendorff, J., Partensky, F., Jacquet, S. J., Bruyant, F., Marie, D., Garczarek, L., Mary, I., Vaulot, D., & Hess, W. R. (2001). Diel expression of cell cycle-related genes in synchronized cultures of *Prochlorococcus* sp. strain PCC 9511. *J. Bacteriol. 183*: 915-920.

Howard, M., & Kruse, K. (2005). Cellular organization by self-organization: mechanisms and models for Min protein dynamics. *J Cell Biol*, *168*, 533-536.

Hu, B., Yang, G., Zhao, W., Zhang, Y. & Zhao, J. (2007). MreB is important for cell shape but not for chromosome segregation of the filamentous cyanobacterium *Anabaena* sp. PCC 7120. *Mol Microbiol*, *63*, 1640-1652.

Huang, F., Fulda, S., Hagemann, M. & Norling, B. (2006). Proteomic screening of salt-stress-induced changes in plasma membranes of *Synechocystis* sp. strain PCC 6803. *Proteomics*, *6*, 910-920.

Ingram, L. O., & Thurston, E. L. (1970). Cell division in morphological mutants of *Agmenellum quadruplicatum*, strain BG-1. *Protoplasma*, *71*, 55-75.

Ingram, L. O., & Van Baalen, C. (1970). Characteristics of a stable, filamentous mutant of a coccoid blue-green alga. *J. Bacteriol.*, *102*, 784-789.

Ingram, L. O., Van Baalen C., & Fisher, W. D. (1972). Cell division mutations in the blue-green bacterium *Agmenellum quadruplicatum* strain BG1: a comparison of the cell wall. *J. Bacteriol.*, *11*, 614-621.

Ingram, L. O., & Fisher, W. D. (1973a). Novel mutant impaired in cell division: evidence for a positive regulating factor. *J. Bacteriol.*, *113*, 999-1005.

Ingram, L. O., & Fisher, W. D. (1973b). Mechanism for the regulation of cell division in *Agmenellum. J. Bacteriol.*, *113*, 1006-1014.

Ingram, L. O., Olson, G. J., & Blackwell, M. M. (1975). Isolation of a small-cell mutant in the blue-green bacterium *Agmenellum quadruplicatum. J. Bacteriol.*, *123*, 743-746.

Jensen, R. B., & Shapiro, L. (2000). Proteins on the move: dynamic protein localization in prokaryotes. *Trends Cell. Biol.*, *10*, 483-488.

Jacobs, C., & Shapiro, L. (1999). Bacterial cell division: a moveable feast. *Proc. Natl. Acad. Sci. USA*, *96*, 5891-5893.

Jones, L. J., Carballido-Lopez, R. & Errington, J. (2001). Control of cell shape in bacteria: helical, actin-like filaments in *Bacillus subtilis. Cell, 104*, 913-922.

Kappock, T. J., Ealick, S. E. & Stubbe, J. (2000). Modular evolution of the purine biosynthetic pathway. *Curr Opin Chem Biol*, *4*, 567-572.

Katayama, T., Kubota, T., Kurokawa, K., Crooke, E. & Sekimizu, K. (1998). The initiator function of DnaA protein is negatively regulated by the sliding clamp of the *E. coli* chromosomal replicase. *Cell, 94*, 61-71.

Kawakami, H., Iwura, T., Takata, M., Sekimizu, K., Hiraga, S. & Katayama, T. (2001). Arrest of cell division and nucleoid partition by genetic alterations in the sliding clamp of the replicase and in DnaA. *Mol Genet Genomics, 266*, 167-179.

Kerner, M. J., Naylor, D. J., Ishihama, Y., Maier, T., Chang, H. C., Stines, A. P, Georgopoulos, C., Frishman, D., Hayer-Hartl, M., Mann, M., & Hartl, F. U. (2005). Proteome-wide analysis of chaperonin-dependent protein folding in *Escherichia coli. Cell, 122*, 209-220.

Kerr, R. A., Levine, H., Sejnowski, T. J. & Rappel, W.J. (2006). Division accuracy in a stochastic model of Min oscillations in *Escherichia coli*. *Proc Natl Acad Sci USA*, *103*, 347-352.

Klint, J., Rasmussen, U. & Bergman, B. (2007). FtsZ may have dualroles in the filamentous cyanobacterium *Nostoc/Anabaena* sp. strain PCC 7120. *J Plant Physiol*, *164*, 11-18.

Koksharova O. A. & Wolk, C. P. (2002a). Genetic tools for cyanobacteria. *Appl Microbiol Biotechnol.*, 58, 123-137.

Koksharova, O. A., & Wolk, C. P. (2002b). A novel gene that bears a DnaJ motif influences cyanobacterial cell division. *J Bacteriol*, *184*, 5524-5528.

Koksharova, O. A., Klint, J. & Rasmussen, U. (2006). The first protein map of *Synechococcus* sp. strain PCC 7942. *Mikrobiologiia*, *75*, 765-774.

Koksharova, O. A., Klint, J. & Rasmussen, U. (2007). Comparative proteomics of cell division mutants and wild-type of *Synechococcus* sp. strain PCC 7942. *Microbiology*, *153*, 2505-2517.

Kondo,T., Mori, T., Lebedeva, N. V., Aoki, S., Ishiura, M., & Golden, S. S. (1997). Circadian rhythms in rapidly dividing cyanobacteria. *Science*, *275,* 224-227.

Kovacs, E., van der Vies, S. M., Glatz, A., Torok, Z., Varvasovszki, V., Horvath, I. & Vigh, L. (2001). The chaperonins of *Synechocystis* PCC 6803 differ in heat inducibility and chaperone activity. *Biochem. Biophys Res Commun*, *289*, 908-915.

Kruse, K., Howard, M., & Margolin, W. (2007). **An experimentalist's guide to computational** modelling of the Min system. *Molecular Microbiology*, *63,* 1279-1284.

Kruse, T., Möller-Jensen, J., Löbner-Olesen, A. & Gerdes, K. (2003). Dysfunctional MreB inhibits chromosome segregation in *Escherichia coli. EMBO J, 22,* 5283-5292.

Kruse, T., Blagoev, B., Løbner-Olesen, A., Wachi, M., Sasaki, K., Iwai, N., Mann, M. & Gerdes, K. (2006). Actin homolog MreB and RNA polymerase interact and are both required for chromosome segregation in *Escherichia coli*. *Genes Dev.*, *20*, 113-124.

Kuhn, I., Peng, L., Bedu, S., & Zhang, C. C. (2000). Developmental regulation of the cell division protein FtsZ in *Anabaena* sp. strain PCC 7120, a cyanobacterium capable of terminal differentiation. *J. Bacteriol.*, *182*, 4640-4643.

Kumar, J. K., Tabor, S. & Richardson, C. C. (2004). Proteomic analysis of thioredoxin-targeted proteins in *Escherichia coli. Proc Natl Acad Sci USA*, *101*, 3759-3764.

Labarre, J., Chauvat, F., & Thuriaux, P. (1989). Insertional mutagenesis by random cloning of antibiotic resistance genes into the genome of the cyanobacterium *Synechocystis* strain PCC 6803. *J. Bacteriol.*, *171*, 3449-3457.

Lamb, J. R., Tugendreich, S., & Hieter, P. (1995). Tetratrico peptide repeat interactions: to TPR or not to TPR? *Trends Biochem. Sci.*, *20*, 257-259.

Laufen, T., Mayer, M. P., Beisel, C., Klostermeier, D., Mogk, A., Reinstein, J., & Bukau, B. (1999). Mechanism of regulation of Hsp70 chaperones by DnaJ cochaperones. *Proc. Natl. Acad. Sci. USA*, *96*, 5452-5457.

Len, A. C., Harty, D. W. & Jacques, N. A. (2004). Stress-responsive proteins are upregulated in *Streptococcus* mutants during acid tolerance. *Microbiology*, *150*, 1339-1351.

Lemos, J. A., Luzardo, Y. & Burne, R. A: (2007). Physiologic effects of forced downregulation of dnaK and groEL expression in *Streptococcus* mutans. *J. Bacteriol.*, *189,* 1582-1588.

Levin, P. A., & Losick R. Asymmetric division and cell fate during sporulation in *Bacillus subtilis*, In Brun YV, & LJ Shimkets, editors. Prokaryotic Development. Washington, DC: Am. Soc. Microbiol.; 2000; 167-189.

Liu, G., Begg, K., Geddes, A. & Donachie, W. D. (2001). Transcription of essential cell division genes is linked to chromosome replication in *Escherichia coli. Mol. Microbiol. 40,* 909-916.

Liu, Y. & Tsinoremas, N. F. (1996). An unusual gene arrangement for the putative chromosome replication origin and circadian expression of *dnaN* in *Synechococcus* sp. strain PCC 7942. *Gene*, *172*, 105-109.

Liu, Y., Tsinoremas, N. F., Golden, S. S., Kondo, T. & Johnson, C. H. (1996). Circadian expression of genes involved in the purine biosynthetic pathway of the cyanobacterium *Synechococcus* sp. strain PCC 7942. *Mol. Microbiol.*, *20*, 1071-1081.

Loose, M., Fischer-Friedrich, E., Ries, J., Kruse, K., & Schwille, P. (2008). Spatial regulators for bacterial cell division self-organize into surface waves in vitro. *Science*, *320*, 789-792.

Löwe, J., & Amos, L. A. (1998). Crystal structure of the bacterial cell-division protein FtsZ. *Nature*, *391*, 203-206.

Löwe, J., van den Ent, F. & Amos, L. A. (2004). Molecules of the bacterial cytoskeleton. *Annu Rev Biophys Biomol Struct*, *33*, 177-198.

Luque, I., Herrero, A., Flores, E., & Madueño, F. (1992). Clustering of genes involved in nitrate assimilation in the cyanobacterium *Synechococcus. Mol. Gen. Genet.*, *232*, 7-11.

Lutkenhaus, J, & Addinall, S. G. (1997). Bacterial cell division and the Z ring. *Annu Rev Biochem*, *66*, 93-116.

Lutkenhaus, J. (2007). Assembly dynamics of the bacterial MinCDE system and spatial regulation of the Z ring. *Annu Rev Biochem*, *76*, 539-562.

Madueño, F., Borrias, W. E., van Arkel, G. A., & Guerrero, M. G. (1988). Isolation and characterization of *Anacystis nidulans* R2 mutants affected in nitrate assimilation: establishment of two new mutant types. *Mol. Gen. Genet.*, *213*, 223-228.

Maple, J., Aldridge, C., & Moller, S. G. (2005). Plastid division is mediated by combinatorial assembly of plastid division proteins. *Plant J*; *43*, 811-823.

Maple, J., Fujiwara, M. T., Kitahata, N., Lawson, T., Baker, N. R., Yoshida, S., Moller, S. G. (2004). GIANT CHLOROPLAST 1 is essential for correct plastid division in *Arabidopsis. Current Biology*, *14*, 776-781.

Maple, J. & Møller, S. G. (2007). Plastid division: evolution, mechanism and complexity. *Annals of Botany*, *99*, 565-579.

Marcus, Y., Altman-Gueta, H., Finkler, A. & Gurevitz, M. (2003). Dual role of cysteine 172 in redox regulation of ribulose 1,5-bisphosphate carboxylase/oxygenase activity and degradation. *J. Bacteriol.*, *185*, 1509-1517.

Margolin, W. (2000). Themes and variations in prokaryotic cell division. *FEMS Microbiol. Rev.*, *24*, 531-548.

Martin, W. & Kowallik, K. V. (1999). Annotated English translation of Mereschkowsky's 1905 paper Über Natur und Ursprung der Chromatophoren im Pflanzenreiche. *Eur J Phycol*, *34*, 287-295.

Martin, W., Rujan, T., Richly, E., Hansen, A., Cornelsen, S., Lins, T., Leister, D., Stoebe, B. , Hasegawa, M. , & Penny, D. (2002). Evolutionary analysis of *Arabidopsis*, cyanobacterial, and chloroplast genomes reveals plastid phylogeny and thousands of cyanobacterial genes in the nucleus. *Proc. Natl. Acad. Sci. USA*, *99*, 12246-12251.

Maruyama, K., Sato, N. & Ohta, N. (1999). Conservation of structure and cold-regulation of RNA-binding proteins in cyanobacteria: probable convergent evolution with eukaryotic glycine-rich RNA- binding proteins. *Nucleic Acids Res*, *27*, 2029-2036.

Mary, I., Tu, C. J., Grossman, A. & Vaulot, D. (2004). Effects of highlight on transcripts of stress-associated genes for the cyanobacteria *Synechocystis* sp. PCC 6803 and *Prochlorococcus* MED4 and MIT9313. *Microbiology*, *150*, 1271-1281.

Mayer, F. (2003). Cytoskeletons in prokaryotes. *Cell Biol Int*, *27*, 429-438.

Mazouni, K., Domain, F., Cassier-Chauvat, C. & Chauvat, F. (2004). Molecular analysis of the key cytokinetic components of cyanobacteria: FtsZ, ZipN and MinCDE. *Mol Microbiol, 52*, 1145-1158.

McAndrew, R. S, Froehlich, J. E, Vitha, S., Stokes, K. D, & Osteryoung, K. W. (2001). Colocalisation of plastid division proteins in the chloroplast stromal compartment establishes a new functional relationship between FtsZ1 and FtsZ2 in higher plants. *Plant Physiology, 127,* 1656-1666.

Mereschkowsky, C. 1905. Uber natur und ursprung der chromatophoren im pflanzenreiche. *Biol Centralbl, 25*, 593-604.

Mercer, K. L. & Weiss, D. S. (2002). The *Escherichia coli* cell division protein FtsW is required to recruit its cognate transpeptidase, FtsI (PBP3), to the division site. *J Bacteriol., 184*, 904-912.

Meroueh, S. O., Bencze, K. Z., Hesek, D., Lee, M., Fisher, J. F., Stemmler, T. L. & Mobashery, S. (2006). Three-dimensional structure of the bacterial cell wall peptidoglycan. *Proc Natl Acad Sci USA, 103*, 4404-4409.

Michie, K. A. & Löwe, J. (2006). Dynamic filaments of the bacterialcytoskeleton. *Annu Rev Biochem, 75*, 467-492.

Mirelman, D. Biosynthesis and assembly of cell wall peptidoglycan. In Inouye M., editor. *Bacterial Outer Membranes*. New York: Wiley; 1979; 115-166.

Miyagishima, S., Wolk, C. P., & Osteryoung, K. W. (2005). Identification of cyanobacterial cell division genes by comparative and mutational analyses. *Molecular Microbiology, 56*, 126-143.

Mizusawa, S., Gottesman, S. (1983). Protein degradation in *Escherichia coli*: the *lon* gene controls the stability of sulA protein. *Proc Nat l Acad Sci U S A, 80*, 358- 362.

Mori, T., Binder, B., & Johnson, C. H. (1996). Circadian gating of cell division in cyanobacteria growing with average doubling times of less than 24 hours. *Proc.Natl.Acad.Sci.USA, 93*, 10183-10188.

Mori, S., Castoreno, A., Mulligan, M. E. & Lammers, P. J. (2003). Nitrogen status modulates the expression of RNA-binding proteins in cyanobacteria. *FEMS Microbiol Lett, 227*, 203-210.

Mukherjee, A., & Lutkenhaus, J. (1998). Dynamic assembly of FtsZ regulated by GTP hydrolysis. *EMBO J., 17*, 462-469.

Mutsuda, M., Michel, K. P., Zhang, X., Montgomery, B. L., & Golden, S. S. (2003). Biochemical properties of CikA, an unusual phytochrome-like histidine protein kinase that resets the circadian clock in *Synechococcus elongatus* PCC 7942. *J Biol Chem, 278*, 19102-19110.

Neidhardt, F. C. & VanBogelen, R. A. Proteomic analysis of bacterial stress responses. In: Storz, G. & Hengge-Aronis, R. editors. *Bacterial Stress Responses*, Washington, DC: ASM Press; 2000; 445-452.

Nimura, K., Takahashi, H. & Yoshikawa, H. (2001). Characterization of the *dnaK* multigene family in the cyanobacterium *Synechococcus* sp. strain PCC7942. *J Bacteriol, 183*, 1320-1328.

Ohtsuka, K., & Hata, M. (2000). Molecular chaperone function of mammalian Hsp70 and Hsp40 - a review. *Int. J. Hyperthermia, 16*, 231-245.

Osteryoung, K. W., Stokes, K. D., Rutherford, S. M., Percival, A. L., & Lee, W. Y. (1998). Chloroplast division in higher plants requires members of two functionally divergent gene families with homology to bacterial *ftsZ*. *The Plant Cell, 10,* 1991-2004.

Paciorek, J., Kardys, K., Lobacz, B., & Wolska, K. I. (1997). *Escherichia coli* defects caused by null mutations in *dnaK* and *dnaJ* genes. *Acta Microbiol. Pol., 46,* 7-17.

Pallen, M., Chaudhuri, R. & Khan, A. (2002). Bacterial FHA domains: neglected players in the phospho-threonine signalling game? *Trends Microbiol, 10,* 556-563.

Pogliano, J., Pogliano, K., Weiss, D. S., Losick, R. & Beckwith, J. (1997). Inactivation of FtsI inhibits constriction of the FtsZ cytokinetic ring and delays the assembly of FtsZ rings at potential division sites.*Proc Natl Acad Sci USA, 94,* 559-564.

Pyke, K. A., Rutherford, S. M, Robertson, E. J., Leech, R. M. (1994). *arc6*: a fertile *Arabidopsis* mutant with only two mesophyll cell chloroplasts. *Plant Physiology 106,* 1169-1177.

Raskin, D. M., & de Boer, P. A. (1999a). Rapid pole-to-pole oscillation of a protein required for directing division to the middle of *Escherichia coli. Proc. Natl. Acad. Sci. USA, 96,* 4971-4976.

Raskin, D. M., & de Boer, P. A. (1999b). MinDE-dependent pole-to-pole oscillation of division inhibitor MinC in *Escherichia coli. J. Bacteriol., 181,* 6419-6424.

Raven, J. A., & Allen, J. F. (2003). Genomics and chloroplast evolution: what did cyanobacteria do for plants? *Genome Biology, 4, 209.1-209.5.*

Raynaud, C., Cassier-Chauvat, C., Perennes, C. & Bergounioux, C. (2004). An *Arabidopsis* homolog of the bacterial cell division inhibitor SulA is involved in plastid division. *The Plant Cell, 16,* 1801-1811.

Rippka, R., Deruelles, J., Waterbury, J. B., Herdman, M., & Stanier, R. Y. (1979). Generic assignments, strain histories and properties of pure cultures of cyanobacteria. *J. Gen. Microbiol., 111,* 1-61.

Rothfield, L., Justice, S. & Garcia-Lara, J. (1999). Bacterial cell division. *Annu Rev Genet, 33,* 423-448.

Sauer, J., Görl, M. & Forchhammer, K. (1999). Nitrogen starvation in *Synechococcus* PCC 7942: involvement of glutamine synthetase and NtcA in phycobiliprotein degradation and survival. *Arch Microbiol., 172,* 247-255.

Sauer, J., Schreiber, U., Schmid, R., Volker, U. & Forchhammer, K. (2001). Nitrogen starvation-induced chlorosis in *Synechococcus* PCC7942. Low-level photosynthesis as a mechanism of long-term survival. *Plant Physiol., 126,* 233-243.

Schmitz, O., Katayama, M., Williams, S. B., Kondo, T., & Golden, S. S. (2000). CikA, a bacteriophytochrome that resets the cyanobacterial circadian clock. *Science, 289,* 765-768.

Shapiro, L., & Losick, R. (2000). Dynamic spatial regulation in the bacterial cell. *Cell, 100,* 89-98.

Sherratt, D. J. (2003). Bacterial chromosome dynamics. *Science, 301,* 780-785.

Shih, Y. L., Le, T. & Rothfield, L. (2003). Division site selection in *Escherichia coli* involves dynamic redistribution of Min proteins within coiled structures that extend between the two cell poles. *Proc Natl Acad Sci U S A, 100,* 7865-7870.

Sikorski, R. S., Boguski, M. S., Goebl, M., & Hieter, P. (1990). A repeating amino acid motif in CDC23 defines a family of proteins and a new relationship among genes required for mitosis and RNA synthesis. *Cell, 60,* 307-317.

Slabas, A. R., Suzuki, I., Murata, M., Simon, W. J. & Hall, J. J. (2006). Proteomic analysis of the heat shock response in *Synechocystis* PCC6803 and a thermally tolerant knockout strain lacking the histidine kinase34 gene. *Proteomics, 6*, 845-864.

Smith, C. A. (2006). Structure, function and dynamics in the mur family of bacterial cell wall ligases. *J Mol Biol, 362*, 640-655.

Soballe, B. & Poole, R. K. (1999). Microbial ubiquinones: multipleroles in respiration, gene regulation and oxidative stress management. *Microbiology, 145*, 1817-1830.

Stokes, K. D., McAndrew, R. S., Figueroa, R., Vitha, S. & Osteryoung, K. W. (2000). Chloroplast division and morphology are differentially affected by overexpression of FtsZ1 and FtsZ2 genes in *Arabidopsis. Plant Physiology, 124,* 1668-1677.

Strepp, R., Scholz, S., Kruse, S., Speth, V. & Reski, R. (1998). Plant nuclear gene knockout reveals a role in plastid division for the homolog of the bacterial cell division protein FtsZ, an ancestral tubulin. *Proceedings of the National Academy of Sciences of the USA, 95,* 4368-4373.

Sullivan, S. M., & Maddock, J. R. (2000). Bacterial division: finding the dividing line. *Curr. Biol., 10*, 249-252.

Susin, M. F., Baldini, R. L., Gueiros-Filho, F., & Gomes, S. L. (2006). GroES/GroEL and DnaK/DnaJ have distinct roles in stress responses and during cell cycle progression in *Caulobacter crescentus. J. Bacteriol., 188*, 8044-8053.

Suzuki, K., Nakanishi, H., Bower, J., Yoder, D. W., Osteryoung, K. W., & Miyagishima, S. (2009). Plastid chaperonin proteins Cpn60alpha and Cpn60beta are required for plastid division in *Arabidopsis thaliana. BMC Plant Biology, 9*, 38 doi:10.1186/1471-2229-9-38

Sweeney, B. M. & Borgese, M. B. (1989). A circadian rhythm in cell division in a prokaryote, the cyanobacterium *Synechococcus* WH7803. *J.Phycol., 25*,183-186.

Tandeau de Marsac, N., Borrias, W. E., Kuhlemeier, C. J., Castets, A. M., van Arkel G. A., & van den Hondel, C. A. M. J. J. (1982). A new approach for molecular cloning in cyanobacteria: cloning of an *Anacystis nidulans met* gene using a Tn*901*-induced mutant. *Gene, 20*, 111-119.

Thomaides, H. B., Freeman, M., El Karoui, M. & Errington, J. (2001). Division site selection protein DivIVA of *Bacillus subtilis* has a second distinct function in chromosome segregation during sporulation. *Genes Dev, 15*, 1662-1673.

van den Ent, F., Amos, L. A. & Lowe, J. (2001). Prokaryotic origin ofthe actin cytoskeleton. *Nature, 413*, 39-44.

van den Ent, F., Vinkenvleugel, T. M., Ind, A., West, P., Veprintsev, D., Nanninga, N., den Blaauwen, T., & Löwe, J. (2008). Structural and mutational analysis of the cell division protein FtsQ. *Mol. Microbiol., 68*, 110-123.

van den Hondel, C. A. M. J. J., Verbeek, S., Van den Ende, A., Weisbeek, P. J., Borrias, W. E., & van Arkel, G. A. (1980). Introduction of transposon Tn*901* into a plasmid of *Anacystis nidulans*: preparation for cloning in cyanobacteria. *Proc. Natl. Acad. Sci. USA, 77*, 1570-1574.

Vitha, S., McAndrew, R. S., Osteryoung, K. W. (2001). FtsZ ring formation at the chloroplast division site in plants. *Journal of Cell Biology, 153*, 111-119.

Vitha, S., Froehlich, J. E., Koksharova, O. A., Pyke, K. A., van Erp, H. & Osteryoug, K. W. (2003). ARC6 is a J-domain plastid division protein and an evolutionary descendant of the cyanobacterial cell division protein Ftn2. *Plant Cell, 15*, 1918-1933.

Wachi, M., Doi, M., Tamaki, S., Park, W., Nakajima-Iijima, S. & Matsuhashi, M. (1987). Mutant isolation and molecular cloning of *mre* genes, which determine cell shape, sensitivity to mecillinam, and amount of penicillin-binding proteins in *Escherichia coli. J. Bacteriol., 169*, 4935-4940.

Wachi, M. & Matsuhashi, M. (1989). Negative control of cell division by *mreB*, a gene that functions in determining the rod shape of *Escherichia coli* cells. *J Bacteriol, 171*, 3123-3127.

Wolk, C. P., Cai, Y., & Panoff, J. M. (1991). Use of a transposon with luciferase as a reporter to identify environmentally responsive genes in a cyanobacterium. *Proc. Natl. Acad. Sci. USA, 88*, 5355-5359.

Wood, Z. A., Schroder, E., Robin Harris, J. & Poole, L. B. (2003). Structure, mechanism and regulation of peroxiredoxins. *Trends Biochem Sci, 28*, 32-40.

Wortinger, M., Sackett, M. J., & Brun, Y. V. (2000). CtrA mediates a DNA replication checkpoint that prevents cell division in *Caulobacter crescentus. EMBO J., 19*, 4503-4512.

Yalowitz, J. A. & Jayaram, H. N. (2000). Molecular targets of guanine nucleotides in differentiation, proliferation and apoptosis. *Anticancer Res, 20*, 2329-2338.

Yoshida, T, Maki, M., Okamoto, H. & Hiroishi, S. (2005). Coordination of DNA replication and cell division in cyanobacteria *Microcystis aeruginosa. FEMS Microbiology Letters, 251*, 149-154.

Zhang, C. C., Huguenin, S., & Friry, A. (1995). Analysis of genes encoding the cell division protein FtsZ and a glutathione synthetase homologue in the cyanobacterium *Anabaena* sp. PCC 7120. *Res. Microbiol., 146*, 445-455.

Zhevner, V. D., Glazer, V. M., & Shestakov, S. V. (1973). Mutants of *Anacystis nidulans* with modified process of cell division. Mikrobiologiya, 42, 290-297 (in Russian).

Zhou H. & Lutkenhaus, J. (2005). MinC mutants deficient in MinD- and DicB-mediated cell division inhibition due to loss of interaction with MinD, DicB, or a septal component. *J. Bacteriol., 187*, 2846-2857.

INDEX

A

B

C

D

E

F

G

H

I

J

K

L

M

N

O

P

R

T

U

V

W

X

Y

Z